Contents

Immunology in Clinical Medicine

Immunology in Clinical Medicine

J. L. Turk, *M D DSc (Lond) FRCP FRCPath*
*Sir William Collins Professor of Human and
Comparative Pathology,
The Royal College of Surgeons of England and
the University of London*

Foreword by
Selwyn Taylor, *DM MCh FRCS*

Third Edition

William Heinemann Medical Books Limited
London

First published 1969
Reprinted 1971
Second edition 1972
Reprinted 1974
Reprinted 1975
Third edition 1978
Reprinted 1980

ISBN 0 433 32852 5

Printed and bound in Great Britain
at The Pitman Press, Bath

Foreword

It has always appeared a strange paradox to me that the word immunology, derived as it is from a Latin word which means exempt, should be associated for the most part with hypersensitivity reactions and have little to do with exemption from anything. Immunology, however, is a science full of paradoxes yet one that grows daily in its importance for the clinician.

It is because immunology is so important to all of us in the medical profession today and because it is such an odd discipline, full of paradoxes, that I welcome this introduction to it by Dr. John Turk. He has that fortunate gift of clear, simple exposition, which is only found in those with complete mastery of their subject, and not always with them.

I bear some responsibility for the pattern of this book as I discussed it at length with Dr. Turk before he wrote it and I was delighted when he let me read the finished manuscript as it seemed to me just what most of us are now looking for. Its title explains precisely what it is all about; "Immunology in Clinical Medicine." I commend it to all who want a good introduction to the subject, Dr. Turk is a splendid guide.

The bibliography is highly selective and well suited to a book of this kind. If I can prophesy there will soon be a demand for a second edition. Certainly the speed with which this new subject is developing will call for it.

SELWYN TAYLOR

Royal Postgraduate Medical School
Hammersmith Hospital
London W12 0HS

Preface to the First Edition

Advances in medical science have progressed so rapidly in the past twenty years that most physicians and surgeons find it very difficult to keep up with changes in the basic concepts of disease which underly the practice of medicine. Although Immunology is one of the oldest branches of pathology, the relation of immunological processes to the causation of diseases other than those initiated by infectious agents, has been little appreciated until recent years. It is now realized that immunological concepts apply to a diverse number of medical conditions ranging at one extreme from the appearance of a simple furuncle in the skin to, at the other extreme, the means whereby the body controls the spread of cancer. Naturally throughout this period of rapid advance in knowledge, there has been a wealth of books, reviews and scientific articles each contributing to our understanding of these processes. Books written at the beginning of the period of rapid expansion of knowledge have been found to be out of date and have been revised. However, as soon as they are revised they appear to double their content to the extent that they cease to be books which can be read by the non-specialist and become encyclopaedias into which one might dig for information on a small aspect of the subject or how to perform a laboratory technique. As these volumes increase in size and scope they leave the practising physician far behind and become incomprehensible to all but the specialist in that particular field.

This is not only so with standard texts on the subject but also with books which were originally written with the medical student in mind. Such is the breadth of the subject that many of these books have now reached the same size as the standard medical student's textbooks of internal medicine and pathology. They have in fact become the textbooks for those taking specialized courses in immunology, rather than being books which can be taken up and read by medical students and practitioners who wish only to be acquainted with the way in which this subject impinges on the practice of clinical medicine.

The purpose of this "small" book is to describe current concepts of immunology and how they affect our understanding of disease processes, for an audience which has been left behind by the advances.

As an immunologist with a wide circle of clinical friends and colleagues I have been impressed by the need for such a book which discusses the immunological concepts underlying disease processes rather than the principles behind laboratory tests. Such a book should I felt be written by one author rather than being, as most of the available texts on the subject, a multi-author book. It should express the opinion of one immunologist on how he thinks diseases are affected by immunological processes, rather than present a confusion of opinions.

It is now known that cell-mediated immunological processes are as important, in disease mechanisms, as those processes involving circulating antibody, both in their initiation and in their control. Most textbooks of immunology tend to place a greater emphasis on circulating antibodies as these are easier to investigate in the laboratory and more knowledge has accumulated about antibodies in disease rather than about cell-mediated immune processes. As far as is possible the present volume attempts to provide a more balanced approach and wherever the knowledge is available cell-mediated immune processes are given full emphasis in proportion to their importance. However, there has been a noticeable movement towards calling any disease process in which an immunological component is suspected, but circulating antibody involvement cannot be proved, cell-mediated. It is hoped that this will not develop in the same way as the recent trend to call diseases "autoimmune", where, for technical reasons, an extraneous antigen cannot be demonstrated.

With these points in mind, this book has been written to present immunology to students and practitioners of clinical medicine. I have started with an exposition of basic immunological concepts as they impinge on disease and then taken a tour through a number of diseases or disease processes in which we know or suspect that immunological processes play a part. These include not only those diseases which result from a heightened immunological activity but also those which develop as a result of a depression of these processes. Throughout the effect of drugs known to suppress immunological processes are considered especially in relation to whether they operate by really suppressing immunological processes or whether they have other actions.

No references are included in the text, but a bibliography is provided at the end of each chapter. This has three parts. The first is a collection of books which would bring the reader, if he so desired, deeper into the subject. The second and third parts consist of two types of references, review articles and actual references to recent scientific or medical publications. The former have been chosen to supplement the books and the latter are only included where the subject is not covered by the books or review articles, and are mainly publications which have occurred within the last two years. These are intended to give a lead to anyone wanting to delve deeper into the subject. References are thus kept to a minimum and are intended only to give material which might help the reader get started, and are intentionally not comprehensive. This book can be used either to give an outline of the subject to those for whom time is at a premium or as an introduction to those clinicians who wish to dig deeper into the subject.

I should like to take this opportunity of thanking Mr Frank Price for drawing the figures for me. I need to emphasize that these by no means depict what is going on accurately, but are intended to give an idea what we think may be going on in as simple a way as is possible, in relation to the information available at the present time. Finally I should like to thank and dedicate this book to my closest clinical colleague, my wife, who has continually indicated the direction in which this book has been written.

J.L.T.

London
March 1969

Preface to the Third Edition

In the five years since the publication of the second edition of this book the subject of Immunology has flourished. Perhaps the greatest advances have been in our knowledge of the genetic control of the immune response and the link up of this with histocompatibility antigen systems. Although much of the early work has been performed with mice, the relevance of these observations has been enhanced by the demonstration of the linkage between HLA antigens and certain diseases, especially ankylosing spondylitis, gluten sensitive enteropathy and multiple sclerosis. Our concept of the role of immune deficiency in disease has enlarged with the definition of variable states of low level deficiency that can result in a considerable degree of morbidity from recurrent infections with ubiquitous micro-organisms. In the field of cancer immunology there has been a shift in emphasis away from enhancing antibody as a modulator of the immune response, to the role of soluble tumour specific transplantation antigens. More notice is now being taken of the role of soluble tumour products that are undoubtedly shed continuously into the circulation. Advances have also occurred in the role of immunological processes in rheumatic disorders and diseases of the gastrointestinal tract. Gastrointestinal immunology is exciting considerable interest at the present moment. However, the greatest advance has probably been the awareness of all clinicians of the degree to which immunological processes play a role in common disease processes. Immunology is no longer an erudite backroom subject, but forms part of the day to day discussion at the bedside. Pathological processes are regularly discussed in immunological terms. The major contribution of immunology would seem to be in the way it has changed thought processes on the mechanism of disease, rather than the tests or therapeutic advances that inevitably stems from this.

J.L.T.

London
October 1977

Chapter I
The Nature of the Immune Response

1. Introduction

The science of immunology began with a study of immunity to infection and can be reckoned to have started with Jenner's classical study in 1798 of the role of vaccination in protection against the virus infection smallpox. The study of immunity was coupled with that of bacteriology throughout the latter part of the nineteenth century. However, a number of observations made about the time of the beginning of this century indicated that similar mechanisms to those involved in protection from microbial infection could produce tissue damage. The terms "hypersensitivity" and "allergy" were introduced at this time to describe the increased reactivity of the body to a foreign substance, after there had been a previous contact with the agent, as compared with the first reaction when the body made its initial contact with this material. Hypersensitivity reactions were first described to foreign serum proteins or bacterial extracts. Eventually such reactions were discovered to occur after contact with a wide range of substances of both plant and animal origin as well as contact of the skin to certain molecules with a very simple chemical structure. Hay fever, asthma, urticaria, anaphylaxis and serum sickness were among the first conditions attributed to allergic or immunological mechanisms. However, it was probably the syndrome of "serum sickness", which developed as a result of repeated treatment of bacterial infections with sera prepared in animals, which first alerted pathologists to the wide range of tissues which could be damaged by immunological reactions.

Throughout the first half of this century research into diseases involving immunological mechanisms was restricted to a study of those involving classical allergic phenomena. Within the last thirty years, however, there has been an increasing awareness that immunological mechanisms in disease were not restricted to those phenomena which had previously been accepted as being "allergic", but were involved in a much wider range of pathological conditions. Perhaps the greatest stimulus to this widening of the scope of immunology was the enormous steps made during and after the second world war in the study of the nature of the homograft reaction. Much of this work was done under the stimulus from practising surgeons who envisaged the need for more knowledge of the nature of this reaction, so that eventually the transplantation of organs and tissues might become a feasible surgical procedure. The demonstration that the rejection of tissue homografts was an immunological phenomenon led to a study of those conditions

1

under which an immune response might be inhibited. The stimulus for research along these lines developed because of the obvious value that an inhibition of the immune response would have in allowing grafts of foreign tissues or organs to "take". Two approaches to this problem were discovered almost simultaneously, one was the production of a specific state of immunological tolerance to a single antigen and the other was the demonstration of the immunosuppressive effect of a wide range of drugs which had been demonstrated both clinically and experimentally to be cancer chemotherapeutic agents. At the same time paediatricians were becoming aware of the fact that in rare cases neonatal death was being caused by a deficiency of immunological mechanisms. It was from a study of these immunological deficiency diseases coupled with an interest in the mechanisms of rejection of tissue homografts that it soon became apparent that the thymus, an organ whose function was until then wrapped in mystery, played an important role in the control of immunological processes.

Another line of investigation occurring again at about the same time was the demonstration of immunological processes directed against the body's own tissues in certain diseased states. Ehrlich at the turn of the century had postulated that although the body would react immunologically against foreign substances, it could not react against components of its own tissues. He thus introduced the concept of *Horror autotoxicus*. This was confirmed as a general principle by the demonstration of blood group *iso-antibodies* in the blood which were always the opposite of and did not react with the individual's own blood group antigens on his red cells. However, it is now known that under certain disease conditions the body can overcome this *Horror autotoxicus* and develops *autoantibodies* against its own tissues. Almost simultaneously it was demonstrated that disease of the thyroid gland could be produced in experimental animals, associated with the presence of *autoantibodies* in the serum directed against the body's own thyroid tissue and that similar *autoantibodies* could be demonstrated in the serum of humans with Hashimoto's thyroiditis, directed against thyroid tissue. Since then autoimmune phenomena have been found to be associated in some way or another with a wide range of tissue disorders.

Another group of disorders in which immunological processes have been implicated or associated are the so-called connective tissue diseases. Of these probably the most important group are those of a rheumatic or rheumatoid nature. Research over the past twenty years into this group of diseases has revealed a complex pattern in which the damaging effects of both infective and immunological processes are intimately interwoven and are often difficult to dissociate. From a study of these and other diseases it has become apparent that tissue damage can result as readily from proximity to an immunological reaction of the body directed against the infective agent, as from the direct toxic effect of the infective agent itself. It is also apparent that the body can react against its own tissues damaged either by an infective agent or by physical or chemical means as though it were a completely foreign tissue.

Perhaps one of the most exciting fields of modern immunology is recent evidence of the role of immunological processes in controlling cancer. It appears that the body recognizes cancer cells as being foreign. In this way an immunological reaction is started in an attempt to control the growth and spread of the malignant cells. In most cases of clinical cancer a fine balance is set up with the scales weighted very slightly in favour of the malignant cells so that the cancer progresses but in a slow but sure manner. It is, however, suspected that malignant clones (colonies) of cells are produced continuously throughout life but are eliminated rapidly by the body's immune processes and it is only in those cases where the immune response is in some way slightly deficient that the cancer can spread throughout the body. The importance of this concept is that a new approach is now being made for the treatment of cancer by attempting to develop means by which it might be possible to enhance the immunological response of the body against cancer and tip the fine balance between the immune reaction and the malignant cells in a more favourable direction.

2. The Nature of Antigens

It can thus be seen that the immunological reaction of the body is concerned with firstly the recognition and secondly the rejection of foreign material. The body has an inborn mechanism for recognizing what is "self" and what is "not self". Damage to tissue can result during the process of rejecting what is "not self" and also on rare occasions from a failure to recognize what is "self" and treat it as "not self". This capacity to recognize "self" and reject "not self" develops at some early stage during foetal life because it is known that certain mammalian foetuses can develop the property of rejecting homografts and of producing circulating antibodies before parturition.

Most immunologists agree that, to become antigenic or be able to immunize, a foreign substance must be of a relatively high molecular weight. However, the actual size the molecule need be to make it antigenic will vary on its chemical nature. Lipids alone are not antigenic, proteins and polysaccharides are and so are lipo-proteins and lipo-polysaccharides. Polysaccharides need to be of a higher molecular weight than proteins to become antigenic. Proteins of molecular weight as low as 5,000 can be found to be antigenic. An example of a low molecular weight protein of clinical importance which is antigenic is insulin (molecular weight approximately 6,000). Polysaccharides need to be far larger to be antigenic. Thus dextran of molecular weight 100,000 is not antigenic, whereas dextrans of molecular weight 600,000 or more are antigenic. (The dextrans used as plasma volume expanders are of molecular weight between 40,000 and 150,000 and are not believed to be antigenic.)

Small chemical molecules such as dinitrochlorobenzene (molecular weight 203) or primulin the active sensitizer from the plant *primula obconica* (molecular weight 210) which bind immediately to protein carriers can convert the body's own proteins into antigens and the specificity of the immunological reaction is directed against these small chemicals themselves. Such small molecular weight chemicals are called *haptens*. However, a small molecular weight chemical can only become haptenic if it binds onto protein spontaneously or if it is bound to a macromolecular carrier artificially in the laboratory. Haptens such as dinitrochlorobenzene and primulin can convert the body's own protein into an antigen which the body will fail to recognize as "self" by virtue of the addition of the small chemical grouping. An immunological response will then be launched directed against proteins carrying this small molecular weight group. This subject will be discussed much more fully in relation to chemical contact sensitivity which is an important cause of industrial dermatitis.

The ability of the body to distinguish between different antigens is remarkably specific. Immunological mechanisms can recognize small molecular weight substances such as aniline and amino-benzoic acid and even distinguish the three stereoisomers of tartaric acid when bound to protein. It can recognize different spatial configurations of the same chemical structure, as well as discriminate between a wide range of simple organic molecules. Study of contact dermatitis has shown moreover that people can develop immunological reactions and become hypersensitive to a number of simple inorganic metal radicals containing nickel, chromium, beryllium and mercury when attached to the body's own proteins, and can thus distinguish between one metal ion and another.

3. Types of Immune Response

The immune response can be divided into two different but fundamentally similar mechanisms (Fig. 1). Rejection of foreign antigen can be produced by means of the action of humoral antibodies (serum proteins—immunoglobulins) or by direct interaction with specifically sensitized lymphocytes producing what is called the cell-mediated immune response (CMI). Cell-mediated immune reactions are responsible for phenomena such as tissue homograft rejection and delayed hypersensitivity. Humoral antibodies are synthesized by plasma cells which are themselves derived from lymphocytes. Lymphocyte precursors of the specifically sensitized lymphocytes of CMI and of plasma cells which synthesize CMI are found in the liver in foetal life and later on in development in the bone marrow. Lymphocytes involved in CMI come under the influence of the thymus in late foetal or early neonatal life and are therefore generally referred to as T-lymphocytes. Lymphocytes which become plasma cell precursors are independent of the thymus. In birds they come under the influence of the bursa of Fabricius in late foetal or neonatal life. In mammalia it has been postulated that the bursal equivalent is provided by lymphoid tissue lining the intestinal

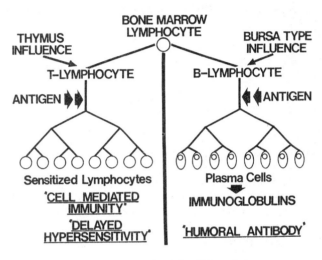

FIG. 1. Pathways of cellular differentiation.

tract—the Peyer's patches and the appendix. Lymphocytes of this pool are therefore often referred to as B-lymphocytes. Lymphocytes in the body may be static or mobile. They may also be long lived or short lived. T-lymphocytes are usually long lived and mobile. They are found circulating in the blood, lymph and through certain areas of the lymphoid tissue referred to as thymus-dependent areas (Figs. 5b, c). In lymph nodes these are the paracortical areas. B-lymphocytes are found in the lymph follicles and at the cortico-medullary junction of lymph nodes as well as in the non-thymus-dependent area of the spleen and in the bone marrow. They tend to be far less mobile than T-lymphocytes. T-lymphocytes may differ from B-lymphocytes in a number of ways. In the mouse T-cells carry specific antigens such as the θ-antigen by which they can be detected. In man they form spontaneous rosettes *in vitro* with sheep erythrocytes, known as E-rosettes. B-cells can be recognised as they bear immunoglobulins on their surface. They also have specific receptors for the Fc part of the immunoglobulin molecule and the C3 component of complement. They form rosettes *in vitro* with sheep erythrocytes coated with antibody and complement, known as EAC-rosettes.

(a) Humoral antibody response

Antibodies are serum proteins which run electrophoretically mainly as γ-globulins and react directly with antigens. Often, if they are in sufficient concentrations and if they have a strong enough binding power, they will specifically precipitate a solution of the macromolecular antigen. If the antigen is on the surface of cells, such as erythrocytes or bacteria, these can be agglutinated by sera containing antibodies specifically directed against the particular antigen. Antibodies belong to the class of serum proteins now known as immunoglobulins, because it is thought that this class of proteins all have an immunological function. Immunoglobulins are made by cells of the plasma cell series. One cell is thought to make only one type of globulin. Plasma cells have all the apparatus within them for synthesizing and secreting proteins. Plasma cells are found under normal circumstances in the medulla of lymph nodes and the red pulp of the spleen. They develop from B-lymphocytes derived originally from the bone marrow. How these cells are influenced to become plasma cell precursors is not known, but the process is thought to be analogous to a similar mechanism by which the thymus is thought to influence other stem cells lymphocytes to become T-lymphocytes (see below) (Fig. 1). To date, immunoglobulins in the human have been divided into five groups known as IgG, IgA, IgD, IgE and IgM. IgG, IgA and IgD have a molecular weight in the range of 150,000, IgE is of molecular weight approximately 200,000. IgM is a macroglobulin of molecular weight of 900,000 and consists of five subunits each similar in structure to that of the lower molecular weight immunoglobulins. The structure of the IgG molecule has been studied extensively and is thought to consist of four polypeptide chains, two of molecular weight approximately 25,000 and two of molecular weight 50,000, which are called the light and heavy chains respectively. These polypeptide chains are joined by disulphide bonds (Fig. 2). The whole immunoglobulin molecule can be split by enzymes into two fragments containing a light chain and the adjacent part of the heavy chain (Fab fragment: ab = antigen binding) and a third fragment consisting of the rest of the heavy chains which can be crystallized (Fc fragment: c = crystallizable). The heavy chains when separated from the light chains can be split into two fragments, the part adjacent to the light chain is known as the Fd fragment. There are two antibody-combining sites on a simple immunoglobulin molecule each on the Fab fragment, involving a light chain and the adjacent Fd fragment of the heavy chain. It has, however, been demonstrated under the electron microscope that when antibodies react with antigens the angle between the Fab fragments widens so that the molecule can react with two antigens and in the same process the Fc fragment contracts (Fig. 3). The specificity of the different antibodies is thought to be due to differences in the sequence of amino-acids in those parts of the polypeptide chains which form the

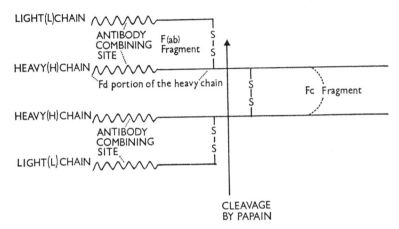

FIG. 2. Diagram of the polypeptide chains of the immunoglobulin molecule. The two antibody combining sites are formed by the end portions of the light chain and the Fd fragment of the heavy chain.

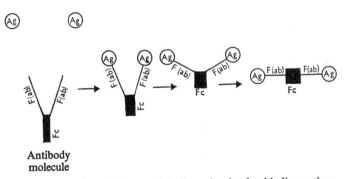

FIG. 3. Behaviour of immunoglobulin molecule after binding antigen. [After Feinstein and Rowe (1965), *Nature*, **205**, 147.]

antibody-combining site. Immunoglobulins differ from all other proteins in that the terminal half of the light chain and the terminal quarter of the heavy chain in the antibody-combining site vary from one protein to another in their amino-acid sequence. In these "variable" regions, 80% of the amino-acids may vary. However, the position of the glycine components is always constant. It has been considered that the glycines can function as a pivot on which the variable regions of the

molecule can move to provide a better fit for the antigen. Most antibodies belong to the class of immunoglobulins IgG, only a small
fraction of serum antibodies belong to the class IgA. IgA antibodies
form, however, most of the antibodies in saliva, nasal secretions, tears,
colostrum and the intestinal secretions. They appear to be derived from
plasma cells in the mucous membranes and around the exocrine glands.
They immunize the individual against antigens found on the surface of
mucous membranes and are involved in local immunity. IgA antibodies
are found against ABO blood group antigens because these develop as a
result of cross reaction with the intestinal flora. However, they are not
found against Rhesus antigens as immunization against these antigens
is caused by transfusion or leakage of foetal red cells across the placenta.
IgA is frequently secreted as a dimer (SIgA) conjugated to an epithelial
glycoprotein of M.W. 50,000 referred to as the "secretory piece". It also
contains a further polypeptide chain, the J-chain of M.W. 25,000 the
function of which is as yet unknown. The concentration of IgA in
parotid saliva is 100 times that of IgG. Antibodies of the IgD class are
not commonly found. However, IgD antibodies have been described
against insulin, bovine proteins, penicillin and diphtheria toxoid as well
as autoimmune antinuclear and antithyroid antibodies. The IgM fraction contains some of the ABO red cell isoantibodies and the saline
agglutinating anti-Rhesus red cell antibodies (although incomplete Rh
antibodies are IgG). Cold agglutinins directed against red cells are also
IgM. Among antibacterial antibodies which belong to the IgM class
are antibodies directed against the somatic antigen of Salmonella. The
rheumatoid factor is also a macroglobulin antibody.

Reagins, the skin sensitizing antibodies, associated with anaphylactic
phenomena such as hay fever and asthma have been classed as IgE
antibodies. They have a number of different physico-chemical properties which distinguish them from other low molecular weight antibodies
and account for their marked difference in behaviour. These antibodies
will be discussed more fully in the chapter on immediate-type hypersensitivity reactions.

Multiple myeloma is a disease where the growth and development
of a colony of plasma cells of one particular type gets out of control
and becomes neoplastic forming tumour-like aggregations consisting
mainly of plasma cells and occurring mainly in bones. These tumours
as they are formed of plasma cells make immunoglobulins which are
all of one type (either IgG, IgA, IgD or IgE). Until recently it was
thought that these cells were programmed to make immunoglobulins
without antibody specificity. However, in a few cases it has been
shown that these myeloma proteins have antibody-like specificity. This
activity has been discovered against streptococcal and staphylococcal
antigens, and even against the dinitrophenol group acting as a hapten.
In experimental animals, the incidence of antibody-like specificity in

myeloma proteins is as high as 5–10%. Many of the antigens with which these proteins react can be shown to be produced by organisms in the gastrointestinal and respiratory microbial flora. Thus it appears that these tumours could develop as a result of somatic mutation in one cell. This then forms a highly neoplastic colony which proliferates and seeds all over the body. Benign proliferation of single colonies of plasma cells can also occur producing what is called a "monoclonal gammopathy". In many cases these have been found to be unassociated with actual tumour formation and the proliferation is not malignant. The proportion of myelomas and benign monoclonal gammopathies of one particular immunoglobulin type is similar to the proportion which that protein forms of the immunoglobulins as a whole in the serum. Multiple myelomas are often associated with abnormal proteins in the urine— Bence Jones proteins. These proteins precipitate on heating and then redissolve on boiling. It has been shown that Bence Jones proteins cross react with the myeloma protein in the serum. However, the serum myeloma protein has the same molecular weight as normal immunoglobulins (150,000), whereas Bence Jones proteins have a molecular weight of 20,000. It has been shown that Bence Jones proteins are light chains of the myeloma proteins which could be a by-product of an abnormal type of immunoglobulin synthesis.

Overgrowth of cells making IgM protein is not quite so malignant but is associated with a high level of IgM in the serum—Waldenström's macroglobulinaemia. Evidence that myelomas and monoclonal gammopathies develop as a result of random mutation among plasma cell precursors is afforded by the fact mentioned above that the myeloma proteins and benign monoclonal gammopathies fall into specific immunoglobulin groups in approximately similar proportions to the distribution of these immunoglobulins in normal human serum. Table I

Table I

Immunoglobulin levels in normal serum. Comparison of the proportion of different immunoglobulins in the serum with the proportion of monoclonal gammopathies[1] carrying the same antigenic specificities.

	Normal range in serum (mg/100 ml)	Percentage immunoglobulins in serum	Percentage immunoglobulins in monoclonal gammopathies
IgG	800–1680	78·0	60
IgA	140–420	16·6	25
IgM	50–190	5·0	15
IgD	0·3–40	0·4	
IgE	0·0001–0·0007		

[1] Including myelomatosis and macroglobulinaemia as well as benign gammopathies.

gives the normal range of these immunoglobulins in serum, the percentage of the total immunoglobulins each protein forms in normal
individuals and the percentage of monoclonal gammopathies, benign
and malignant, formed by each immunoglobulin type.

It is considered that circulating antibodies are produced in response
to antigen in a soluble form, whereas cell-mediated immunity may
develop in response to an antigen fixed in the tissues. The soluble
antigen passes down to the medulla of the lymph node or the red pulp
of the spleen where it is taken up initially by macrophages. These cells
then appear to pass on a message to the plasma cell precursors. Whether
this is in the form of antigenic fragments caused by digestion of the
antigen by the macrophages or soluble ribonucleic acid (RNA) formed
within these macrophages is not yet understood. The plasma cell precursors (probably small lymphocytes) exist at the cortico-medullary
junction and are stimulated to proliferate into antibody-producing cells
here and in the medullary cords of lymph nodes as a result of the
antigenic message received from the macrophages, which lie in close
proximity to them.

After first contact with an antigen a person produces what is known
as a primary antibody response. This is a limited response of low
intensity and short duration (Fig. 4), often the production of IgG

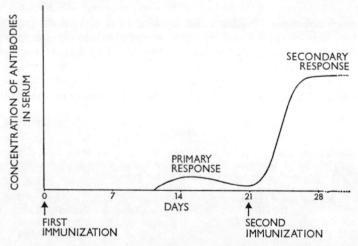

Fig. 4. Primary and secondary response to immunization with an antigen.

antibodies is preceded by the production of high molecular weight
antibodies of the IgM class. During the primary antibody response
germinal centres develop in localized collections of lymphocytes in the
lymphoid tissue called lymph follicles at the same time as plasma cells

begin to proliferate at the cortico-medullary junction and in the medullary cords.

On second and subsequent contacts with the antigen a secondary response (Fig. 4) occurs; antigen is now localized in the germinal centres as well as the medulla of the lymph nodes affected and a much more extensive proliferation of plasma cells occurs. This secondary or anamnestic response is much more extensive and of greater intensity than the primary response, and antibody may be produced as a result for many months or years. This response is of molecules of the IgG type. IgM antibodies are produced on secondary contact with antigen but at the same low intensity and for the same limited period as in a primary response. The extensive secondary response is thought to occur as a result of "immunological memory" and this is believed to reside within cells of the small lymphocyte class.

(b) Cell-mediated immune response

Humoral antibodies are formed in response to stimulation with antigens in a soluble form, or if particulate, in a form in which they can travel to the lymph nodes or spleen and be ingested by macrophages in the medulla of lymph nodes or red pulp of the spleen. If antigen is, on the other hand, fixed in the tissues such as a solid tissue homograft or is in fact a modified part of the body's own tissues, such as the skin treated with a simple chemical sensitizing agent, the response is of a different type (Fig. 1). It has been suggested that T-lymphocytes passing through the tissues are sensitized in the periphery and then pass down to the local lymph node where they enter the free area of the cortex between the lymph follicles. Here they find the right milieu for proliferation and in the process of proliferation enlarge this region into what is known as the "paracortical area" of the lymph node or the corresponding area in the spleen (Figs. 5a, b, c). The sensitized lymphocytes first differentiate into large cells with easily identifiable characteristics which reach a peak in concentration four days after sensitization. On this day they begin to divide into a new population of lymphocytes some of which are immunologically active and which leave the local lymphoid tissue to pass to other lymph nodes, where they can propagate into other immunologically active lymphocytes. From this time immunologically active cells can be found in the peripheral blood and pass to the graft where they can initiate the process of graft rejection or react with the antigen deposit in the periphery to produce an inflammatory response such as that which occurs in chemical contact sensitivity. It is not known what changes occur in the lymphocyte once it has become sensitized but these cells have now developed the property of being able to recognize antigen and react with it in a way which is probably not very different from that in which a soluble immunoglobulin molecule will react with antigen. This would suggest that antigenic recognition and reaction is a function related to the F(ab) fragment of immunoglobulin, embedded in the cell membrane of the T-lymphocyte. Macrophages interact with lymphocytes in the production of cell-mediated immune lesions.

The cell-mediated immune response is known to be dependent on the integrity of the thymus during embryonic and early neonatal life (Fig. 1). The role of the thymus which is one of the major lymphoid tissues in the body is still wrapped in mystery. However, it is known that if the thymus is removed from experimental animals (mice or rats) in early neonatal life, these animals will be unable to develop cell-mediated immune responses. Among other things they will not be able to reject tissue homografts. At the same time the lymphoid tissue will be depleted of lymphocytes and the areas affected are those in which cells proliferate during the development of a "cell-mediated immune response" (Figs. 5b, c). These areas in the lymph node are the paracortical areas,

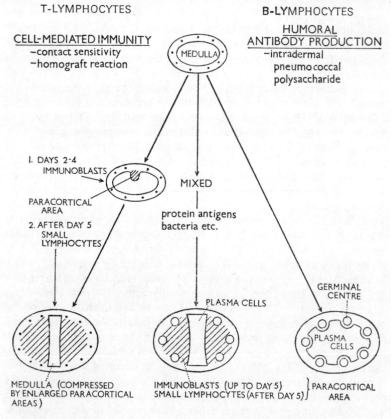

FIG. 5a. Primary response of lymph node to antigenic stimulation.

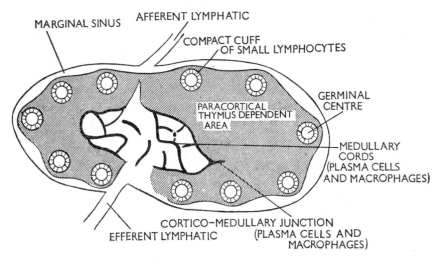

FIG. 5*b*. Diagram of immunologically active lymph node.

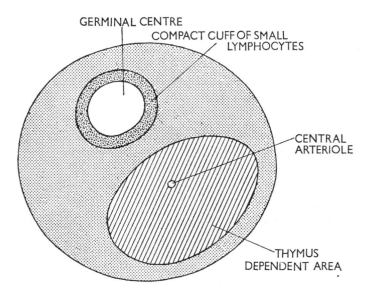

FIG. 5*c*. Diagram of a spleen follicle.

described above, and proliferation of lymphocytes in these areas will be prevented when the animal is presented with a fixed antigenic stimulus. The paracortical area of the lymph node can thus be considered to be functionally a "thymus dependent area" within the lymph node. It can also be shown that the area of white pulp in the spleen, immediately surrounding the central arteriole, is also an area of lymphoid tissue dependent on the integrity of the thymus in embryonic and early neo-natal life. Neonatally thymectomized animals are still able to respond to stimulation with a soluble antigen by the proliferation of plasma cells at the cortico-medullary junction and in the medullary cords of lymph nodes or in the red pulp of the spleen and to develop germinal centres within lymph follicles in the cortex of lymph nodes or the white pulp of the spleen. These animals have normal levels of immuno-globulins and can produce certain antibodies, although there is some inhibition of formation of other antibodies. An analogy to the condition produced by neonatal thymectomy in mice is found in the condition of congenital thymic aplasia and will be described more fully in the chapter on immunological deficiency diseases. A T-cell response may also act synergistically in the production of certain humoral antibodies. The level of these antibodies is low in animals which have been thy-mectomized in early neonatal life. The mechanism by which T-lym-phocytes amplify the production of antibody by B-lymphocytes is poorly understood. Such T-cells are often referred to as "helper" cells and it has been suggested that they act by focusing antigen on B-lymphocytes. Another possibility is that they act by the production of a specific soluble substance that is cytophilic for macrophages, which then binds antigen and presents it to the B-cells. Other factors involved appear to be non-specific and could promote B-cell differentiation and proliferation once it has been initiated. As well as being "helper" cells, T-cells may act as suppressor cells and be involved in the maintenance of a state of immunological unresponsiveness.

Another class of lymphocyte are the so-called K-cells. These cells are involved in cytotoxicity *in vitro* to target cells already coated with antibody. These cells cannot be identified with any other known group of lymphocytes, although they might bear some relation to immature cells of the mononuclear phagocyte series. Their role *in vivo* has not yet been clearly defined.

(c) Trigger mechanisms

The immune response can be considered to consist of three phases (i) recognition of antigen (ii) amplification by clonal proliferation and differentiation (iii) rejection of that which is foreign. In the past there was much discussion as to the nature of the trigger mechanism. It is now accepted that there exist in the body lymphocytes carrying re-ceptors on their surface that will recognise individual antigens. One cell will carry only one receptor specifically. When such a cell recognises antigen it will then be stimulated to clonal proliferation to produce either T-cells carrying similar membrane receptors or B-cells capable of becoming plasma cells and secreting immunoglobulins. These have receptors forming part of the Fab fragment with a peptide sequence the same as that of the original pre-existing receptor. The aminoacid sequence of the antibody combining site can be shown to have a specific antigenicity. As a result, antibodies can be produced in a foreign species specific for the site. These antibodies are referred to as anti-idiotypic antibodies. These antibodies are also specific for the idiotypes of the pre-existing receptors on lymphocytes. Moreover anti-idiotypic antibodies can be shown to take the place of antigen in stimulating specific clonal proliferation and thus the immune response. This demonstration that these receptors can be triggered by anti-idiotypic antibody, indicates that the pre-existing receptors for antigen on circumalting lymphocytes have the same antigenicity and thus chemical structure as the antigen-combining site of the antibody that is subsequently produced as part of the immune response.

4. Control Mechanisms in the Immune Response—Immunological Unresponsiveness

Until recently it was useful to think of a primary immune response as if it was a unidirectional force involving the stimulation of a single mechanism. The concept of a simple immune response was that of a stimulation of a single clone of lymphocytes which would proliferate and differentiate into plasma cells making humoral antibody or into the specifically sensitized lymphocytes of cell-mediated immunity. The later idea that initial contact with antigen could result in a balance between a positive immune response and a similar, but related negative force has been slow to develop, although indications of such a homeo-static mechanism have been inherent in studies for many years. With the introduction of the concept of "immunological enhancement" this approach has had increasing popularity. However it might be con-sidered to have been inherent in early studies of densensitization in clinical allergy and in the nature of blocking antibodies. Such a negative feedback can be provided by suppressor cells of either the T or the B class of lymphocytes as well as by "enhancing antibody".

Immunological unresponsiveness may be *antigen specific* or, as in a number of disease states *antigen non-specific*. The latter conditions are frequently referred to as primary or secondary immuno-deficiences. These will be discussed in further detail in later chapters and similar states can be induced by the action of immunosuppressive drugs. Specific immunological unresponsiveness occurs as a result of an upset in the normal balance of immunological control. A number of terms are used to describe the different processes that can produce such changes. It is now accepted that every immune response develops to a greater or lesser extent as a result of a balance between conventional reactive immunocytes which may be referred to as "effector cells" and cells that specifically block the immune response which are referred to as "suppressor cells". These cells would appear to act either by direct competition for antigen or by producing a soluble mediator that can inhibit other immunological mechanisms. Thus immunological unresponsiveness can develop as a result of the elimination of active clones of "effector" cells or from an increase in the activity of these "suppressor" cells.

The elimination of specifically responsive clones of effector lymphocytes is referred to as *immunological tolerance*. This form of unresponsiveness is more readily produced in neonatal than in adult life and is best demonstrated with transplantation antigens. Neonatal individuals injected with a large amount of transplantation antigen from an unrelated donor will subsequently accept skin grafts that would under normal circumstances be rejected.

It is thought that the reason that we recognise "self" antigens and do not normally produce an immune response against our own tissues is because we develop immunological tolerance to our own tissues during embryonic life at a stage before we develop the ability to produce an immune response. Red cell isoantibodies appear in the circulation during the second half of the first year or during the second year of life. It is thought that these antibodies are developed as an immune response to bacteria in the intestinal tract which carry antigens that cross react with A or B blood group substances carried on red cells. If an individual carries A or B or both antigens on the surface of his red cells he will have become tolerant to these antigens during embryonic life and will not then be able to develop the isoantibodies which appear in the serum of those who do not carry these antigens.

Another way in which immunological unresponsiveness can be produced, particularly in respect of cell-mediated immunity is known as *immunological enhancement*. The term immunological enhancement has been coined by cancer research workers to describe the "enhanced" or increased growth of tumours in animals whose cell-mediated immunity is specifically inhibited from developing by the presence of certain types of humoral antibody directed against the same antigen. These antibodies either alone or complexed with soluble tumour specific transplantation antigen (TSTA) in the form of soluble circulating immune complexes will then compete with T-cells for the antigenic sites on the tumour cells. This then blocks the development or action of cell-mediated immune processes directed towards tumour rejection. The phenomenon of immunological enhancement can also be used to allow the retention of tissue homografts. Antibody is produced against the transplantation antigen and transfusion of this antibody will prevent cell-mediated immune processes developing to the specific antigen.

To recapitulate, it is now recognised that a number of mechanisms exist that can account for a disturbance in the homeostatic balance as a result of which a state of specific immunological unresponsiveness may occur. These include:

1. Elimination of specifically responsive clones of lymphocytes.
2. Suppressor T-lymphocytes.
3. Suppressor B-lymphocytes.
4. Suppression of lymphocyte response by humoral (enhancing) antibody.
5. Suppression of lymphocyte response by circulating immune (antigen–antibody) complexes.

Decreased host resistance to a tumour or infective organism may result from any of these five processes, upsetting the homeostatic balance. Increased host resistance can therefore be achieved by restoring the balance through a selective inhibition of suppressor cells or the B-cells producing enhancing antibody.

5. Genetic Control of the Immune Response—The Role of the Major Histocompatibility Complex (MHC)

Perhaps the greatest advance in immunological thinking in the past five years has been on the role of the major histocompatibility complex (MHC), especially its effect on the control of the immune response. Much of the work on the MHC has been in the mouse and it is therefore important to discuss this using the mouse as the main model, drawing analogy to the human system as far as possible.

The MHC or H2 system in the mouse was first shown to be associated with the development of transplantation antigens that were responsible for the rapid rejection of skin grafts between different strains of highly inbred histocompatible mice. The H2-region is a limited area on the 17th chromosome of the mouse. The genes carried by this area form what is known as the H2 haplotype. (The term haplotype is used to describe a set of genetic determinants carried on a single chromosome.) The H2 haplotype has four regions (Fig. 6). These are known as the K, I, S and D regions. The K and D regions control the expression of the two major groups of glycoprotein transplantation antigens that can be found on the surface of most cell types including lymphocytes. The I region is associated with particular antigenic determinants found on B rather than T-cells known as the Ia antigens. Three subregions have been described I-A, I-B and I-C. The fourth region is the S region which controls the expression of the fourth component of complement (C4) and the levels of the first and second components (C1 and C2).

Table 2

The role of the major histocompatibility complex (MHC)
1. Control of expression of membrane glycoprotein antigens that result in strong histocompatibility differences.
2. Expression of Ir genes.
3. Regulation of lymphocyte development and interaction.
4. Expression of complement components.
5. Susceptibility to certain diseases.

The immune response of mice to certain specific antigens are controlled by the Ir genes and these are also located in the H2-complex, particularly in the I-A and I-B subregions of the I region. Histocompatibility-linked immune response genes have now been demonstrated in a number of species including guinea pigs, mice, rats and rabbits. These are all autosomal dominant genes which are inherited in a strictly Mendelian fashion. Ir genes may under certain circumstances be expressed by T or B cells. Much of the work has been done with the ability to express an immune response to artificially prepared peptide antigens with a known aminoacid sequence such as (T,G)-A—L or (Phe,G)-A—L. However genetic differences can also be found in the ability of experimental animals to develop chemical contact sensitivity to metals. There are two inbred strains of guinea pigs that differ in the MHC, strain 2 and strain 13. Strain 2 can be sensitized with chromium and beryllium but not mercury, whereas strain 13 can be sensitized to mercury but not to chromium or beryllium.

In man the MHC is situated on chromosome 6 and is called the HLA region. There are four loci controlling four groups of histocompatibility antigens. These are referred to as HLA-A, HLA-B, HLA-C and HLA-D. The HLA-A region is the equivalent of the D region in the mouse and the HLA-B the equivalent of the K region. The antigens controlled by the A and B regions can be detected serologically on the surface of leucocytes by the standard dye exclusion tests using suitably absorbed sera from multitransfused people, multiparous women or those who have rejected grafts. These are the antigens detected by standard tissue typing procedures and each person has four, one each of the A and B groups inherited from the father and one each of the A and B groups from the mother. The D locus controls a set of antigens known as lymphocyte activating determinants that initially were not detected serologically and can be demonstrated by the mixed lymphocyte reaction (MLR). The D region is also considered to be equivalent to the I region in the mouse.

The role of Ir genes in man has not been defined to the same extent as in experimental animals. However there is definite data to suggest that HLA-linked Ir genes are involved in the expression of IgE antibody against ragweed antigen E. Data is also accumulating demonstrating an association between HLA antigens and certain diseases. These

GENETIC STRUCTURE OF THE MAJOR HISTOCOMPATIBILITY COMPLEX OF MICE AND MEN.

a. MOUSE. (chromosome 17)

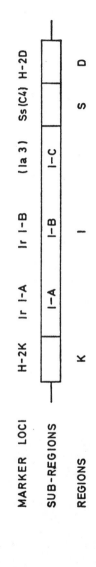

MARKER LOCI	H-2K	Ir I-A	Ir I-B	(Ia 3)	Ss(C4)	H-2D
SUB-REGIONS		I-A	I-B	I-C		
REGIONS	K		I		S	D

b. HUMAN. (chromosome 6)

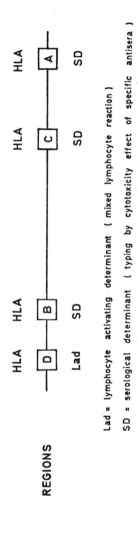

	HLA	HLA	HLA	HLA
REGIONS	D	B	C	A
	Lad	SD	SD	SD

Lad = lymphocyte activating determinant (mixed lymphocyte reaction)

SD = serological determinant (typing by cytotoxicity effect of specific antisera)

FIG. 6.

include ankylosing spondylitis, acute anterior uveitis, Reiter's syndrome, coeliac disease and multiple sclerosis. The association of HLA antigens with certain disease states in which immunological mechanisms had so far not been defined, raises a number of points for speculation. These come out particularly in a discussion of the high incidence of HLA antigen B27 in patients with ankylosing spondylitis, which may be

Table 3

Positive associations between HLA and disease

Hodgkin's disease	A1, B8
Acute lymphatic leukaemia	A2, B12
Ankylosing spondylitis	
Acute anterior uveitis	
Psoriasis	B27
Reiter's syndrome	
Coeliac disease	
Dermatitis herpetiformis	
Thyrotoxicosis	B8
Myasthenia gravis	
Chronic active hepatitis	
Systemic lupus erythematotus	BW15
Multiple sclerosis	A3, B7, DW2
Paralytic poliomyelitis	A3, B7
Ragweed allergy	HLA linked Ir gene

as high as 96%. There is also a high incidence of B27 among patients with arthritis associated with defined infectious agents such as Yersinia, gonococci or salmonella. It could well be that HLA linked Ir genes control the expression of cell-mediated immunity and antibody production to these and other organisms. In such a situation the possession of the B27 antigen could be associated with a decreased host resistance and increase in the potential to develop immune complex arthritis. Recently there has been an increased interest in the association of antigens controlled by the D locus. These antigens have lymphocyte activating determinants and can be detected by the mixed leucocyte reaction. A number of diseases which had previously been shown to be associated relatively weakly with B locus antigens, can be shown to have a stronger association with D locus antigens. These include multiple sclerosis, gluten sensitive enteropathy and dermatitis herpetiformis, and more recently rheumatoid arthritis.

Another role that the MHC plays is to act as the basis for antigenicity in immunological surveillance, particularly in tumour and virus systems. In certain virus infections in mice it has been found that the immune response can be demonstrated only against virus infected cells of the same histocompatibility type. This has been extended to show a similar restriction in chemical contact sensitivity where sensitized lymphocytes will only react with hapten linked cells of the same histocompatibility type. This would indicate that the histocompatibility antigen of the individual or a structure coded for in close proximity must form part of the antigen. The implication therefore exists that the immune response to virally infected cells or chemically altered cells is to "altered" self and particularly products of the major histocompatibility complex. This has suggested that an important function of the MHC is to signal changes in self to the immune system and that the development of such strong antigens may be important in the evolutionary development of the immunological surveillance mechanisms.

Bibliography

Books

Dresser, D. W. (ed.) (1976), "Immunological Tolerance." *Brit. med. Bull.*, **32**, 2.

Gell, P. G. H. & Coombs, R. R. A. (eds.) (1975), *Clinical Aspects of Immunology*. Oxford: Blackwell. Third edition.

Haurowitz, F. (1968), *Immunochemistry and the Biosynthesis of Antibodies*. New York: Interscience.

Hobart, M. J. and McConnell, I. (eds.) (1975), *The Immune System. A course on the molecular and cellular basis of immunity*. Oxford: Blackwell.

Humphrey, J. H. & White, R. G. (1970), *Immunology for Students of Medicine*. Oxford: Blackwell. Third edition.

Kabat, E. A. (1976), *Structural Concepts in Immunology and Immunochemistry*. New York: Holt, Rinehart Winston. Second edition.

Landsteiner, K. (1945), *Specificity of Serological Reactions*. Harvard University Press.

Manning, M. J. and Turner, R. J. (1976), *Comparative Immunobiology*. Glasgow: Blackie.

Roitt, I. M. (1974), *Essential Immunology*. Oxford: Blackwell. Second edition.

Steward, M. W. (1974), *Immunochemistry*. Chapman and Hall.

Thompson, R. A. (1974), *The Practice of Clinical Immunology*. London: Edward Arnold.

Turk, J. L. (1975), *Delayed Hypersensitivity*. Amsterdam: North Holland Publishing Company. Second edition.

Weir, D. M. (ed.) (1973), *Handbook or Experimental Immunology*. Oxford: Blackwell Scientific Publications. Second edition.

Articles

Burnet, F. M. (1968), "Evolution of the immune process in vertebrates." *Nature*, **218**, 426.

Doherty, P. C. and Zinkernagel, R. M. (1975), "A biological role for the major histocompatibility antigens." *Lancet*, **i**, 1406.

Hobbs, J. R. (1967), "Paraproteins, benign or malignant." *Brit. med. J.*, **3**, 699.

"Nomenclature for factors of the HLA system." *Bull. Wld. Hlth. Org.*, **52**, 261 (1975).

Chapter II
Reactions in the Tissues Mediated by Humoral Antibodies

The type of tissue damage caused by antigen–antibody interaction depends on the physical nature of the antibody involved, and the site where the antigen–antibody reaction takes place. Broadly, antibodies can be divided into conventional antibodies, which belong to the immunoglobulin classes: IgG, IgA and IgM and antibodies which fix rapidly to tissues. In the human these antibodies are known as reagins and belong to the group of immunoglobulins known as IgE. It is this latter group of antibodies which are thought to be responsible for the different manifestations of anaphylaxis. Whereas conventional antibodies can be detected in the serum by standard *in vitro* laboratory procedures such as precipitation, agglutination and complement fixation, reagins can only be detected with ease by their reaction *in vivo*. These antibodies can only be detected *in vitro* by complex radioactive assay procedures. Reagins differ from other antibodies by their increased ability to adhere to tissues and thus any reactions between antigen and reagins takes place on the surface of tissues and it is these tissues which respond with anaphylactic phenomena. The type of reaction produced by conventional antibodies (such as IgG antibodies) depends on the site in the tissue where the antigens and antibodies interact. Whereas reagins always interact with antigen on mucosal or other cell surfaces, IgG antibodies will react with antigen within tissue spaces. One of the commonest sites of such a reaction is in the wall of small blood vessels as antibody is present within the circulation and the antigen often lies in the extravascular space. The antigen and antibody then diffuse towards one another and reaction occurs in the vessel wall. However, if the antigen is present in the circulation as well, antigen and antibody will interact intravascularly and immune complexes will be present in the circulation and be able to lodge in small blood vessels in the kidney glomerulus, synovial membranes, skin, cardiac muscle and other sites where they produce areas of localized tissue damage.

1. Passive Sensitization with Humoral Antibodies

As humoral antibodies are serum proteins, passive sensitization can be produced by the transfer of serum from one individual to another. Passive transfer can produce a generalized state of sensitization if the serum from a sensitized individual is injected intravenously. However, if the serum is injected intradermally, only a local state of sensitization is produced in the area of skin into which the serum has been injected. A state of generalized passive sensitization will last as long as the

Reactions Mediated by Humoral Antibodies   23

antibody is present in the circulation. If the serum is homologous (i.e. from the same species) the level of antibody in the circulation will fall off exponentially, with a half life of about 20 days. However, if the serum is from another species (such as horse antitoxin against tetanus toxin injected into a human), elimination will start off with a half life of 8 days, but after 7 days antibodies will be produced against the foreign serum which itself acts as an antigen and the foreign antiserum will begin to be eliminated very rapidly from the circulation. If antibodies are already present in the circulation against the foreign serum, foreign antiserum will be eliminated rapidly from the beginning.

As reagins adhere strongly to tissues, they are often called tissue sensitizing antibodies. If serum containing reagins are injected intradermally the area injected will remain responsive for over 48 hours. This is the fundamental basis of the Prausnitz-Küstner reaction for the demonstration of the presence of these anaphylactic antibodies in the human. Antibodies that produce anaphylaxis in other species can be demonstrated by classical *in vitro* methods such as precipitation or agglutination of erythrocytes in which the antigen has been artificially stuck to their surface. In the human, anaphylactic antibodies can be demonstrated by the technique of passive transfer to an individual who has not been previously sensitized. Twenty-four to forty-eight hours after the transfer, the antigen is pricked into the area of skin which has been sensitized. Within 15–20 minutes a typical weal and flare similar to that produced by histamine develops in the skin (Prausnitz-Küstner reaction). Serum transfers in the human carry a strong risk of transferring serum hepatitis and should not be undertaken lightly. Serum should not be used for Prausnitz-Küstner transfers unless the patient has been a blood donor and has thus been proved not to be a carrier of the virus of serum hepatitis. Whereas the concentration of other antibodies injected into the skin drops off within 24–48 hours to about half of that injected originally, there is little diminution in the concentration of reagins injected into the skin, over the same period of time. Reagins also differ from other antibodies in being heat labile, the reaginic activity of a serum can be destroyed by heating at 56°C for 20 minutes, whereas the activity of more conventional antibodies is not affected by similar treatment. The identification of reaginic antibodies as belonging to the class of immunoglobulin IgE has been confirmed by experiments in the human where prior injection of IgE globulin into the skin, blocks the tissue sites to which reagins can bind and produce a Prausnitz-Küstner reaction. Reaginic antibodies have been detected in the IgG class of immunoglobulins. These antibodies are not common. They are classified as reagins because they induce histamine mediated increased vascular permeability in the skin. They differ from IgE reagins in that they are heat stable and do not produce the long-term anaphylactic sensitization of skin, typical of the

IgE antibody. They also appear to need complement for their action, whereas IgE antibodies act independently of complement. Reaginic antibodies can be detected *in vitro* in the serum of patients with allergies by a two-stage test (RAST: Radioallergosorbent test). In the first stage the antibody (IgE globulin) can be made to react with the antigen (animal dandruff, pollen, fungal extracts, extracts of shellfish or house dust) bound to an insoluble dextran carrier. These antibodies can then be detected specifically as reagins in the second stage of the test in which the immune complex on the insoluble carrier is reacted with a radio-actively-labelled antiserum directed specifically against IgE globulin. The amount of IgE globulin (reagin) taken up by the insoluble antigen-carrier complex will then be proportional to the amount of radioactive anti-IgE bound in the second stage of the test. A further method that has been used is to link the antigen to a red cell and then react the antigen-red cell complex with reaginic serum (containing IgE anti-bodies). The red cells will then have the specific reaginic antibodies (IgE) on their surfaces and can be agglutinated by antisera prepared specifically against the IgE immunoglobulin. This latter technique could eventually prove suitable for routine *in vitro* testing for reaginic activity.

2. Reactions Mediated by Anaphylactic Antibodies (Fig. 1)

Although it is possible to produce anaphylactic phenomena with human IgG antibodies in experimental animals, only reagins (mainly IgE antibodies) are able to produce these phenomena in man. However, human IgE antibodies will not produce these phenomena in experimental animals. There is a direct analogy to this in experimental animals, the guinea pig produces two types of antibody belonging to the class of γ_1 and γ_2 globulins. γ_1-globulin antibodies will produce anaphylactic phenomena in guinea pigs but not in other species and are analogous in this respect to reagins in the human. Guinea pig γ_2 globulin antibodies will however produce anaphylactic phenomena in other species of experimental animals in the same way as human IgG antibodies.

Anaphylactic phenomena are caused by the antigen–antibody reaction activating a series of enzymes leading to the release of certain pharmacological agents from cells or activating precursors of pharmacological agents which are free in the circulation. In man anaphylactic reactions are of two types depending on the portal of entry of the antigen. The first group of milder reactions occur when antigen–antibody reactions occur at an exposed mucosal surface. These reactions occur most commonly to pollens or animal dander and the reactions may be limited to a simple rhinorrhoea and conjunctivitis. If the state of allergy is more intense, bronchospasm may also be produced as a result of inhalation of the antigen. Patients with allergic asthma have been found to have levels of IgE immunoglobulin (which contains reaginic antibody) up

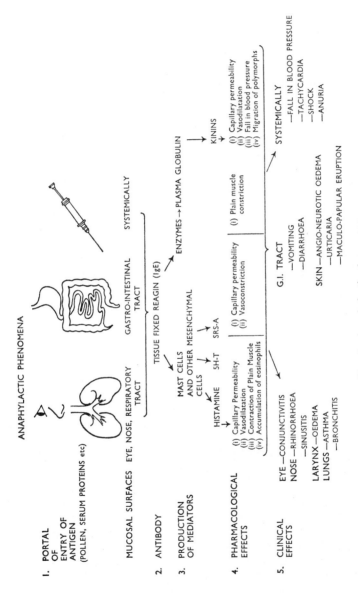

Fig. 1. Anaphylactic phenomena.

to six times higher than that found in patients with "non-allergic" asthma, confirming the relation between these antibodies and this condition.

If the antigen is injected parenterally as in the case of a drug such as penicillin, foreign sera or the saliva of biting insect, systemic anaphylaxis may supervene rapidly. This is manifested in man by bronchospasm, laryngeal oedema resulting in extreme dyspnoea with cyanosis, and a marked fall in the blood pressure. There may also be nausea, vomiting and diarrhoea. Systemic anaphylaxis is a potentially fatal condition if not treated promptly. Cutaneous urticaria, the formation of weal and flare lesions in the skin, is an anaphylactic phenomenon which may develop from the absorption of antigen through the intestinal tract. It more often occurs alone, but may be associated with other signs of generalized anaphylaxis. Not all urticaria is caused by an immune reaction. It is known that the pharmacological agents which cause urticaria can be released by other means especially physical agents such as trauma or cold. Most of the reactions found in anaphylaxis can be attributed to the release or activation of pharmacologically active agents. Five groups have so far been recognized. These are histamine, slow reacting substance (SRS-A), serotonin, the group of related agents known as the plasma kinins and the prostaglandins. These will be described separately.

(a) Histamine

Histamine is released from the mast cells and basophil leucocytes distributed throughout the tissues. It exists in the form of its precursor L-histidine and is formed by the action of the enzyme histidine decarboxylase. Histidine is often associated with heparin in the mast cells. Release of histamine is accompanied by degranulation of tissue mast cells or the basophil leucocytes. Histamine injected into the skin causes a typical weal surrounded by a flare. The weal is caused by increased capillary permeability and the flare of local vasodilatation. Histamine also causes contraction of plain muscle, hence the bronchospasm. The action of histamine can be inhibited by anti-histamine drugs such as Mepyramine (Anthisan) and Promethazine (Phenergan).

(b) Serotonin

Serotonin or 5-hydroxytryptamine also causes contraction of plain muscle and increased capillary permeability. It is however a capillary vasoconstrictor. In some species serotonin occurs mainly in the platelets. An antagonist to serotonin is lysergic acid diethylamine. The role of serotonin in human anaphylactic phenomena is not yet fully understood, although it is known to play a role in certain anaphylactic phenomena in experimental animals, such as the rabbit.

(*c*) *Slow reacting substance*

Slow reacting substance (SRS-A) is released during anaphylaxis especially in the lung, though it is released at a later stage than histamine. It is not blocked by antihistamine drugs. It is recognized mainly by its ability to contract plain muscle, and could be one of the main causes of bronchial constriction in the human.

(*d*) *Plasma kinins*

The plasma kinins—bradykinin and kallidin are simple peptides consisting of nine and ten amino acids respectively, they are formed from plasma globulins by the plasma kinin forming enzymes, kallikrein, plasmin or trypsin. Kallikrein is released from basophils during anaphylaxis. Kinins cause increased capillary permeability, vasodilatation and a fall in blood pressure. Bradykinin produces pain when injected in the human. Another effect is to cause migration of polymorphonuclear leucocytes from blood vessels and their accumulation in the tissues. Kinins once they are formed are rapidly broken down by kininases, enzymes also present in the blood. Thus their accumulation at any site is controlled.

(*e*) *Prostaglandins*

The prostaglandins are fatty acids of Molecular Weight between 300 and 400. They are secondary mediators released from plain muscle as a result of the action of other mediators. Prostaglandin E and F are antagonistic in inflammation. PGE increases vascular permeability and potentiates the effect of other mediators, whereas PGF inhibits these effects. There are fourteen known prostaglandins and one, prostaglandin E_1, has been shown to be released in anaphylactic shock.

Reagins and comparable anaphylactic antibodies in experimental animals are thought to cause the release of these pharmacologically active agents through a number of stages which are far from being completely worked out. Some work has, however, been done on the release of histamine from mast cells. It appears that the antigen/antibody reaction probably takes place on the surface of the mast cell. By studying the inhibitors of histamine release *in vitro*, it has been suggested that the intermediate steps involve a number of esterases one of which has a substrate specificity similar to that of the enzyme chymotrypsin.

Blocking antibodies. Desensitization of anaphylactic individuals can be produced by multiple subcutaneous injection of antigen. This is most commonly done with pollen antigens to prevent the development of hay fever and asthma. Up to 50 subcutaneous injections are given increasing the dose of antigen gradually. Another technique is to suspend the antigen in an oily base. As a result of this treatment the patient develops

IgG antibodies against the antigen. These antibodies have a higher avidity for the antigen than the reagins and are able to compete successfully with the reagins for the antigenic sites of the allergenic molecule. As reaction with the IgG antibody does not take place at a cell surface, anaphylactic phenomena are not produced, and reaction with the IgG antibody does not have any harmful effect as the level present should be below the high level of IgG antibody necessary to produce an Arthus type of reaction.

Eosinophil leucocytes. Eosinophil leucocytes play a considerable role in anaphylactic reactions, though the exact part they play is still controversial. Eosinophils are formed in the bone marrow and are released into the circulating blood as required. There is no doubt that infiltration of the tissues with eosinophils is a common denominator of many anaphylactic reactions and that these reactions are generally associated with an eosinophil leucocytosis in the peripheral blood. Most workers agree that eosinophils are attracted in the human by antigen–antibody complexes and in experimental animals they have been shown to phagocytose these complexes. Eosinophils may be found in the skin in urticarial reactions whether these have an immunological or a pharmacological basis. Eosinophil chemotactic factor (ECF-A), a simple tetrapeptide, has been shown to be released in anaphylaxis. Eosinophils are also attracted by concentrations of histamine and that the eosinophils have the property of being able to detoxify histamine. It has been found that the phagocytosis of immune complexes can be potentiated by the presence of histamine. The intradermal injection of histamine into ponies has been shown to cause an accumulation of eosinophils at the site of the weal which developed from the histamine. Moreover equine eosinophils have been shown to inactivate histamine and serotonin both *in vivo* and *in vitro*. It has been suggested that the detoxification of histamine by eosinophils could be due to their having a potent peroxidase enzyme. Experiments have been performed which show that the accumulation of eosinophils in the periphery can be inhibited by antihistamine drugs.

3. The Arthus Reaction—Complement

Anaphylactic antibodies produce tissue reaction within 15 minutes of contact with antigen on cell surfaces. The Arthus reaction on the other hand is an allergic reaction which only occurs when there is a very high concentration of conventional antibody such as IgG in the circulation and a high concentration of soluble antigen lying extravascularly in the tissue spaces. A lot can be learnt of the nature of the Arthus phenomenon from a study of the reaction as it occurs in the skin of experimental animals such as the rabbit or guinea pig following intradermal injection of the antigen once the animal has become sensitized. The

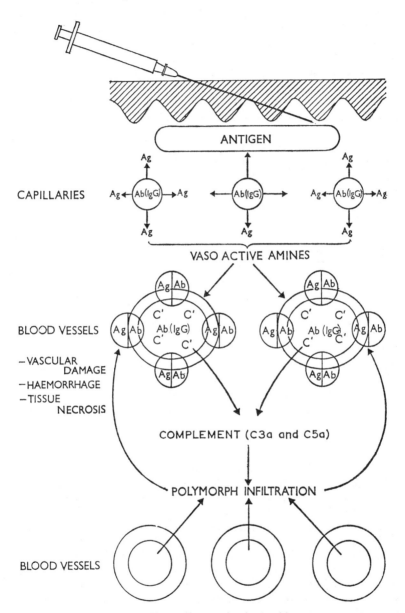

Fig. 2. The Arthus reaction in the skin.

reaction occurs primarily in the wall of small blood vessels as a result of antibody from the circulation meeting antigen diffusing inwards from the extravascular space. The lesion found is a vasculitis. Antigen–antibody complexes can be demonstrated in the vessel wall. Polymorphonuclear leucocytes are attracted in large numbers to the site of reaction, where they can be shown to be phagocytosing antigen, both within and outside the vessel walls. The vessel wall then becomes damaged. Some vessels can be found to contain thrombi consisting of platelets and leucocytes whereas others are so damaged that there is marked leakage of red cells. The tissues also become oedematous due to increased permeability from the damaged blood vessels. In experimental animals, the Arthus reaction takes 2–8 hours to develop persisting for 12–24 hours and macroscopically there is oedema of the site often with petechial haemorrhages. Much of the damaging effects of an Arthus reaction can be reduced by lowering the number of circulating polymorphonuclear leucocytes. This can be done especially with an antiserum directed against these cells prepared in another animal. There is no doubt that polymorphs play a vital role in the development of the lesions found in Arthus reactions (Fig. 2).

As mentioned in the previous section the reaction between anaphylactic antibody and antigen activates a series of esterases in the process of releasing pharmacological agents to produce tissue damage. The reaction between conventional IgG antibody and antigen also appears to activate a similar but not identical system of enzymes. This system has been known for a long time as it is involved in the lysis of bacteria and red cells and in the phagocytosis of foreign antigens in the presence of antibody. It is known as the *complement* system and was first described as a group of factors present in fresh serum that was necessary to be present for antibody to lyse red cells *in vitro*. Complement is recognised as a system of factors that occur in normal serum, which are activated characteristically by antigen–antibody interaction and subsequently mediate a number of biologically significant functions (Fig. 3). Complement is normally studied in its role in immune haemolysis. Immune haemolysis is associated with the development of lesions in the erythrocyte membrane. These circular lesions (100 $A°$ diameter) develop as the end result of a sequence of events involving all nine components of complement reacting in five stages. Homeostasis of complement action is controlled by a series of inhibitors or inactivators. The classical pathway of complement is generally considered to be activated by IgG or IgM antibody complexed with antigen. Complement does not appear to play a role in IgE-mediated anaphylactic reactions, nor is it activated by IgA antibody under normal conditions. Activation of the classical pathway of complement plays a central role in the development of Arthus and similar immune complex reactions. Apart from the membrane lytic effect of C9, the main direct biological

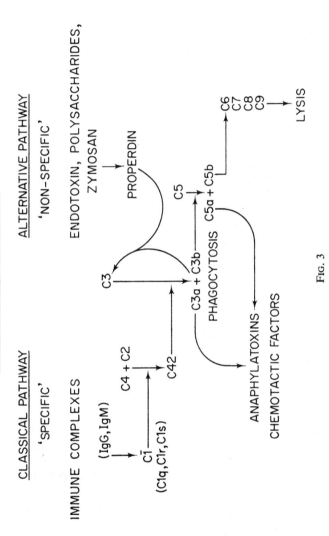

FIG. 3

effect of complement is through C3 and C5. C3 plays a major role through the immune adherence phenomenon by which antigens adhere to membrane receptors. This is important in phagocytosis by macrophages and polymorphs. A small fragment of C3 produced by the action of C3 convertase known as C3a has a series of biological actions that have been grouped together under the title of *anaphylatoxins*. C5a produced during the activation of C5 by C5 convertase is also an anaphylatoxin as well as being chemotactic for polymorphonuclear leucocytes. C3a and C5a are peptides of 7,500 and 17,000 M.W. respectively. *In vitro* they can be demonstrated by their action in contracting guinea pig ileum. However the intradermal injection of C5a into human skin will also cause pruritus and wheal and erythema associated with mast cell degranulation and polymorphonuclear leucocyte accumulation. These effects have been shown to be associated with release of histamine and 5-hydroxytryptamine. C5a is also a potent neutrophil chemotactic agent. This action is independent of its anaphylatoxin activity and is due to another peptide breakdown product. A similar peptide fragment derived from C3 is also chemotactic.

Evidence for an *alternative pathway* of complement action comes from studies showing that complement can be inactivated by yeast or zymosan, an insoluble carbohydrate derived from yeast. This is due to a two stage reaction in which zymosan reacts non-specifically with a protein called properdin and a glycine rich glycoprotein called Factor B or C3 proactivator (C3PA) as well as C3 itself. The resulting complex then inactivates C3. This inactivation is independent of the classical pathway through C1, C4 and C2 that is activated by immune complexes. C3 can also be inactivated by a wide range of bacterial and other polysaccharides including bacterial endotoxins and carageenan. Inactivation of C3 by the alternative pathway is also associated with the production of anaphylatoxin in the serum and activation of the rest of the stages of complement pathway down to C9. The alternative pathway of complement activation can also interact with the blood coagulation system. It has been suggested that endotoxin causes platelets to release platelet factor 3 (PF3). Platelets are disrupted in large numbers releasing PF3 which accelerates coagulation once it has already developed. This is associated with basophil and mast cell degranulation induced by anaphylatoxin, which results in increased vascular permeability leading to haemoconcentration and stasis. Both together may then result in widespread small vessel vasculitis and diffuse intravascular coagulation. Activation of the alternative pathway by the injection of endotoxin into the skin will result in the development of a local inflammatory reaction with marked polymorphonuclear leucocyte infiltration, resembling the Arthus phenomenon. Intravenous injection of endotoxin or another polysaccharide 24 hours later will result in massive haemorrhage at the local site of injection. This is referred to as the *local*

Shwartzman reaction. An intravenous injection of endotoxin followed 24 hours later by a further intravenous injection of endotoxin or similar polysaccharide will result in generalised haemorrhages throughout the body including the suprarenal glands. This reaction is referred to as the *generalised Shwartzman reaction.*

It is thought that the massive infiltration of the tissues with granulocytes in the Arthus reaction is due to the activation of complement. Moreover, animals which are genetically deficient in respect of one of these components of complement do not appear to be able to develop Arthus reactions. Complement components have been shown to accumulate at the site of an Arthus reaction. The third component of complement (C_3) which is electrophoretically identical with β_{1c} globulin, has been demonstrated together with IgG or IgM by immunohistological techniques in the tissues at the site of tissue damage by immune complexes, e.g. in glomerulonephritis and cutaneous vasculitis. Glomerulonephritis due to immune complex deposition is sometimes associated with reduced circulating levels of complement, especially C_3 (β_{1c} globulin), presumably as a result of fixation during the disease process.

The factors which cause the localization of immune complexes in blood vessels are very important in determining the mechanism of the Arthus reaction and other similar reactions caused by the deposition of these complexes in blood vessel walls. The development of these lesions has been found to be associated with an increased permeability of the vessel walls. This is thought to be due to the release of vasoactive amines such as histamine and 5-hydroxytryptamine. Inhibition of this increased permeability can be produced by treatment with suitable antagonists and this causes a decrease in the deposition of immune complexes in the blood vessel walls and a marked diminution in the intensity of the lesion produced.

In summary it has been suggested that reactions of the Arthus type result from the deposition of immune complexes as a result of increased vascular permeability due to the release of vasoactive amines. After deposition the immune complexes cause the activation of complement and especially C3a and C5a which attract polymorphonuclear leucocytes. These then accumulate and release hydrolytic enzymes from their granules which in turn cause the irreversible vascular damage which is the hall mark of the Arthus reaction (Fig. 2). The Arthus reaction can be induced in the human by the intradermal injection of antigens if there is a high level of circulating IgG antibodies. Arthus sensitivity has been detected by the intradermal injection of fungal antigens in pulmonary aspergillosis, and to thermophilic actinomycetes in patients with the disease "Farmer's lung". Other pulmonary diseases due to the inhalation of foreign antigens such as serum proteins have been found to be associated with a high degree of Arthus sensitivity, when the patients are skin tested. Arthus reactions in the human are red and oedematous reaching maximum intensity between four and twelve hours after intradermal injection. Immune complexes and complement may be detected in the blood vessels of the skin. The infiltration has a strong mononuclear component in the human, the degree of polymorphonuclear leucocyte infiltration being proportional to the amount of tissue damage. In the human it has also been suggested that an earlier anaphylactic component is necessary for the proper development of an Arthus reaction. This is similar to the demonstration in experimental animals that the release of vasoactive amines is necessary to produce increased vascular permeability before immune complexes can localize in the blood vessel wall.

Whereas immune complexes formed in antigen excess produce acute Arthus reactions and other lesions associated with blood-vessel damage, the subcutaneous injection of immune complexes formed at equivalence cause the local development of a granuloma in the tissues.

The fixation of complement components from fresh guinea pig serum is used by clinical pathologists as a means of detecting low levels or antibody in the serum. This is used especially in the Wassermann reaction for syphilis or in the demonstration of antibodies against certain viruses. An indicator system is used consisting of sheep red cells coated with horse or rabbit antibody against the red cells. If an antigen–antibody reaction has occurred, fixing the complement, complement is no more available and the sheep cells in the indicator system are not lysed. If either antigen or antibody are absent the complement is not fixed and is available for lysing the sheep red cell indicator system. This reaction is depicted diagrammatically in Fig. 4.

4. Serum Sickness

Much can be learnt about the damaging effect of immunological reactions on the body from a study of the condition known clinically as serum sickness. This condition was first described soon after the introduction of the treatment of diphtheria with antitoxin serum prepared in the horse. It was later reproduced by the injection of normal horse serum, not containing antitoxin, showing that the condition was a reaction to the injection of the foreign serum and was not related to the reaction between the toxin and antitoxin. The first observations made were of skin eruptions, but later anaphylactic reactions such as bronchial asthma and sudden death were more and more frequently associated with the injection of foreign sera in the human. The syndrome known as serum sickness is now known to be caused by a wide range of different antigens especially drugs such as penicillin, streptomycin, sulphonamides and the thiouracils. Serum sickness can be divided into two types. The first type can be called primary serum sickness and occurs in those who have not had any previous contact with the antigen and therefore have no pre-existing circulating antibodies

INDICATOR SYSTEM

E = sheep erythrocytes; A = antibody against sheep erythrocytes; C' = complement (fresh normal guinea pig serum)

E + A → EA → No LYSIS (of erythrocytes)

EA + C' → LYSIS (of erythrocytes)

TESTS

POSITIVE TEST

Stage 1   Immune complexes fixing complement.

[Ag + Ab + C']   [Ag + Ab + C']
          [Ag + Ab + C']

Stage 2   Addition of Indicator System   NO LYSIS

[Ag + Ab + C']   EA   [Ag + Ab + C']
EA   [Ag + Ab + C']   EA

NEGATIVE TEST

Stage 1   No formation of immune complex. No fixation of complement.

NO ANTIGEN			NO ANTIBODY IN SERUM		
Ab	C'	Ab	Ag	C'	Ag
C'	Ab	C'	C'	Ag	C'

Stage 2   Addition of Indicator System

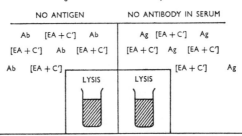

NO ANTIGEN			NO ANTIBODY IN SERUM		
Ab	[EA + C']	Ab	Ag	[EA + C']	Ag
[EA + C']	Ab	[EA + C']	[EA + C']	Ag	[EA + C']
Ab	[EA + C']		[EA + C']		Ag

LYSIS   LYSIS

FIG. 4.   COMPLEMENT FIXATION TEST

directed against the particular antigen. The other group of reactions
occur in those who have had a previous injection of the serum or have
circulating antibodies directed against the antigen from other causes.
These more severe reactions may occur in an individual allergic against

horse serum, as a result of contact with horse dander which is known to be contaminated with horse serum proteins. The reactions which occur in serum sickness are a result of the production of both anaphylactic and conventional circulating antibodies (IgG or IgM). The lesions which develop will depend on the relative amounts of each class of antibody produced. If most of the antibodies produced are anaphylactic antibodies (IgE), the symptoms, which develop, will be mainly anaphylactic as a result of reactions taking place on the cell surface. If the antibodies produced are mainly IgG or IgM, soluble antigen–antibody complexes will be found in the circulation and the lesions produced by these complexes will dominate the clinical picture. Often the condition is a result of a mixture of anaphylactic type reactions and those due to the presence of circulating immune complexes.

(i) *Primary serum sickness*

If a person is injected with a foreign serum, the proteins will initially be eliminated from the circulation at a slow rate with a half life of the order of eight days. As soon as the serum is injected an immune response will develop against the antigenic determinants of the foreign serum. The latent period of such an immune response is between six and twelve days depending on the strength of the immune response. Antibody against the foreign serum will begin to be present in the circulation after the seventh day and will combine directly with antigen. Symptoms of serum sickness are often found between the seventh and twelfth day after the injection of the foreign serum. The condition which develops will depend on the amounts of both anaphylactic and conventional antibody produced. The illness may be mild, lasting two to four days or may be more severe and lasting many weeks. The degree of severity will also depend both upon the amount of each type of antibody produced and upon the amount of foreign serum present in the circulation.

(a) *Anaphylactic symptoms* (Table 1).

The anaphylactic symptoms found in serum sickness are those described at the beginning of this chapter in the discussion of the effect of anaphylactic antibodies. Patients may develop swelling of the mucous membranes of the nose, throat and upper respiratory tract causing difficulty in breathing. Bronchial asthma is not uncommon and a diffuse urticarial or maculo-papular rash may develop all over the body. The face and eyelids might also become swollen due to the development of angio-neurotic oedema. Patients may also complain of itching all over the body probably due to the release of histamine. Contraction of plain muscle throughout the body can cause abdominal cramps, and painful contractions of the bladder have also been described.

An increase in the number of circulating eosinophils may be found

Table 1

Symptoms and signs of serum sickness

(a) *Acute symptoms*	(b) *Chronic symptoms*
Anaphylactic	Deposition of *Immune Complexes* in blood vessels
IgE antibodies → release of vasoactive amines → plain muscle and mucous membranes	IgG antibodies + Complement → acute vasculitis

(a)	(b)
(i) RESPIRATORY TRACT —laryngeal oedema —bronchospasm	(i) KIDNEY —acute glomerulonephritis —renal failure —anuria
(ii) GASTRO-INTESTINAL TRACT —vomiting —diarrhoea	(ii) HEART —myocarditis —valvulitis
(iii) URINARY BLADDER —spasm	(iii) JOINTS —arthritis
(iv) PERIPHERAL VASCULAR SYSTEM —pooling of blood in mesenteric vessels —low blood pressure —shock	(iv) SKIN —allergic vasculitis "Arthus-like" lesions
(v) SKIN —urticaria —maculo-papular eruptions	(v) FEVER (vi) LEUCOCYTOSIS

in the circulating blood and in experimental animals an increase in the number of circulating basophil leucocytes has been described coincidental with the fall in circulating eosinophils. The rise in both circulating eosinophils and basophils is probably a result of an increased production of these cells in the bone marrow to make up for the increased concentration of these cells in the tissues which are the site of the anaphylactic reaction.

Fever is a general concomitant of serum sickness but the cause of this is not known.

(*b*) *Reactions due to the presence of soluble antigen-antibody complexes* (Table 1). A number of lesions classically associated with serum sickness are not typically due to anaphylactic antibody. These lesions which are often transient are carditis and swelling of the joints resembling that found in rheumatic fever, glomerulo-nephritis and multiple lesions due to inflammation of the small arteries similar to that found in polyarteritis nodosa. These lesions have been shown in experimental animals to occur at a time when soluble complexes formed by antigen with IgG antibody can be detected in the circulation. Moreover, they tend to resolve as soon as these complexes are eliminated from the circulation.

Similar lesions in the kidney and heart can be reproduced in experimental animals by injecting soluble antigen-antibody complexes intravenously. Such complexes are prepared in antigen excess so that they can be injected in solution. The lesions that can be seen are proliferation of the glomerular endothelium in the kidney and thickening of the mitral valve of the heart with infiltration with neutrophils, mononuclear cells and Anitchkow myocytes. The lesion in the heart is very similar to that seen in rheumatic fever. Many arteries show inflammation in all the layers and often there is a typical necrosis of the media. Fluorescent techniques have been used to identify the site at which the soluble complexes are localized in both the human and experimental animal and they are found typically in the media of small arteries such as the coronary arteries and also in the glomeruli of the kidney. In severe serum sickness urinary output may be nil in the first 24 hours followed for many days by an oliguria. The urine may contain masses of cellular debris, numerous hyaline and granular casts and some red cells.

Although anaphylactic symptoms may be relieved by antihistamine drugs, these will not have any effect on the lesions due to the localization of soluble antigen–antibody complexes in the tissues.

(ii) *Accelerated serum sickness reactions*

If the patient has been previously sensitized to the antigen, either by injection of the foreign serum, some years before, or from inhalation of dander or from contact with a cross-reacting antigen, the symptoms of serum sickness will develop more rapidly than in the case of primary serum sickness. In primary serum sickness the earliest symptoms are found seven days after first contact with the antigen. If there has been previous contact with the antigen, even if no circulating antibody remains from the primary sensitization, antibody will be produced as a result of a secondary response. In this case symptoms will develop between one and three days after this second contact with antigen. If however, residual antibody is present in the circulation from the primary sensitization, anaphylactic symptoms may occur as early as twenty minutes after injection and symptoms due to lesions caused by circulating antigen–antibody complexes can occur within two to four hours. Symptoms are generally more severe in accelerated serum sickness reactions and may last as long as two to three weeks after provocation. If the anaphylactic state is severe the patient might actually die as a result of vasomotor collapse. Severe accelerated reactions are more common in patients with an inherited atopic state than in normal subjects. The nature of the inherited atopic diathesis will be discussed in a later chapter. However, at this stage it should be mentioned that one of the concomitants of the atopic state is an increased ability to produce anaphylactic type antibody on even minimal antigenic stimulation.

Immune complex disease. Lesions due to the deposition of immune complexes, together with complement in blood vessels throughout the body, have been found to be the basis of a large number of pathological processes (in addition to those in serum sickness). These range from glomerulonephritis to many of the lesions found in infectious diseases. Although glomerulonephritis, diffuse vasculitis, arthritis and uveitis frequently occur together forming a typical symptom complex, they are more often found singly or in pairs. The antigen causing immune complex deposition may be derived from a drug taken during the course of treatment or may be a soluble antigen of bacterial origin. Antigen derived from the infecting microorganisms have been demonstrated in immune complexes in the glomeruli in the nephrotic syndrome found in children with *Plasmodium malariae* infection and in the skin in the cutaneous vasculitis found in patients with lepromatous leprosy (erythema nodosum leprosum). Circulating immune complexes containing the surface antigen of Hepatitis B virus (HBsAg—Australia antigen) have been found in this disease. Similar complexes containing Hepatitis B antigen IgM and complement ($C_3–\beta_{1c}$ globulin) have also been found in the serum of four patients with polyarteritis nodosa. Rarely, as in the nephritis of systemic lupus erythematosus the complexes may be formed by autoantibodies reacting with the body's own intrinsic antigens such as those associated with nucleoprotein.

As well as serum sickness multiorgan immune complex lesions would appear to underly many of the features of defined bacterial diseases such as subacute bacterial endocarditis and chronic meningococcal septicaemia. However, a number of symptom complexes have been given a distinctive diagnostic label such as Henoch-Schonlein purpura and polyarteritis nodosa under situations where the causative antigen has not been identified. The symptom complex of fever, arthritis and lymphadenopathy with or without glomerulonephritis following meningococcal and gonococcal infection, *Sh. shigæ* dysentery and probably also Reiter's syndrome, are further examples of this state. However, similar symptom complexes are seen following the more common viral exanthemata. "Immune complex disease" is thus a common "complication" of infection due to complexes formed with antigens derived from the infecting organisms or the drugs used to treat the disease. Although the full symptom complex of arthritis, diffuse vasculitis, glomerulonephritis and uveitis are seen in serum sickness, in other situations only one or two features of the disease may be obvious. The reason for this is not known. Two factors may contribute to this. One may be the size of the complexes formed in the circulation, the other the different physico-chemical nature of the antigens involved. In most immune complex diseases, immunoglobulin and complement may be found by immunohistological techniques deposited in the vessel walls in affected tissues.

In a number of infectious diseases the development of "immune complex disease" could be related to a failure in cellular immunity under conditions in which there is no parallel failure in humoral antibody production. Such a process could underlie immune complex disease in infections in which the organism such as a virus or mycobacterium needs cell-mediated immunity for its elimination. The infecting organism will proliferate as a result of a specific failure of T-cell function and soluble bacterial antigen or viral antigen will be released into the circulation. This will stimulate further B-cell activity and humoral antibody production. The large amount of antigen released will then react with antibody in antigen excess and lead to the deposition of immune complexes causing arthritis, glomerulonephritis, cutaneous vasculitis and uveitis (Fig. 5).

Many laboratories have been struggling in the past few years to develop a technique for the detection of soluble immune complexes in the circulation in immune complex diseases. In rare situations these conditions may be associated with low levels of complement or β_{1c} globulin (C3). One test that has been introduced has been to demonstrate material in the circulation that will react with C1q the major component of the trimolecular complex that forms C1. However C1q is also precipitated by biological polyanions and endotoxin. Thus, despite good results in the demonstration of soluble DNA–anti DNA complexes in systemic lupus erythematosus, this test has not found general applicability.

Anti-immunoglobulin antibodies—cryoglobulins, rheumatoid factor.
Soluble immune complexes formed between IgG and antibodies directed against it (IgG, IgA or IgM) together with complement are found in the circulation in a number of chronic immune complex diseases. Such complexes come out of solution when left in the refrigerator at 4°C from between 24 hours and one week. Higher levels of anti-immunoglobulin antibodies are found in the serum of patients especially with rheumatoid arthritis. These autoantibodies are referred to by the generic term "rheumatoid factor". Rheumatoid factor antibodies are directed against antigenic groups present on the Fc fragment of the IgG molecule of certain individuals. These antigenic groups are genetically inherited and are referred to as the Gm groups. Rheumatoid factor will also react with rabbit immunoglobulin which have reacted with sheep erythrocytes.

It is suspected that cryoglobulins are immune complexes in which the anti-immunoglobulin reacts with immunoglobulin molecules which have had their tertiary structure modified either by reaction with antigen or by non-specific aggregation. In most cases, it has not been possible to detect a specific antigen in the cryoglobulin aggregate, other than IgG. However, DNA has been detected in cryoglobulins in a few cases of

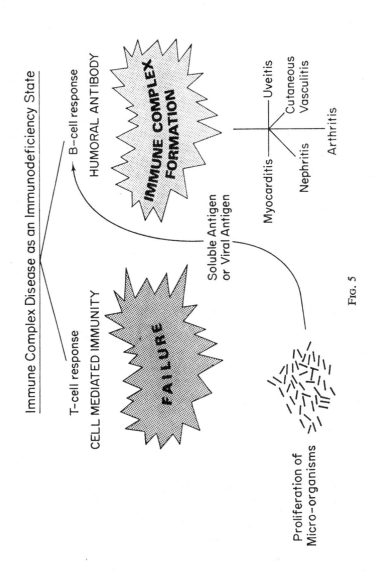

Fig. 5

systemic lupus erythematosus. The frequent occurrence of cryoglobulins in chronic infectious diseases associated with lesions caused by immune complex deposition, such as leprosy and syphilis suggest that an extrinsic antigen may be present in these complexes.

Drug allergy. Certain drugs are broken down *in vivo* into compounds which are capable of binding onto the body's own proteins. These compounds act as haptens and the resulting hapten–protein complex may become highly antigenic, although the drug in its native form is not itself an antigen. Drug allergy is basically of two types depending on whether sensitization produces humoral antibody or a cell-mediated immune response. If the drug induces a cell-mediated immune response, the individual will develop contact sensitivity whenever he comes in contact with the drug. The subject of contact sensitivity will be dealt with at more length in the next chapter. If however, the immune response incurs the production of humoral antibody the reaction will either be anaphylactic or may take the form of serum sickness with all its manifestations. Thus patients with drug allergy can develop an urticarial or maculo-papular rash, joint swelling and even on occasions there might be renal involvement, or polyarteritis nodosa.

One drug that produces allergic reactions and has been studied extensively is Penicillin. Penicillin is broken down in the body to ten or more groups which can become haptenic. However, it is the penicilloyl group which is thought to be the most important group involved in penicillin allergy. It is often difficult to decide before giving penicillin whether a patient is allergic to penicillin. In many cases the subjects may not react to a skin test with penicillin itself, although a certain number of people who are allergic to penicillin develop a weal and flare reaction, to the intradermal injection of penicilloyl polylysine, which develops within 15 to 20 minutes. It is estimated that about 40% of patients with a positive history of penicillin allergy will react to the intradermal injection of penicilloyl polylysine.

Other drugs which produce immediate type hypersensitivity reactions are organic iodides, local anaesthetics such as procaine, mercurials, vitamin K oxide, bromsulphalein and sodium dehydrocholate. A serum sickness like syndrome can be produced against streptomycin, sulphonamides and thiouracils as well as with penicillin. It appears that all antibiotics are potential sensitizers. Other drugs affect blood platelets and can cause agranulocytosis, aplastic anaemia and haemolytic anaemias, but these will be discussed in a later chapter.

There is a great need for some *in vitro* test for the presence of allergy to drugs in clinical medicine. *In vivo* tests such as intradermal testing with the particular drug can give both false positive and false negative results. Moreover, intradermal injection of the drug into a patient, who is allergic, carries the risk of precipitating anaphylactic shock.

A number of tests have been introduced over the past few years. However, as a whole these have given inconsistent results. An example of one of these tests is the basophil degranulation test. In this test the patient's serum is mixed with a fresh preparation of human or rabbit basophils which are stained supravitally and then a solution of antigen is added. The test was considered positive if over 30% of the basophils became degranulated. This test was recommended for penicillin and other drug allergies as well as for the diagnosis of food and insect allergies. Although the author of this test correlated positive results with the presence of an allergy to the particular antigen, subsequently it has not been found to be reproducible in the hands of a number of other reputable workers.

Another system that is being tried currently is the transformation of peripheral blood lymphocytes into lymphoblasts over 5–6 days in the presence of the specific antigen to which the patient is hypersensitive. A number of workers have shown a positive correlation between transformation of lymphocytes *in vitro* by antigen and a hypersensitive state. Transformation of lymphocytes by sulphonamides, penicillin and tetracycline has been described. However, as yet, the number of patients in whom this test has been tried are too small to assess whether this test will be of use in routine clinical practice. Moreover, the techniques used are somewhat specialized as the cells have to be cultured for many days and it is doubtful whether this technique could be used in routine clinical laboratories, even if it were found to be reproducible. Also present information indicates that, although a response can be demonstrated in certain cases of drug allergy, in other cases of proved allergy the test is negative and thus in its present form cannot be used as a routine test for the presence of drug allergy.

In addition to acting as haptens certain drugs may contain unsuspected contaminants which can act as sensitizers. It has recently been found that resident in certain pharmaceutically marketed penicillins there is often a protein contaminant to which penicillin derivatives are already attached. Such penicillinated proteins have the full capacity of inducing sensitivity to penicillin without the necessity of attaching to the body's own tissue proteins. It has been found that the protein is often of bacterial origin derived from organisms providing products used in the preparation of the drug. Penicillin preparations rendered free of such contaminants can be given to certain patients who are allergic to the contaminant only. However, this does not rule out the fact that a considerable amount of penicillin allergy is due to penicillin acting as a hapten and is not due to reaction to the contaminant. Similar contaminants may account for allergic reactions to other antibiotics such as cephalosporins.

Bibliography

Books

Amos, H. E. (1976), *Allergic Drug Reactions.* London: Edward Arnold.
Bonomo, L. & Turk, J. L. (eds.) (1970), "Proceedings of the International Symposium on Immune Complex Diseases." Milan: Carlo Erba Foundation.
Keller, R. (1966), *Tissue Mast Cells in Immune Reactions.* Monographs in Allergy, **2.** Basel: Karger.
Lepow, I. H. and Ward, P. A. (eds.) (1972), *Inflammation: Mechanisms and Control.* New York: Academic Press.
Movat, H. Z. (ed.) (1971), "Inflammation, Immunity, and Hypersensitivity." New York: Harper and Row.
Samter, M. (ed.) (1971), *Immunological Diseases.* 2nd edition. Boston: Little, Brown.
Stanworth, D. R. (1973), *Immediate Hypersensitivity.* Amsterdam: North Holland Publishing Company.

Articles

Cochrane, C. G. (1967), "Mediators of the Arthus and related reactions." *Progr. Allergy,* **11,** 1.
Cochrane, C. G. and Ward, P. A. (1966), "The role of complement in lesions induced by immunologic reactions." *Immunopathology IVth International Symposium.* Ed. P. Grabar and P. A. Miescher, p. 433. Basel: Schwabe.
Czekalowski, J. W. (1965), "A case of serum sickness in man." *J. Path. Bact.,* **90,** 607.
Feinberg, J. G. (1968), "Allergy to antibiotics. I. Facts and conjectures on the sensitizing contaminants of penicillins and cephalosoprins." *Int. Arch. Allergy,* **33,** 439.
Gocke, D. J., Hsu, K., Morgan, C., Bombardieri, S., Lockshin, M. & Christian, C. L. (1970), Association between polyarteritis and Australia antigen. *Lancet,* **ii,** 1149.
Levine, B. B. (1966), "Immunochemical mechanisms of drug allergy." *Ann. Rev. Med.,* **17,** 23.

Chapter III

Reactions in the Tissues Caused by the Cell-mediated Immune Response

The term "specific cell-mediated immunity" has recently been introduced to cover those immunological conditions in which the antibody-like activity is performed by circulating T-lymphocytes and are related to allergic conditions known generically as "delayed hypersensitivity". The term delayed hypersensitivity has been used for many years for a group of allergic reactions, especially in the skin, which, once the individual is sensitized, take 24–48 hours to develop on subsequent contact with the specific antigen. This longer period of development is in marked contrast to that of reactions mediated by humoral antibody. As mentioned in the last chapter, reactions mediated by humoral antibody occur between 15 and 30 minutes after contact with antigen in the case of anaphylactic reactions or between 4 and 8 hours in the case of Arthus reactions.

1. Microbial Allergies

Historically the first group of reactions in the group of delayed hypersensitivities to be studied in any depth were the so-called microbial allergies. Of these the tuberculin reaction has probably been studied in greatest depth.

Table 1 gives a list of some of the reactions which are now generally accepted to result from cell-mediated immune reactions. Table 2 shows the main differences between the tuberculin reaction and the Arthus

Table 1

Examples of cell-mediated Immunity (CMI)

A. *INFECTIOUS AGENTS* (Obligate and facultative intracellular parasites)

CELLULAR IMMUNITY		DELAYED HYPERSENSITIVITY TESTS
BACTERIA:		
Mycobacteria	M. tuberculosis	Tuberculin
	M. leprae	Lepromin (Fernandez)
Brucella		Brucellin
CHLAMYDIA:	Lymphogranuloma venereum	Frei test
	Psittacosis	
VIRUSES:	Vaccinia	"Reaction of immunity"
	Paramyxoviruses, Herpes etc.	Measles, mumps, Herpes simplex
FUNGI:	Candidiasis	Candidin
	Histoplasmosis	Histoplasmin
	Coccidiomycosis	Coccidioidin
PROTOZOA:	Leishmaniasis	Leishmanin

Table 1—continued

B. FIXED TISSUE ANTIGENS
   Organ and tissue graft rejection
   Immunosurveillance against tumours
   Contact sesitivity to simple chemicals
   Organ specific autoimmune diseases (thyroiditis, encephalitis, adrenalitis)

C. MISCELLANEOUS
   Insect bites
   Pseudo-Schick reaction to diphtheria toxoid
   Delayed hypersensitivity reactions to heterologous serum proteins (following
   small doses of foreign antigen).

reaction. Apart from the difference in time which these two reactions take to develop, they also differ in their morphological and histological appearance as seen in the skin. The Arthus reaction is mainly oedematous but it is also associated with haemorrhage into the skin as a result of an acute vasculitis. The blood vessels are damaged as described in the previous chapter and there is a marked emigration of polymorphonuclear leucocytes from them.

Table 2

*Differences between the tuberculin reaction (cell-mediated)
and the Arthus reaction*

	Tuberculin	Arthus
Time of maximum response	24–48 hours	4–8 hours
Macroscopic appearance	Erythema, Induration	Oedema, Haemorrhage
Microscopic appearance	Mononuclear cell infiltrate	Polymorphonuclear leucocyte infiltrate
Passive sensitization	Suspension of lymphoid tissues (containing sensitized lymphocytes)	Serum (containing antibodies—immunoglobulins)
Systemic manifestations	Fever	Deposition of "immune complexes" in organs

The tuberculin reaction can be induced by the intradermal injection of 0·1 ml of a dilution of Koch's old tuberculin or the protein purified derivative of tuberculin (PPD) in dilutions of 1:100, 1:1,000 or 1:10,000 depending on the degree of sensitivity of the individual. The reaction begins to develop in the human after a few hours increasing in strength during the first 24 hours after injection reaching a peak at 48 hours, sometimes taking a week or more to resolve. If the reaction is severe it forms what is known as a cocarde with a central nodule separated from a peripheral halo by an intermediary zone. In children the tuberculin reaction may be induced as a patch test by applying Koch's old tuberculin to an area of skin on the back which has been gently abraded. When fully developed it is erythematous and indurated rather than oedematous, sometimes, but rarely, with petechial haemorrhages in the centre. The oedema of the Arthus reaction is due to exudation of fluid into the tissues, whereas the induration of the tuberculin reaction is caused by changes in the collagen. In the human, the tuberculin reaction is the site of an intense infiltration with mononuclear cells, 80–90% of these are lymphocytes but 10–20% are active macrophages. At the peak of the reaction between 24 and 48 hours after skin testing, the histological findings are mainly in relation to blood vessels. Mononuclear cells are found surrounding small capillaries and venules and many of these vessels are packed with these cells. They are also found in the connective tissue and in the fatty tissue at some distance from the blood vessels. In experimental animals polymorphonuclear leucocytes and macrophages appear to play a much greater role in the tuberculin reaction, than in the human. In the human polymorphonuclear leucocytes are found only rarely in delayed hypersensitivity reactions and appear only when there is severe tissue damage.

Initially it was thought that the tuberculin reaction was an anaphylactic reaction or related to the Arthus reaction. However, it will be remembered that anaphylactic sensitivity can be transferred from a sensitized individual to a non-sensitized person by serum in such a way that a localized area of the recipient's skin can be sensitized and that Arthus type sensitivity can be transferred systemically by serum in the experimental animal. After a number of years it became apparent that there was a marked difference in the nature of the tuberculin reaction in that all attempts to transfer this reaction passively with serum were consistently negative. The microbial allergies were thus formally separated from anaphylactic reactions and the Arthus reaction in that they could not be transferred with serum. Eventually it was shown that tuberculin allergy could be produced passively in experimental animals by the injection of cells of lymphoid origin from sensitized donors. These cell suspensions could be derived from peripheral blood, spleen, lymph nodes, thoracic duct or mononuclear cell exudates induced in the peritoneal cavity. All the cell suspensions used have consisted of macrophages as well as lymphocytes, but it is the lymphocyte rather than the macrophage that is the active cell which transfers the passive sensitization state. It is probable that a suspension of lymphocytes which is injected to sensitize an animal passively contain only a small proportion of cells which are sensitized. These cells are derived by proliferation of T-lymphocytes in the thymus-dependent areas of lymph nodes and spleen under specific antigenic stimulus as described in the first chapter. Moreover, it is known that in a tuberculin reaction developing as a result of passive sensitization with lymphocytes, over 90% of the cells forming the infiltrate in the reaction when fully developed are derived from the host and the injected cells form somewhat less than 10% of the infiltrating cells. Thus most of the cells infiltrating a delayed hypersensitivity lesion arrive there non-specifically and are not the specifically sensitized lymphocytes produced as a result of the initial antigenic stimulus. It is probable that sensitized lymphocytes react directly with the antigen. The way in which they react is not known as yet, but it is thought that a receptor group must exist on the surface of the lymphocyte which has a molecular configuration similar to that of the receptor group on an immunoglobulin molecule. Such a "recognition factor" might actually form part of the structure of the cell wall or be secreted by the cell onto its surface in a soluble form. Active lymphocytes are passing through the tissues all the time. Once a sensitized lymphocyte arrives at the site of antigen deposition, probably as a random event, a sequence of events is set up as a result of which further cells are brought into the area, a small number of which are also sensitized and capable of reacting with antigen. Delayed hypersensitivity reactions consist of two stages. The first is the reaction of antigen with sensitized lymphocytes and then a chain of events is set up as a result of which the reaction site becomes an area of non-specific inflammation in which the cells are not attracted in any specific way but behave as though they were taking part in any subacute inflammatory process. (Fig. 1.)

The reaction between sensitized lymphocytes and antigen results in the production of a group of pharmacological agents by these cells. These substances, sometimes called "lymphokines", are proteins with molecular weights in the region of 40,000. A number of actions have so far been attributed to these substances. The main action that has been defined so far is the ability to inhibit the migration of macrophages *in vitro*. This activity is therefore referred to as "Migration inhibition factor" or "M.I.F." A further action of this family of molecules is that when injected intradermally they produce a skin reaction similar to a tuberculin reaction. Further properties are a mitogenic effect on lymphocytes in culture, stimulation of chemotaxis of macrophages and polymorphonuclear leucocytes, and cytotoxicity for certain types of target cell in tissue culture. The lymphocyte chemical mediators probably act firstly by being chemotactic for macrophages and then act directly by causing a decreased electrostatic charge on the surface of these cells, as a result of which they tend to aggregate in the lesion. The chemical mediators of delayed hypersensitivity contain all the ingredients necessary to produce a delayed hypersensitivity reaction, so that when the cell-free supernatant from the reaction between sensitized lymphocytes and antigen is injected intradermally, the result is an inflammatory reaction which resembles many features of delayed hypersensitivity. Most of the lymphoid cells infiltrating a delayed hypersensitivity reaction are not specifically sensitized to antigen but are derived from the bone marrow directly. It is probable that these cells are related to the enzymically active macrophages which can be found to a varying degree in different types of cell-mediated immune reaction. To summarize, it is the bone-marrow-derived macrophages which produce the inflammatory reaction

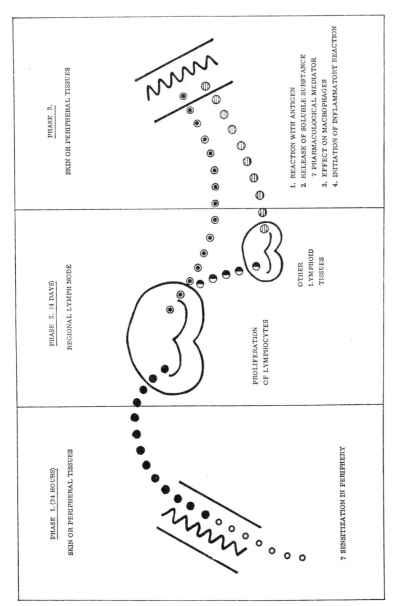

FIG. 1. The mechanism of cell-mediated immunity.

of cell-mediated immunity and these cells are activated by chemical mediators produced by the interaction between antigen and a small number of specifically sensitized lymphocytes.

Experimental animals can be passively sensitized by injecting lymphocytes from sensitive animals either intravenously or intraperitoneally so that they enter the circulation and are distributed throughout the body in the same way as the recipient's own lymphocytes. The animal is then sensitized immediately and remains sensitive as long as the cells remain in the circulation. Sensitivity will be lost, however, as soon as these cells are rejected by a homograft reaction. Sensitivity can only be transferred within a species and generally only if there is some degree of genetical identity between the donor and the recipient. Local passive transfer analogous to the Prausnitz-Küstner transfer of anaphylactic sensitivity can be effected by mixing sensitized cells and antigen and injecting them intradermally into an unsensitized animal, in which case a reaction develops in the skin resembling a tuberculin reaction in an actively sensitized animal. In this case the animal does not become sensitized systemically and will not develop a tuberculin reaction if tested at a different site. In the experimental animal both systemic and local passive transfer can only be produced with live cells, dead cells or cell extracts are invariably ineffective.

Transfer factor. This discussion of sensitization in the experimental animal is necessary to understand and interpret experiments which have been designed to demonstrate passive transfer of delayed hypersensitivity in the human. In the adult human, generalized sensitization can be produced by injecting peripheral blood leucocytes derived from an actively sensitized donor by the intradermal route. These cells need not be alive as similar results can be produced by the injection of cells which have been killed either by ultrasonication or by freezing and thawing. Sensitization, produced in this way, often takes up to six days to develop fully and, once it has developed, lasts for many months. The intradermal route is known to be the best route for inducing an active state of delayed hypersensitivity. It is therefore possible that such transfers are not analogous to passive transfers in the experimental animal but would appear to be more analogous to active sensitization. This could be by producing an anamnestic response in an individual who already has a latent or subliminal sensitivity. This latent sensitivity could be due to actual contact with the antigen or to some weak sensitivity caused by contact with a weakly cross-reacting antigen. Attempts at characterization of this human "transfer factor" show that it is not an immunoglobulin or a fragment of immunoglobulin or of a related protein. A strong possibility exists that it may be a highly degraded fragment of antigen extracted from circulating macrophages and which is present in a form which could be more active than the whole antigen.

No demonstration of "transfer factor" activity in the human has been made under conditions where a latent sensitivity has been completely excluded.

"Transfer factor" has now been purified by a number of methods and has been shown to be a dialysable substance of molecular weight <10,000. It does not have any antibody-like action and can be considered to act on the afferent side of the immunization arc. It is thought that transfer factor is produced by antigen-responsive lymphocytes and acts by conveying "information" or "derepressing" unsensitized lymphocytes. In some experiments it has been shown that the addition of "transfer factor" from sensitized cells will cause unsensitized lymphocytes to respond to antigen as though they had previously been sensitized. It is also being suggested that transfer factor can cause lymphocytes in a number of specific and non-specific immuno-deficiency states to respond to antigens under conditions where they would normally be unresponsive. However, in many of the situations where this has been claimed transfer has been with live leucocyte suspensions and not with purified transfer factor, suggesting that the transfer of sensitivity might have been a function of the injection of live sensitized lymphocytes. Transfer factor has been used therapeutically with some success in the treatment of muco-cutaneous candidiasis. The effect appears to be non-specific. As a result it is now considered that much of the effect is that of a T-cell adjuvant.

As well as the tuberculin reaction delayed hypersensitivity reactions in the skin can be produced to a wide range of microbial antigens. The bacterial antigens include typhoidin from *Salmonella typhi*, abortin from *Brucella abortus* and mallein from *Pfeiferella mallei*. The intra-dermal injection of mixtures of Streptokinase and Streptodornase (Varidase—Lederle) produce a high incidence of reactions of this type due to the high incidence of delayed hypersensitivity to *Streptococci* in the population, which is always in contact with these organisms.

An important delayed hypersensitivity reaction is the "pseudo-Schick" reaction produced by the intradermal injection of diphtheria toxin or toxoid. This reaction occurs within 24 hours of injection and disappears within six days. This is in marked contrast to the Schick reaction which is caused by the diphtheria toxin itself and which is maximal between the fourth and seventh days after injection. The pseudo-Schick reaction develops equally to the toxin and the control heat incubated toxin (toxoid).

Delayed hypersensitivity reactions in the skin can be induced by extracts of a number of fungi which infect man. These extracts include coccidioidin, histoplasmin, trichophytin and candidin. Similar reactions can be induced to a suspension of heated organisms, both fungal and bacterial.

Delayed hypersensitivity reactions to protozoal parasites are rarer. The Montenegro test for cutaneous leishmaniasis is a tuberculin-like hypersensitivity which can be induced by an intradermal injection of a suspension of dead organisms or an alkaline extract of *Leishmania tropica*.

Delayed hypersensitivity reactions to viruses and chlamydia can be seen quite often. The commonest of these is the "reaction of immunity" to vaccinia virus. This is a papular erythematous lesion reaching its maximum 24–72 hours after vaccination and disappears without passing through the pustular stage and leaving a scar. Delayed hypersensitivity reactions have been used in the diagnosis of lymphogranuloma venereum and have been demonstrated to measles virus, mumps virus and the virus of Herpes simplex.

2. Insect Bites

The red indurated reaction in the skin which occurs 24 hours after a mosquito bite is another manifestation of delayed hypersensitivity and is directed towards an antigen present in the saliva of the mosquito. The usual pattern of reactivity is that delayed hypersensitivity is the first form of allergic reaction to develop. As the person becomes more allergic this is then accompanied by an anaphylactic immediate weal and flare reaction. Finally the patient loses his state of delayed hypersensitivity and only reacts with the immediate type reaction. After a large number of bites the patient may become completely desensitized. Delayed hypersensitivity reactions are also seen to flea bites.

Reactions to stings from bees, wasps and hornets are generally anaphylactic, and severe and fatal systemic anaphylaxis can develop as a result of stings from these insects in sensitized individuals.

3. Chemical Contact Sensitivity

Another form of cell-mediated immunological response is the allergic reaction produced in the skin by contact with simple chemical compounds. One of the first reports of this was of contact sensitivity to mercury. This was followed by reports of sensitivity to East Indian satinwood and then to the plant *Primula obconica*. Other metals which cause contact sensitivity are nickel and chromium. Sensitivity to potassium dichromate occurs commonly among workers in the cement industry. The property of being able to cause contact sensitivity appears to be related to the ability of the simple chemical to bind onto proteins, especially those of the epidermis. Thus many dye-stuffs are sensitizers, since their ability to colour fabrics permanently is also dependent upon their ability to bind to proteins. Other common sensitizers are dinitrochlorobenzene, picryl chloride, p. phenylenediamine and phenylhydrazine. Sensitizers derived from plants are primulin from *Primula obconica* and poison ivy. Simple chemicals which can cause contact sensitivity can also be found in simple animal forms. Thus the bryozoan

Alcyonidium gelatinosum which is found in the North Sea off the Dogger Bank carries a substance as yet unidentified of molecular weight between 250–350 which is a potent cause of contact sensitivity among fishermen in the area.

As in all forms of cell-mediated immunity there is a minimum latent period of at least five days between first contact with the allergen in this case the chemical sensitizer, and the ability to react at a distant site to further contact with a non-irritant concentration of the agent (Fig. 1). Sensitivity may be demonstrated by the conventional patch test. Reactions take between 24 and 48 hours to develop and if severe may persist for a week or longer. The skin is erythematous and indurated as in the tuberculin reaction. However, if the reaction is severe, vesiculation may develop and the epidermis can break down. As the lesion resolves the area may be replaced by scaling.

The histological appearance of the lesion when fully developed is similar to that of the tuberculin reaction. The cellular infiltrate is mononuclear with very little infiltration with polymorphonuclear leucocytes and the infiltrating cells tend to be localized round blood vessels. The epidermis shows marked spongiosis leading to vesiculation with some thickening of the Malpighian layer and some intracellular oedema. The earliest changes probably occur in the sweat ducts and hair follicles. The cellular infiltrate in the dermis in primary irritant dermatitis looks little different from that seen in allergic eczematous contact sensitivity.

As with the tuberculin reaction sensitivity cannot be transferred passively with serum. However, it can be transferred systemically in experimental animals by cells of the lymphoid series, as can tuberculin sensitivity. The cells need to be alive and sensitivity cannot be transferred with dead cells or extracts of cells. It is thought that the mechanism of contact sensitivity is identical to that of other forms of cell-mediated immunity. The development of contact sensitivity is associated with pro-liferation of T-lymphocytes in the thymus-dependent areas of the drain-ing lymph node in the same way as other forms of cell-mediated immunity.

Whereas passive transfer of contact sensitivity in the experimental animal is an acceptable and reproducible procedure, reports of the passive transfer of contact sensitivity in the human are open to a considerable amount of criticism. There have been a number of reports of failure to transfer contact sensitivity passively in the human. In those few cases where it appeared that passive transfer was successful (*a*) persistence of sensitivity lasted 2–8 months, (*b*) positive transfers were to those compounds which were strongest sensitizers, (*c*) most of the recipients had had a previous patch test to show that they were negative reactors or did not show sensitivity until four days after the beginning of patch testing, at a time when it could have been possible for active sensitization to have occurred, (*d*) finally, the possibility was not excluded that the cells used for transfer did not contain antigenic material.

Other reports have been criticized on the grounds that the skin test dose used was above the level which could cause non-specific irritant reactions. Finally in reports of transfer of sensitivity to poison ivy, the question still remains as to whether it might have been due to the boosting of a pre-existing subliminal sensitivity as in the case of reports of similar transfers of tuberculin sensitivity.

Sites of previous contact with a chemical sensitizing agent can "flare up" under two types of circumstance. The first contact with a non-irritant but sensitizing dose can flare up as soon as the individual becomes sensitive. Reaction in this case is with residual sensitizer remaining at the site of sensitization. This type of flare up is generally considered to be a cell-mediated reaction. The other situation in which a flare up can occur is when a sensitizer is absorbed systemically in an already sensitive individual. This will result in the flare up of old cell-mediated contact sites caused by the same sensitizer. This type of reaction is believed to be mediated by locally produced humoral antibodies reacting with the absorbed antigen.

3. Allograft (Homograft) Reaction

The role of immune reactions in the rejection of organ and tissue grafts has been known for many years. Early observations of the histological nature of grafts in the process of rejection noted that the cellular infiltrate was mononuclear with an almost complete absence of polymorphonuclear leucocytes. This suggested that the mechanism behind graft rejection was a cellular immune reaction rather than involving humoral antibodies. This was confirmed by a consistent failure to transfer transplantation immunity with serum. It was found, however, that transplantation immunity could be passively transferred by the injection of lymphocytes derived from lymph nodes or the peripheral blood. Moreover, the same cellular events have been observed in the lymph nodes draining a skin allograft, as occur in lymph nodes draining the site of first contact with a chemical sensitizing agent on the skin. These changes described in the first chapter are typical of the cell-mediated immune reaction and are those of T-lymphocyte proliferation. Before division, lymphocytes in the paracortical or thymus-dependent area of the lymph node, which lies between the true compact cortex and the medulla, transform into large cells containing a substantial amount of ribonucleic acid in their cytoplasm. These cells which have a very typical appearance and are often referred to as immunoblasts reach a peak in concentration just before the graft is about to be rejected. At this time they divide into further small lymphocytes and they begin to fall off in numbers very rapidly. The changes in the cortex of the lymph node are completely different from those found in lymph nodes involved in pure humoral antibody production where the changes are those of B-cell proliferation in the germinal centres and cortico-medullary junction leading to plasma cell differentiation in the medulla. Although similar changes may be found in lymph nodes during antibody production, needing thymus-bone marrow interaction, they do not occur if the T-lymphocyte population is reduced by neonatal thymectomy, treatment with anti-lymphocyte serum or following chronic thoracic duct drainage.

If lymphocytes from an individual who has rejected a graft are injected intradermally back into the donor, being sensitized by the graft they will react with the donor's skin and produce a strong delayed hypersensitivity reaction which resembles a tuberculin reaction very closely. Similar though not so intense reactions can be produced by injection of lymphocytes from a normal person intradermally into another normal person. This normal lymphocyte transfer (NLT) reaction occurs more strongly the greater the genetic difference between the two individuals. The reaction may be due to a state of "natural immunity" as it occurs within 24 hours in someone who has not been previously sensitized. Another possible explanation is that the lymphocytes become sensitized within the 24 hours it takes for the reaction to develop.

Humoral antibodies are usually produced at the same time as "sensitized lymphocytes" against an allograft. They can be involved in allograft rejection as well as the cell-mediated immune reaction and probably act synergistically with it. Changes attributable to the effects of circulating antibody may be seen strikingly in renal allograft rejection, especially following immunosuppressive therapy. The changes produced by antibody and complement under these conditions are in the blood vessels of the graft and are typically those of an acute vasculitis.

5. The Possible Role of the Cell-mediated Immune Reaction in Auto-immunity

In experimental animals organ specific autoimmune conditions such as thyroiditis, encephalomyelitis, aspermatogenesis and adrenalitis are associated with development of a state of delayed hypersensitivity against tissues of the target organ. This can be demonstrated by skin testing the animals with extracts of the tissues and the reaction they show is just like a tuberculin reaction reaching its peak 24 hours after the intradermal injection of the extract. Thus there is no doubt that the animals have developed a state of cell-mediated immunity against the target organ and this skin reactivity can be transferred from animal to animal in the same way as tuberculin sensitivity. One of the arguments, in favour of the implication of cell-mediated reactions in autoimmune diseases, is that these conditions are usually associated with perivascular collections of mononuclear cells. Moreover, in experimental animals, it has not been possible to transfer the autoimmune state passively with serum alone except under rather special conditions. However, in experimental autoimmune encephalitis and aspermatogenesis, increased vascular permeability or tissue damage can be demonstrated before the development of the cellular infiltrate, indicating that some other process is also involved. It is possible to transfer autoimmune encephalitis and thyroiditis passively in experimental animals with cells. However, these cell suspensions contain both "sensitized lymphocytes" and plasma cells capable of secreting humoral antibody. Recently it has been found that it is possible to transfer allergic autoimmune aspermatogenesis with cells, but only to recipients which are already making humoral antibody. Thus there is a very strong suggestion that in experimental animals organ specific autoimmune states are produced by the action of cell-mediated immune mechanisms and humoral antibodies acting synergistically. The way in which these two independent processes act together to cause the pathological lesions is not known. However, it has been suggested that the "sensitized cells" cause an increased permeability of the cells of the target organ as a result of which the humoral antibodies can enter and cause direct damage to the tissue.

6. Cellular Immunity

Cellular immunity processes against microorganisms are very important in the defence of the body against organisms such as mycobacteria, fungi and certain protozoa which have a cell wall constituted in such a way that they are resistant to the effects of humoral antibodies. Cellular immune processes may play a role in the defence of the body against certain viruses, e.g. variola, vaccinia, measles and mumps. Microorganisms that need cell-mediated immunity for their elimination from the body are generally obligate or facultative intracellular parasites. Overwhelming and fatal infection with fungi or with these viruses occurs in patients whose cellular immunity has been decreased by thymic dysfunction or by immunosuppressive therapy with, for example, antilymphocyte serum. A state of immunity to tuberculin develops about the same time as the individual becomes tuberculin-sensitive. Moreover, the reaction of immunity to vaccinia virus which is also a delayed hypersensitivity reaction is associated with the development of a state of immunity to smallpox. There has also been a consistent failure to transfer the acquired resistance, produced by BCG vaccine, passively to normal animals by the injection of serum from an actively immunized individual. The role of cells from hypersensitive animals in defence against infection has been studied extensively. Macrophages from immunized animals are capable of inhibiting the growth of tubercle bacilli *in vitro*, to a greater extent than those from normal animals. Cellular immunity has now been studied against a wide range of organisms.

Although transfer of resistance to tuberculous infection has not been transferred with serum, transfer of resistance from immunized to normal animals can be demonstrated using either exudate cells (containing both macrophages and lymphocytes) or lymph node cells. Many years ago doubt was cast on whether there was any connection between delayed hypersensitivity reactions and the development of cellular immunity, as it is possible to desensitize BCG-immunized animals, as far as sensitivity to intradermal injection of tuberculin is concerned, without reducing their state of immunity. Moreover, animals can be made sensitive to tuberculin without developing any immunity, by injecting a waxy extract of bacteria. Animals can also be made allergic to vaccinia virus without showing any signs of resistance to infection.

It would appear that cellular immunity to infection and the cell-mediated immune reactions concerned in microbial allergy, contact sensitivity and transplantation immunity could be independent phenomena. However, a number of parallels exist between these states and differences may not be in the mechanism of the reaction but in the antigens to which the two forms of reaction are directed. Thus differences between delayed hypersensitivity in the skin and cellular immunity to infection with the tubercle bacilli could be explained on the basis of the skin reaction being against one antigen (contained in tuberculin) and immunity to infection being against another antigen in the cell wall of the microorganism.

Another possibility is that both delayed hypersensitivity and cellular immunity involve a two-cell system. T-lymphocyte sensitization is common to both systems. The T-lymphocyte then would activate one other cell type for the production of immunity and another cell type for the manifestation of hypersensitivity. In this way both cellular immunity and hypersensitivity would have a common pathway part of the way but their final pathways would be different. This could also explain why animals desensitized for delayed hypersensitivity still contain cells which can confer sensitivity on normal animals, as well as the lack of correlation between cellular immunity and hypersensitivity.

The relative lack of specificity of cellular immunity as compared with that of cellular hypersensitivity needs further discussion. It has been found that animals immunized with BCG vaccine are more able to eliminate *Listeria monocytogenes*. This has been found to be due to an increased activation of the tissue macrophages. Specific increased activation of macrophages can be transferred passively with lymphocytes to the same extent and in parallel with the development of specific hypersensitivity to tuberculin. However, the non-specific resistance to infection with *Listeria monocytogenes* is not transferred in parallel. This would indicate that the specific cellular immunity is mediated by the same process as delayed hypersensitivity. The temporary rise in non-specific immunity is due to a transient change in macrophage function probably due to some as yet unknown unrelated mechanism. BCG vaccine has also been used to induce a similar state of non-specific immunity in patients with leukaemias and certain other tumours.

Granuloma formation. A granuloma may be defined as a focal collection of histiocytes and macrophages in the tissues. Granulomas may develop as a result of an immunological process. However, granuloma formation commonly occurs in the absence of an immunological reaction following the deposition of certain toxic materials in the tissues. Non-immunological granulomas can develop following the injection of mineral oils, colloidal aluminium hydroxide or silica. Granuloma formation by various silica compounds parallel their direct cytotoxic effects on macrophages. Silica is taken up by lysosomes and the first effect that can be demonstrated is a diffuse release of lyosomsal enzymes into the cytoplasm as a result of an increased permeability of the lysosomal membrane. Silica can also act as an adjuvant to immunoglobulin synthesis. However, this probably does not have much relation to its granuloma-forming capacity. Macrophages in a granuloma may be long lived or short lived. Macrophages are derived mainly from cells in the bone marrow, and in granulomas, due to chronic immunological stimulation, initially have a relatively quick turnover. Macrophages can under certain circumstances aggregate and form giant cells. Immunologically-stimulated granulomas can develop from cell-mediated immune reactions, antibody-induced reactions or the action of both. Recently it has been found that granuloma formation can be induced in tissues following the subcutaneous injection of immune complexes formed when antigen and antibody are precipitated at "equivalence". The presence of lymphocytes round a tissue granuloma would indicate that this is the site of an immunological reaction. Plasma cells in the infiltrate may be derived from B-lymphocytes arriving as part of the cell-mediated reaction and develop from these cells in response to a local antigenic stimulus.

Granulomas due to the deposition of inorganic substances may be immunologically derived as in the case of those caused by zirconium, which only form in people who have previously been sensitized to the metal. However, despite beryllium being a very powerful contact-sensitizing agent, there is no evidence that the granulomas formed by this substance in the lungs are due to a sensitization process.

Cell-mediated immune processes play a role in granuloma formation in chronic mycobacterial infections such as tuberculosis and tuberculoid leprosy. Tuberculoid leprosy is associated with a positive lepromin test which is itself a granuloma occurring maximally three weeks after the intradermal injection of dead bacilli. The lepromatous nodules of lepromatous leprosy are also granulomas which consist of accumulations of macrophages which have ingested large aggregates of mycobacteria. These form without any lymphocytic infiltration indicating that cellular immunity against the infecting organism is absent. The macrophages forming such granulomas, usually called "lepra cells", are undifferentiated and similar to those seen in other non-immunological granulomas associated with a foreign-body response to a colloidal substance such as aluminium hydroxide. In tuberculoid leprosy and tuberculosis the granulomas are immunologically induced. Under these conditions, the macrophages become differentiated into "epithelioid cells" which are associated an increased capacity to eliminate the mycobacteria. There is evidence from experimental studies that the epithelioid appearance of macrophages is related to their participation in cell-mediated immune reactions and that the formation of similar cells can be induced by the pharmacological mediators of cellular immunity.

Helminthic infections are frequently associated with granuloma formation, which can be the cause of such severe pathological changes as pipe stem fibrosis in the liver, in schistosomiasis, which leads to increased portal pressure and oesophageal varices. Under experimental conditions granulomas due to schistosomes can be inhibited from developing by immunosuppressants, antilymphocyte serum and neonatal thymectomy which indicate that cell-mediated immune processes are involved in their formation. However, this does not exclude the coexistence of immune complexes which might also be necessary for their development.

Inhibition of cell-mediated immune responses in certain diseases. A reduced capacity to manifest cell-mediated immune responses has been shown consistently in a proportion of patients with neoplastic and granulomatous diseases of the reticulo-endothelial system. Sarcoidosis and Hodgkin's disease have been among the diseases most studied. Failure to manifest cell-mediated immune reactions also occurs in lepromatous leprosy. In these conditions there is progressive replacement of the reticulo-endothelial system by pathological tissue. Often this process can be shown to start in the paracortical areas, those parts of the lymph node involved in the proliferation of lymphocytes which is associated with the development of a cell-mediated immune response. In Hodgkin's disease where impairment of delayed hypersensitivity has been studied most extensively, this does not occur until the later stages of the disease when a large amount of the total body lymphoid tissue has been affected by the disease process and shows lymphocytic depletion and when there is a marked reduction in the circulating lymphocyte count. It would therefore appear that impairment of delayed hypersensitivity in these diseases is the result of a defect in T-lymphocytes, due to replacement by pathological tissue of those areas of the lymphoid tissue associated with lymphocyte proliferation in cell-mediated immune reaction. As a result of this, the patient may be unable to produce sensitized T-lymphocytes involved in hypersensitivity reactions or immunity.

T-lymphocytes can be identified particularly by their ability to be transformed into lymphoblasts by phytohaemagglutinin (PHA). In many of these conditions T-lymphocyte deficiency can be detected by a reduced transformation of these cells by PHA. Functionally cell-mediated immunity can be tested for by the ability to reject skin grafts or to be sensitized to a contact agent such as 2.4 dinitrochlorobenzene. If the patient has been previously actively sensitized, skin tests with tuberculin, streptokinase-streptodornase (containing ubiquitous streptococcal antigens), trichophytin or mumps antigen may be used as a battery of skin tests to detect delayed hypersensitivity. In some cases of muco-cutaneous candidiasis it has been found that there is a non-specific defect in cellular immunity in the presence of apparently normal levels of reactive T-lymphocytes. These cells respond to PHA and specific antigen stimulation *in vitro*. However, there is a failure on the part of the patient to develop normal delayed hypersensitivity reactions in the skin. This has been found to be associated with an inability of the lymphocytes to produce the chemical mediators of delayed hypersensitivity when reacting with specific antigen *in vitro*.

Bibliography

Books

Bloom, B. R. & Glade, P. R. (1971) *"In Vitro* Methods in Cell-Mediated Immunity". New York: Academic Press.
Jennings, J. F. & Ward, D. J. (1970). "Impaired Cell-Mediated Hypersensitivity in Man; Clinical and Immunological Aspects." Oswestry: Robert Jones and Agnes Hunt Orthopaedic Hospital Management Committee.
Lawrence, H. S. & Landy, M. (1969). "Mediators of Cellular Immunity". New York: Academic Press.
Turk, J. L. (1975), *Delayed Hypersensitivity—North-Holland Research Monographs, Frontiers in Biology*, Vol. 4. Amsterdam: North-Holland. Second edition.

Articles

Arnason, B. G. & Waksman, B. H. (1964), "Tuberculin sensitivity. Immunologic considerations." *Advances in Tuberculosis Research*, **13**, 1.
Bloom, B. R. & Chase, M. W. (1967), "Transfer of delayed type hypersensitivity. A critical review and experimental study in the guinea pig." *Progr. Allergy*, **10**, 151.
Brown, R. S., Haynes, H. A., Foley, H. T., Goodwin, H. A., Berard, C. W. & Carbone, P. P. (1967), "Hodgkin's disease. Immunologic, clinical and histologic features of 50 untreated cases." *Ann. Int. Med.*, **67**, 291.
Epstein, W. L. (1967), "Granulomatous hypersensitivity." *Progr. Allergy*, **11**, 36.
Salvin, S. B. (1963), "Immunologic aspects of the mycoses." *Progr. Allergy*, **7**, 213.

Chapter IV
Immunological Processes in Infectious Diseases

It is probable that in part immunological processes have developed phylogenetically as a means of ridding the body of foreign substances which might harm it. There is no doubt that parasitic organisms and their products form one of the greatest dangers from which the body has to protect itself throughout life. Whether or not one accepts the teleological argument that immune mechanisms were developed by a process of natural selection as a protection against infection, there is no doubt that the beneficial effects of the immune response far outweighs the damage which these processes can produce in the host. Although the greater part of this book is dedicated to the cynical trick of nature that those processes that protect us from our environment can also cause havoc within ourselves and be the instigators of a wide range of pathological processes, this particular chapter will discuss in part the more beneficial aspects of the immune systems.

Immunity against infection with parasitic organisms and against damage caused by their metabolic by-products results from a fine interaction of specific humoral and cell-mediated immunological mechanisms with those mesenchymal cells which are present even in the most primitive of multi-cellular creatures and which have the power of ingesting and digesting foreign material. The action of these cells, whether polymorphonuclear leucocytes or macrophages, depends on their ability to ingest foreign matter by a process of invagination of the cell membrane, known as pinocytosis. These cells also contain a number of subcellular organelles known as "lysosomes" which are the site of synthesis of a wide range of hydrolytic enzymes capable of digesting proteins and other macromolecules which the cell has ingested. It is probable that these cells are not themselves capable of recognizing foreignness of their own accord but depend on interaction with humoral and cell-mediated immune processes for identification of foreignness in a macromolecule or microorganism. An example of this process is the well known fact that microorganisms are more readily phagocytosed by these cells when coated with antibody and after interaction with the series of enzymes and cofactors present in the tissue fluids, known as complement.

It is well known that immunity as any process involved in natural selection is genetically controlled. Much of our immunity against infection is in fact innate or inborn, although immunity to certain microorganisms and toxins develops, as any other immuno-logical process, following actual contact with the antigens in the microorganisms, or their toxic metabolic by-products. Immunity whether innate or secondary to an initial contact with the toxic or infective agent will in most cases be boosted by further contact with these antigens.

Innate or Natural Immunity

Each species may differ from other species in its innate immunity to certain infections. However, within a species, individuals will also differ one from another in their degree of innate immunity to different organisms. The strength of immunity at any particular time, whether innate or acquired, will depend on a number of environmental factors. These include the dietary state of the individual and can be modified from time to time by the balance of hormones within the body. There is no doubt that the balance of hormones secreted by the different endocrine glands has a marked influence on all aspects of the immunological processes. Immunological processes depend on protein synthesis which are susceptible to both the dietary and endocrine state of the individual at any particular time. The reaction of the body to one antigen can also be modified as a result of its reaction at the same time to other antigens.

There are many examples in the animal world of the innate resistance of certain species or strains of species to different infections. However, mention should be made of the association of certain genetic traits in man with an increased resistance to malaria. These are sickle cell anaemia, thalassaemia, the production of haemoglobin C and a deficiency of the enzyme glucose-6-phosphate dehydrogenase in the red cells. These conditions are fatal in homozygotes, but there is no doubt that heterozygotes carry an increased resistance to malaria. It has also been suggested that people of blood group O or B are more resistant to smallpox than those with blood group A.

As examples of differences in resistance between species mention should be made of the often quoted examples that the rat is relatively resistant to diphtheria whereas the guinea pig and human are more susceptible to this infection. Within species, it is always quoted that Algerian sheep are more resistant to anthrax than European sheep. Moreover, it is possible to breed selected strains of the same species in the laboratory which are more resistant or more susceptible to a particular infection.

Natural Antibodies

Innate immunity depends on a number of different factors of which environmental features such as diet, climate and hormonal influences no doubt play a major role. Of the immunological factors involved both humoral antibody and cell-mediated immune reaction play a varying part depending on the nature of the organism or toxin involved. Whereas our knowledge of cell-mediated mechanisms in immunity is unfortunately at the present time poorly developed, there has been a considerable amount of study of so-called "natural" antibodies against bacteria present in the sera of "normal" individuals. Examination of the sera of normal subjects will reveal the presence of humoral antibodies both agglutinating and bactericidal against a wide range of pathogenic and non-pathogenic organisms. It is true that many of these antibodies are directed against organisms which live saprophytically within the intestines or on the surface of the skin. However, antibodies may also be found against such pathogens as *Shigella* and *Salmonella*, organisms which are associated with dysentery and gastroenteritis, and even against the cholera vibrio. These natural antibodies are present at birth since they pass across the placenta from the mother. However, it can be shown that they are not actually produced by the individual himself until a few months after birth. Much controversy has occurred in the past as to whether these antibodies develop as a genetic function, especially as the spectrum of antibodies present and the level found in the serum appears to be very specific to a particular species. However, animals brought up in a "germ-free" environment fail to develop these antibodies. They also show a greater susceptibility to infection than normal animals. They have a low level of circulating immunoglobulin in their serum and their lymphoid tissue is poorly developed as a result of insufficient antigenic stimulation. Natural antibodies develop as a result of antigenic stimulation in early infancy from antigens present in the intestinal bacterial flora or in the food. It would also appear that natural antibodies against pathogenic organisms develop as a result of stimulation of the lymphoid tissue with cross-reacting antigens present on the surface of non-pathogenic organisms present in the intestinal flora. The degree and extent of the response of lymphoid tissue to these ubiquitous organisms is considerably dependent on the genetic make-up of the individual, as can be seen from the different spectra of antibodies and the different levels found in animals of two different species living under identical environmental conditions.

A discussion of the origin of blood group isoantibodies is of interest in connection with the origin of natural antibacterial antibodies in the serum. Antigens cross-reacting with human A and B blood group antigens are present on the surface of a wide range of intestinal bacteria and blood group isoantibodies do not develop until well into the postnatal period. Studies on germ-free animals have elucidated the formation of these antibodies. Antibodies directed against human blood group antigens are absent from the serum of germ-free animals. However, if these animals are fed *Escherichia coli* 086 which carries an antigen on its surface which cross-reacts with human blood group B substance, they will develop anti-human B agglutinins in their serum.

Although antigens cross-reacting with human blood group antigens are widely distributed in plants and bacteria a person of blood group A will not develop anti-A antibodies, due to a tolerance to A antigens which are already present in his tissues from early embryonic life. Similarly a person of blood group B will not develop anti-B. However, a person of blood group O who has neither A or B antigens on his red cells develops both anti-A and anti-B.

The significance of natural antibacterial antibodies in protection from infection will vary from bacterium to bacterium. It is probable that in certain cases they contribute significantly to natural protection from infection. However, there are recorded examples of animals which are highly susceptible to infection with a particular organism despite the presence of a relatively high concentration of natural antibodies in the serum against the organisms in question. This could be either because the antibodies are not capable of activating the complement pathway or because the organism needs cell-mediated immunity for its elimination.

The Development of Immunity After Infection

Immunity to Bacteria

The immunity which develops to bacteria after infection may be lasting, as that to a particular strain of pneumococcus after pneumonia caused by that organism, or after one attack of pertussis. However, immunity to diphtheria may be only temporary unless there have been further subclinical infections with the organism.

The state of immunity which develops following infection can be graded from one of complete immunity, through various stages of partial immunity, to one where no immunity develops. Absence of any form of immunity to a highly invasive organism would result in a generalized bacteraemia and death from generalized toxaemia. The frequency of bacteraemia and death decreases as the state of immunity increases. Also where there is a state of partial immunity lesions will tend to be more localized and there will be an increasing frequency of the infection actually being clinically latent. It is probable that immunity is never complete in the true sense of the word, but in the highest state of immunity the organisms which invade the body are rejected so rapidly by the immune mechanisms that no symptoms develop.

In the case of enteric infections such as those caused by *Salmonella typhi* or *Vibrio cholerae*, once the individual is immune, antibodies are secreted into the lumen of the intestines. These will tend to kill the organisms within the crypts of the intestinal tract, before damage can be caused to the intestinal mucosa.

Many organisms release toxins into the host during infection. The commonest example of this is in diphtheria, tetanus and gas gangrene. These toxins are in many cases known to be enzymes which can damage tissues in various ways. It has been shown that these toxins not only damage the tissues directly but also promote infection with the bacteria in the early stages by inhibiting the cellular elements which might normally keep the infection in check. During infection antitoxins are developed which have the property of neutralizing these toxins.

With other organisms such as the typhoid bacillus or the pneumococcus the toxic substance is an integral part of the cell wall or capsule of the bacteria. In cases where a previous infection has occurred but immunity has to some extent waned over a period of years, further infection will cause a very rapid rise in immunity over a period of two to three days (secondary response). This is in marked contrast to the development of immunity during a first infection which may take seven to ten days to develop and is associated with a far lower level of antibody in the circulation (primary response).

Whereas humoral antibodies play a major role in the defence of the body against most bacteria, by neutralizing toxins, promoting phagocytosis or actually killing the organisms, they appear to play little part in the defence of the body against *Mycobacteria* such as the tubercle bacillus and the leprosy bacillus. Defence of the body against these organisms appears to be dependent on a state of specific cellular immunity. The relation of this state to the other forms of cell-mediated immune reactions has been discussed in the previous chapter. In infection with other organisms defence would appear to be a synergism between specific humoral antibodies, specific cell-mediated immune mechanisms and non-specific cellular reactions involving macrophages and polymorphonuclear leucocytes. Protection against reinfection with mycobacteria appears to develop about the time the person begins to develop delayed type allergy. Originally it was thought that it was the allergic reaction which brought about the expulsion of the bacilli with the exudation. It has, however, been shown that cellular immunity to mycobacteria can exist in the absence of the allergic state following desensitization and that a high degree of allergy can be produced without the development of cellular immunity. The development of the cellular immune state appears to be associated partly with the activation of certain enzymes in macrophages which could be involved in killing the organism.

BCG Vaccination Against Tuberculosis

Vaccination against tuberculosis with an attenuated strain of the tubercle bacillus (Bacille Calmette et Guerin) was first introduced in 1921. It is, however, only in the last few years that the true efficacy of this treatment could be assessed scientifically. In England a single vaccination is given at the age of 13 to individuals who are still at that age tuberculin negative. The criterion of negativity used is a reaction of less than 5 mm to 100 T.U. of tuberculin (equivalent to 0·1 ml of

1/100 dilution of old tuberculin). In a controlled trial over a period of twelve and a half years the British Medical Research Council found this treatment to be 79% effective in reducing the incidence of tuberculosis in such tuberculin negative individuals when compared with originally tuberculin negative unvaccinated individuals. However, in a parallel trial over a period of 14 years the United States public health service found that BCG vaccination was only 14% effective. The discrepancy in these findings is thought to be due to the fact that the American trial was conducted on a population which had already a considerable amount of low grade sensitivity probably due to infection with atypical mycobacteria. The criterion of tuberculin negativity used by the Americans was a reaction of less than 5 mm to 5 tuberculin units (equivalent to 0·1 ml 1/2000 old tuberculin), and thus would have included a number of people rejected by the British trial as being tuberculin positive. It is possible that the control group in the American trial showed a greater degree of immunity to start with, than the control group in the British trial. This is confirmed by the fact that the average rate of disease in the American control group was one-tenth of that in the British control group. Thus the chances of finding a statistically significant decrease in disease after BCG vaccination was very much less. It has also been suggested that the vaccine used in the American trial might not have been as effective as that used in the British trial. Despite these differences the results of the British trial have been fully accepted for a number of years by the World Health Organization, and the use of BCG in protection from tuberculosis is now standard treatment.

The Immunological Spectrum in Chronic Infectious Diseases

In a number of chronic infectious conditions, the clinical manifestation of the disease is dependent on the degree of host resistance. The extent of host resistance is related to the intensity of the cell-mediated or humoral antibody response. In addition, hypersensitivity reactions can develop due to tissue reactions at the site of immune rejection of the infecting organism or to the deposition of immune complexes formed with soluble antigens derived from the infecting organism. In a number of these diseases the organism is not of itself highly pathogenic. However, as a result of either a specific or a non-specific immunological defect, the organism is allowed to proliferate to a greater extent than would be expected in an individual with an intact immune response. Failure of host resistance is frequently a result of a defect in cell-mediated immunity. However, hypersensitivity reactions resulting in tissue damage can occur as readily from cellular immune reactions as from the deposition of immune complexes involving humoral antibody. Such a differential interaction between immune processes and the infecting microorganism can result in a wide spectrum of pathological processes, which in turn leads to the markedly different ways in which a disease due to the same microorganism can manifest itself clinically.

Much of the increased interest in diseases where there is such a spectrum of clinical manifestation has derived especially from the recent elaboration of the varied clinical patterns seen in leprosy. A similar pattern may be found in the other common mycobacterial disease—tuberculosis, in the systemic mycoses and candidiasis and in those viral infections where host resistance is dependent mainly on cellular rather than on humoral immune processes. In other bacterial diseases such as brucellosis and syphilis in which it is suspected, although not proved, that cellular immunity plays an important role in the disease, there also appears to be a similar spectrum of clinical appearances depending on differential immunological processes. Deficiency in cellular immunity forms one pole of the immunological spectrum. The other pole is formed by a hyper reactivity of cellular immunity. At this extreme, there is a very high degree of host resistance to the infecting organism but at the same time there is marked allergic hyper reactivity so that a strong delayed hyper sensitivity reaction will occur at the site of immunological rejection of the infecting organisms. Between these two poles there will be a spectrum of clinical appearances depending on the strength of the cell-mediated immune reaction that can be mounted against the infecting organism.

Leprosy, resulting from infection with the organism *Mycobacterium leprae*, takes on two polar forms—the lepromatous form, in which there is a specific immunological unresponsiveness to *M. leprae*, and the tuberculoid form, in which there is a high degree of host resistance associated with a strong state of delayed allergic reactivity directed against mycobacterial antigens. The role of cell-mediated immunity against this organism is highlighted by the ability to reproduce a lepromatous form of the disease in experimental animals in which cellular immunity has been suppressed by thymectomy and irradiation. In lepromatous leprosy, the tissues are infiltrated with sheets of macrophages which are packed full of leprosy bacilli that cannot be eliminated. Failure to eliminate the infecting organism is associated with a relative absence of small lymphocytes from the lesions. At the tuberculoid pole, where there is a high degree of cellular immunity, it is often difficult to detect the infecting organism in the tissues and the lesions are the site of a dense infiltration with small lymphocytes. Between these two points there is a spectrum of clinical and histological appearances in which the number of infecting organisms varies inversely with the number of infiltrating lymphocytes. The more cell-mediated immunity is present the more the lesions will have a "tuberculoid" appearance both macroscopically and microscopically.

The lepromin reaction can be taken as another indication of the extent of the involvement of cell-mediated immunity in the disease process.

Lepromin is an extract of skin containing whole leprosy bacilli which have been killed by autoclaving. The intradermal injection of this substance produces a typical tuberculoid-like reaction which then fades and is followed after about seven days by a nodular granulomatous lesion which reaches its peak about three to four weeks after injection; 90% of normal people who react to tuberculin react to the cross-reacting lepromin. Patients with tuberculoid leprosy are lepromin positive. People with lepromatous leprosy are always lepromin negative even if they are tuberculin positive. Lepromin is therefore used to determine specific immunological unresponsiveness in respect to cell-mediated immunity in lepromatous leprosy. The specificity of this unresponsiveness is underlined by the fact that many of these patients are tuberculin positive. As patients cross the spectrum of leprosy from the tuberculoid to the lepromatous pole, patients will show varying degrees of lepromin positivity in proportion to the extent of the existing cell-mediated immunity.

Although patients with lepromatous leprosy show no evidence of cell-mediated immunity against *M. leprae*, they have no defect in humoral antibody formation. Very high levels of humoral antibody are found in the serum of patients at this pole of the disease. The level of specific antibody is low in tuberculoid leprosy, despite there being a high level of host resistance. This indicates that in lepromatous leprosy immunological unresponsiveness is split involving cell-mediated immunity only. Such a failure of cellular immunity may be due to the high level of antigen present in the tissues suppressing this aspect of the response. Other possibilities are immunological enhancement by the high level of antibody or soluble immune complexes or the generation of a specific population of suppressor lymphocytes. As patients are treated with specific chemotherapeutic agents, the level of antigen in the tissues will drop, and the patient will move both clinically and histologically across the leprosy spectrum from the lepromatous end of the spectrum towards the tuberculoid pole. In this process, as they regain their cell-mediated immunity, they will develop delayed hypersensitivity reactions wherever there is residual antigen. This is especially common in the skin and peripheral nerves. Such patients often develop a severe peripheral neuritis. These reactions, which are associated with an intense lymphocytic infiltration in the tissues, are often referred to as "reversal reactions". Conversely, patients at the tuberculoid end of the spectrum may lose cell-mediated immunity as the antigen load in the tissues increases as a result of lack of therapy. These reactions are known as "downgrading reactions" and are associated with a relative absence of lymphocytes in the lesions. A similar return of lymphocyte responsiveness has been demonstrated in syphiltic patients, following chemotherapy.

A further type of reaction which occurs in patients with lepromatous leprosy is known as "erythema nodosum leprosum". This may occur in as many as 50% of patients with this form of the disease within the first year of treatment with sulphones, at a time when one would expect a high level of soluble antigen to be released as a result of the massive destruction of organisms. As its name implies, the condition is associated with the development of crops of red nodules in the skin. These nodules last 24–48 hours and the condition is frequently accompanied by fever. In severe cases, there may be other systemic manifestations such as arthritis, iridocyclitis, orchitis and an acutely painful neuritis. The fever is frequently associated with proteinuria. The skin lesions may become haemorrhagic. Histologically they differ from those seen in "reversal reactions" in that they are the site of an intense polymorphonuclear reaction and the blood vessels in the dermis show an acute fibrinoid necrosis. This appearance is highly suggestive of an Arthus reaction and these lesions can be shown to be the site of deposition of immune complexes containing immunoglobulin, complement and mycobacterial antigens. The systemic manifestations associated with the skin lesions are also suggestive of an "immune complex disease".

Despite the fundamental specificity of the immunological unresponsiveness in polar lepromatous leprosy, there have been a number of reports of a non-specific depression of cell-mediated immunity in this condition. These include a failure to be sensitized to contact sensitizing agents such as 2·4 dinitrochlorobenzene and an increased retention of skin allografts. It is unlikely that this depression which is far from complete is related to the inability of the body to eliminate *M. leprae*. Such patients generally have little depression of cellular immunity against other organisms which need cell-mediated immunity for their elimination, nor do they have a higher incidence of tumours as is found in patients whose cell-mediated immunity has been depressed by immunosuppressive therapy.

Although there is generally a high degree of host resistance, dependant on cell-mediated immunity to *M. tuberculosis* a spectrum similar to that in leprosy can be detected. A number of instances have been recorded of a depression of cell-mediated immunity in this disease in which the organism is allowed to proliferate in a relatively uncontrolled manner in the tissues in a manner similar to that found in lepromatous leprosy. This is associated with negative tuberculin reactivity. Many instances have been recorded of familial low resistance to tuberculosis, indicating that the ability to produce varying degrees of cell-mediated immunity to a particular infecting organism is under genetic control. Similarly, it has been demonstrated that the reason why some people develop lepromatous rather than tuberculoid leprosy is a host determined genetic characteristic.

A spectrum of immune response producing a number of varied clinical patterns similar to those found in leprosy has been delineated in infections caused by *Leishmania sp*. The normal self-healing oriental sore found in cutaneous leishmaniasis is associated with a high degree of cellular immunity. However, a nodular granulomatous form of this disease, generally called diffuse cutaneous leishmaniasis, has been found under circumstances where there is a depression of cellular immunity. The lesions consist of macrophages loaded with parasites which cannot be eliminated and lymphocytes may be scanty or absent. As in lepromatous leprosy, this depression is specific to the infecting organism. In Kala-azar, there is a similar depression of cellular immunity as the leishmanin delayed hypersensitivity skin test is also negative. However, the organism produces a severe systemic disease rather than being localized to the skin. In both diffuse cutaneous leishmaniasis and Kala-azar there is no parallel failure of humoral immunity, which as in lepromatous leprosy is exaggerated with high levels of circulating immunoglobulins. A similar spectrum of clinical appearances can be found in the systemic mycoses. For example, in South American blastomycosis. In this disease, there is a localized self-healing skin infection associated with a positive delayed hypersensitivity reaction to paracoccidioidin and a low level of circulating antibody. A number of patients however have a generalized granulomatous skin infection with little lymphocytic reaction or a systemic infection frequently affecting the lungs. These patients who cannot eliminate the infecting organisms have negative skin tests and high levels of circulating antibodies. In all these conditions where there is a specific failure of cellular immunity, treatment with specific chemotherapeutic agents may eliminate the infecting organism but cessation of treatment is frequently associated with a recurrence of the disease, as the infecting organism may not be completely eliminated. Cellular immunity is necessary for the complete elimination of the organism from the body. Where this occurs, it is usually associated with a return of cellular immunity as indicated by a return of delayed hypersensitivity to the specific antigen.

Generalized infection of the skin and mucous membranes with *Candida albicans* occurs in states where there is a non-specific lowering of cellular immunity. This can occur in babies with neonatal thymus dysgenesis or during prolonged immunosuppressive therapy. It can also occur associated with diseases of the endocrine system such as hypoparathyroidism, hypoadrenocorticism, hypothyroidism or diabetes mellitus. Failure of cellular immunity, resulting in chronic mucocutaneous candidiasis, is usually genetically determined, and can be shown to be an autosomal recessive characteristic. In some patients, it has been shown to develop as a result of a failure on the part of the circulating lymphocytes to produce the chemical mediators of cellular immunity when stimulated with specific antigen. Chronic muco-cutaneous candidiasis develops more frequently as a result of a non-specific defect of cell-mediated immunity than as a result of a specific immunological unresponsiveness.

A spectrum of clinical appearances dependent on a differential cell-mediated immune response has as yet to be shown to occur in other forms of infection. However, indications that it can occur in other chronic infections can be found, if sought. Thus, in patients with suspected brucellosis, 60% of those with titres of anti-brucella antibodies of 80 or more have negative brucellin delayed hypersensitivity skin tests, whereas 50% of those with positive brucellin skin tests have low titres of circulating antibody. This would suggest that two forms of host response can occur in brucella infection. Moreover, one of the more common chronic bacterial infections which shows a spectrum of clinical appearances dependent on host resistance is syphilis. In the three stages of syphilis the clinical picture is dependent on the interaction of different aspects of the immune response of the host. Thus, in primary syphilis, the chancre is a localized area of vasculitis with a polymorphonuclear leucocyte infiltrate, an appearance reminiscent of the Arthus reaction. At this time there is a widespread dissemination of the organism despite there being a powerful humoral antibody response, which suggests that there is a specific unresponsiveness of cellular immunity. The secondary stage of the disease has many of the features of an immune complex disease, generalized rash, fever, lymphadenopathy, and occasionally arthritis, nephritis and iridocyclitis. Although the infecting organism is known to disseminate long before the development of secondary features of the disease, it is possible that this phase can only develop when immune complexes can form in the correct proportions. Eventually the patient develops the ability to show a delayed hypersensitivity skin reaction to treponemal antigens. At this time the patient becomes asymptomatic and goes into what is referred to as the latent phase of the disease, when a balance is struck between the infecting organism and the specific cellular immune processes. This balance is somewhat disturbed at a later stage in the disease when the tertiary manifestations become apparent, possibly as a result of intercurrent infection or just as a function of ageing. It could be that the features of the tertiary disease are the result of a further decrease in cellular immunity followed by immune complex deposition. In congenital syphilis there is also evidence of a failure of cellular immunity, as in this condition there is depletion of the thymus-dependent lymphocytes in the spleen in babies dying of this condition under the age of one year. Some of these features have been studied using lymphocyte responsiveness *in vitro*. Occasionally patients with primary syphilis have lymphocytes that can be transformed by *T. pallidum*. However in the secondary stage of the disease all patients are unreactive. Reactivity however develops after treatment. Failure of lymphocyte reactivity to specific antigen in secondary syphilis has been found to be associated with the presence of a non-specific suppressor factor in the circulation.

Malaria and Trypanosomiasis

A strong degree of immunity to malaria parasites is developed by people living in endemic areas. Immunity is mediated by humoral antibodies of the IgG class which can confer protection when transferred in serum from person to person or across the placenta from mother to foetus. However, acquired immunity of this type is effective only against the parasite in the stage when it is within the erythrocyte and only in the later stage of this part of the life cycle, when, it is thought, the red cell membrane becomes more permeable, allowing the entrance of the immunoglobulin molecules. Even in a highly immune subject the exo-erythrocyte stage of the cycle is inaccessible to the immune processes. Thus immune mechanisms can operate only at a very short stage in the life cycle of the organism. In endemic areas children are immune up to six months of age as a result of the continuous presence of maternal antibody. Primary infection occurs during this time and is often asymptomatic. Between six months and two years of age the children go through a stage when they have a severe clinical illness while they are building up their own naturally acquired immunity, which results in clinical improvement. From this stage onwards the number of parasites present in the body drops and the subject lives in a state of tolerance between the parasites and his immune processes which keep the parasites under control.

The role of the various factors involved in immunity to malaria have been studied more fully in plasmodial infections of mice and rats. There is no doubt that protective immunity can be conveyed in these infections by the IgG fraction of serum from infected or hyperimmunized animals. However, recently there has been discussion of the possible role of cell-mediated immunity in these infections. This has derived from two sources. In the first, there has been evidence of more severe infections occurring in animals in which the mobile pool of long-lived lymphocytes have been depleted by neonatal thymectomy or treatment with anti-lymphocyte serum. Secondly, there have been reports that protective immunity could be transferred passively with preparations of lymphoid cells. One should be careful of taking either of these findings as evidence that the infecting parasite is eliminated by cellular rather than humoral immunity. Depletion of the mobile pool of small lymphocytes by neonatal thymectomy or antilymphocyte serum treatment can cause a lowering in the amount of circulating antibody produced (*see* Chapter I: thymus and bone marrow interaction) and plasma cell precursors can also be transferred in cell-suspensions used for the transfer of cellular immunity.

The chronicity of malarial infection results from the number of ways the parasite has for avoiding the host's immune response. Apart from its intracellular localization, inherent immunosuppressive properties (*vide infra*) and ability to interfere with macrophage function, the malarial parasite has an added property that it can change its antigenic structure and thus avoid the immune response.

Malarial infections have been found to cause a drop in certain forms of immune response to other antigens. In this connection an increased growth of certain tumours has been found to develop in mice infected with plasmodia. It is thought that this may have a bearing on the higher incidence of Burkitt's lymphoma in malarial endemic areas. It has been suggested that the syndrome of "tropical splenomegaly" which occurs in malaria endemic areas in patients in whom there is no obvious malarial infection may be the result of plasmodial infection in a situation where there is a high state of cell-mediated immunity. In this condition there is marked infiltration of the liver sinusoids with lymphocytes. It could be that these patients eliminate their organisms particularly effectively and the infiltration of the hepatic sinusoids with lymphocytes is evidence of a delayed hypersensitivity reaction in the liver. The absence of obvious parasites could be similar to the absence of leprosy bacilli which sometimes occurs in the lesions of tuberculoid leprosy. A nephrotic syndrome occurs in children infected with *P. malariae*. This has been shown to be associated with the deposition of immune complexes containing plasmodial antigen, immunoglobulin and complement on the basement membrane of the glomeruli and in the tubules. This is another example of tissue damage developing as a result of an immune reaction in an infectious disease.

Recent advances have been made in the development of a vaccine against malaria, using irradiated sporozoites. Individuals immunised by repeated bites from X-irradiated *P. falciparum* infected mosquitoes were found to be resistant to challenge with sporozoites of *P. falciparum*, but not *P. vivax*. However at the present time there are immense practical problems in producing a sporozoite vaccine, as *P. falciparum* cannot be grown adequately in experimental animals or in tissue culture.

In African trypanosomiasis the problem is more difficult as the organism changes its antigens during the various phases of its life cycle. Thus a positive balance is never really struck between the patient's adaptive immune responses and the organism. In long standing infections the organism eventually enters the central nervous system, causing the classical clinical picture. African trypanosomiasis is associated with high levels of IgM immunoglobulins in both the blood and the cerebrospinal fluid. The level of IgM in the blood may be as high as 8–16 times the normal level.

Chagas disease due to infection with *T. cruzi* has a number of features that suggest an immunological disease with progression from low resistance through high resistance that is exemplified by the pattern found in syphilis. The acute form of the disease is followed by a long latent period which may last 10–20 years before entering the third or chronic stage of the disease. Thus there is a continuous progression through an acute illness in which there is marked proliferation of parasites to a state of balance between the organism and host resistance. Disturbance of this balance after 10–20 years results in the development of a chronic immunopathological lesion in the heart in which there is diffuse fibrosis of the myocardium and infiltration with lymphocytes, macrophages and plasma cells.

Helminthic Infections

The response of the body to different helminth parasites is very variable. Whereas microfilariae, the cause of filariasis, are considered to be poorly antigenic and do not appear to induce much of an immune response, schistosomes, the helminths causing Bilharzia appear to induce a certain degree of immunity in the host. The protective immune mechanisms however only appear to act at an early stage in the life cycle of the worms in man, preventing infection from parasites entering the body through the skin and their dissemination through the blood stream. The main immunogenic stimulus appears to be the adult worm, and the continuous presence of adult worms in the host is necessary for the maintenance of a persistent immune state. However, immunological processes also appear to play an adverse role in these infections, especially causing severe granuloma formation.

Granuloma formation leading to "pipe-stem fibrosis" of the liver may occur in up to 10% of patients infected with *Schistosoma mansoni* in highly endemic areas. This is generally associated with marked splenomegaly due to hyperplasia of the lymphoid elements. Such patients have a marked hypergammaglobulinaemia. Granulomas form in the liver around the eggs of the worm. Lymphoid cells are found around the periphery of the granulomas. Immune complex formation has been described round the egg. However, there is evidence also of cell-mediated immune processes involved in the formation of these granulomas. Schistosome granuloma formation in experimental animals can be accelerated by transfer of lymphoid cells, and not by serum, and can be depressed by neonatal thymectomy or treatment with anti-lymphocyte serum. Patients with hepatosplenic schistosomiasis may also develop a form of glomerulonephritis in which the glomeruli contain IgG, IgM and complement, indicating that the lesions could be due to immune complex deposition.

A striking feature of helminth infections is the frequency of the occurrence of anaphylactic (IgE) antibodies against the parasites which can be demonstrated by the development of immediate weal and flare reactions to the intradermal inoculation of extracts from the worms. Infestation with *Ascaris lumbricoides* in children is associated with attacks of urticaria, maculo-papular rashes, asthma and other allergic manifestations, and it has been found that children infested with these worms have a higher level of IgE immunoglobulins in their serum than children who are not infested with the worms. Peripheral blood eosinophilia is common in all helminthic infections. Migration of helminth larvae through the lungs is sometimes associated with severe pulmonary infiltration with eosinophil leucocytes, resulting in a pneumonia which can prove fatal. This is thought to be a result of an allergic reaction to the larvae antigens. In view of the association of eosinophil leucocytes with histamine release and the knowledge that IgE antibodies are potent causes of the release of histamine, it is possible that this condition could be the result of a chronic anaphylactic reaction in the lungs. Despite the high level of IgE antibodies in ascaris and hookworm infections, it is not considered that these antibodies form the only immune mechanisms that protect the body from worms. It is now accepted that the immune mechanisms that cause the rejection of these parasites require sensitized lymphocytes as well as antibody.

Little attention has been paid to the immunology of filarial infections. However the clinical features of onchocerciasis suggest that this disease has distinct immunological features resembling the low resistance forms of leprosy, cutaneous leishmaniasis and some of the chronic mycoses. There are a number of indications that the form of onchocerciasis seen generally in Africa is a low resistance form of the disease. The presence of large numbers of microfilariae in the tissues without gross cellular infiltration in the presence of high circulating antibody levels would indicate a possible failure of cell-mediated immune mechanisms necessary for the elimination of the organism. Under these conditions ocular changes such as iridocyclitis and sclerosing keratitis could be due to immune complex reactions in which the high level of antibody reacts with traces of antigen left by the microfilariae during their migration through the tissues. These changes could have some analogy with those of erythema nodosum leprosum in lepromatous leprosy patients.

Immune Mechanisms in Virus Infections

Whereas circulating antibody acts against bacteria to promote phagocytosis of the organism, the effect of antibody against viruses is mainly one of neutralization so that virus can no longer infect cells. It must be remembered in this connection that viruses can only reproduce within cells and need to enter the cells of the body for replication to take place. Antibody, however, can only attack the virus outside the body's cells. Once virus is within cells it is protected from antibody. Antibody cannot thus interfere with intracellular virus replication. Moreover, virus can under certain circumstances spread from cell to cell without passing through the extracellular fluid where it is susceptible to neutralization by humoral antibody. Thus virus can exist in the body in the presence of a high concentration of circulating antibody.

It is probable that although the humoral antibody response is more important in the protection from reinfection, it is not the major factor involved in the control of a primary virus infection. Thus certain children with congenital hypogammaglobulinaemia can recover from virus infections without producing any neutralizing antibody against virus. These children however, cannot cope with bacterial infections for which they need the production of circulating antibody. The protective mechanisms involved in recovery from a primary virus infection are not clearly known. It is thought by some that a non-specific antiviral agent "interferon" produced as a result of stimulation of cells with even an unrelated virus (the virus interference phenomenon) might be involved. It has been observed that those children who are congenitally deficient in thymus tissue at birth are unable to cope with certain viruses such as vaccinia due presumably to a defect in cell-mediated immune mechanisms. "Interferon" has been found to be produced by lymphocytes as a result of antigenic stimulation *in vitro*. This would indicate that cell-mediated immune processes could act to control virus infection through the production of "interferon". However, it is known that there are many viruses which can be eliminated from the body without the production of detectable amounts of "interferon". Other viruses known to need cell-mediated immunity for control of infection are herpes simplex, yellow fever, lymphocytic choriomeningitis and certain adenoviruses.

Immunity to viruses differs from immunity to bacteria in that it is almost always long lasting. It is thought that this might be due to the fact that after infection and recovery virus is not completely eliminated from the body and traces remain protected within cells. Periodically small amounts of virus are released into the lymphoid tissue where it can continue to boost the immune response. Most effective immunity is associated with a high titre of antibody secreted outside the body into the possible portals of entry of virus. Thus high immunity to influenza is associated with high antibody level in the nasal secretions, and the most effective way to produce immunity to poliovirus is by feeding an attenuated virus culture by mouth so that antibody production is stimulated in the intestinal lymphoid tissue and antibody is secreted into the intestinal contents to neutralize the virus before it can gain entry through the gastrointestinal tract by infecting the lining cells of the intestinal mucosa. Such antibodies are of the class IgA and their concentration may not in any way be related to the concentration of antibody in the serum which is mainly IgG. Conversely the concentration of IgG antibodies in the circulation may not necessarily be related to the degree of overall immunity against the particular virus. Following the success of orally administered attenuated live poliovaccine in the production of local immunity against poliovirus, other attenuated viruses have been used to produce local immunity by stimulating local IgA antibody formation. An example of this is the intranasal administration of live attenuated influenza virus which has proved a most successful method of vaccination in both Russia and America. Live attenuated virus has also been used by subcutaneous injection in vaccination against measles and mumps, although the result of these trials has yet to be evaluated over a long period.

Infection with many viruses in embryonic or neonatal life confer a partial immunological tolerance in which the organism may fail to be eliminated although the foetus itself may be producing antibody *in utero* against the virus. An example of such a foetal infection is rubella. The foetus can be infected with rubella as early as the fourth to twelfth week of embryonic life. Such infection may be associated with foetal death or if the foetus is not killed it will develop a chronic infection as a result of which a number of congenital malformations may occur. Examination of the sera of such infants at birth will show the presence of neutralizing antibody against rubella virus. Some of this is IgG antibody which can pass across the placenta. However, a considerable amount of the antibody is IgM which cannot pass across the placenta and must have been made by the foetus itself *in utero*. In congenital rubella a situation exists similar to that seen in a number of other infectious diseases. Immunological tolerance is in respect of cell-mediated immunity only, antibody production being unaffected. As a result, the organism fails to be eliminated. Whether this is a true example of split tolerance or is another example of "immunological enhancement" has yet to be determined.

Not all the effect of antibody or cell-mediated immune mechanisms against viruses is protective. The reaction between viruses and either antibody or cell-mediated immune mechanisms can produce harmful hypersensitivity phenomena. The natural history of many virus infections is biphasic and the development of gross clinical phenomena is often preceded for five days or more by a non-specific febrile illness. The febrile illness is possibly due to the direct action of virus. However, the rash can be due to the combined effect of delayed hypersensitivity and humoral antibody on the virus. Thus, in poxvirus infections, it is considered that the pock itself is caused by virus multiplying in the skin, destroying cells, and interacting with a cell-mediated immune response, while the erythema probably depends on the formation of immune complexes with humoral antibody. In a simple exanthematous disease such as rubella other signs often associated with diseases due to circulating immune complexes such as arthritis may be seen occasionally. Another aspect of immune complex disease in virus infections is the glomerulonephritis which occurs in chronic virus infections where there may be a deficient cell-mediated response. An example of this occurs in lymphocytic choriomeningitis of mice and Aleutian disease of mink. Immune complexes have been observed in the serum of patients infected with hepatitis virus and it is thought that these may be the cause of liver damage in this disease. Encephalitis following vaccination, measles and mumps is thought to result from a cell-mediated immune reaction developing against virus in the brain and occurs about ten days after infection. It is associated with perivascular accumulation of mono-nuclear cells in the brain and the demyelination which occurs is thought to be tissue damage resulting from local immune reaction between virus and immunologically active lymphocytes. It is also thought that the encephalitis resulting from infection with arthropod-born viruses such as Dengue is due to hypersensitivity mechanisms. The illness is biphasic. First, there is a febrile illness associated with a viraemia and this may be followed one to fourteen days later by the encephalitis. The onset of encephalitis is often associated with the appearance of antibody in the circulation. A more severe form of this disease is "Dengue haemorrhagic fever" which occurs in children in areas such as South East Asia where they might have had repeated infections with this virus. It is likely that the fulminating aspects of this disease are due to massive deposition of immune complexes in the vessel walls causing haemor-rhagic Arthus-like reactions throughout the body. The pneumonia associated with infection with *Mycoplasma pneumoniae*, the so-called "Primary atypical virus pneumonia" is also believed to be due to hypersensitivity against the organism as it occurs more frequently following vaccination than during a primary infection.

Bizarre clinical manifestations in virus infections may result from abnormalities in the immune response. Thus measles may be the cause of a giant cell pneumonia in children with leukaemia treated with steroids, as a result of suppression of cell-mediated immunity. Another abnormal manifestation of measles virus infection is the condition known as Subacute sclerosing panencephalitis. This condition is associated with measles virus intranuclear inclusion bodies in the brain cells and a diffuse infiltration of the brain with glial cells and plasma cells. There is also a high titre of measles antibodies in the serum and cerebro-spinal fluid. It has been suggested that, following a normal attack of measles, tolerance with respect to cell-mediated immunity develops, while there is still infectious measles virus left in the brain. This allows the measles virus to proliferate slowly and maintain a slow encephalitis. At the same time, antibody will be produced which can react to form immune complexes without being able to eliminate the virus. Other adverse reactions may follow either exposure to natural measles or live measles virus vaccina-tion in children who had previously received two or three inoculations of inactivated alum precipitated virus vaccine by injection. Such children developed high fever (105°F) and marked local reaction to the subsequent injection of live virus vaccine. Other observations were of an abnormal disease developing during exposure to natural measles, often associated with severe and atypical pulmonary complications. The rash which developed was often unusual in character, sometimes vesicular. It was found that children immunized with dead measles vaccine developed tuberculin-like reactions when skin tested by intradermal injection with the virus, suggesting that these untoward reactions on further exposure were due to the presence of a high degree of delayed hypersensitivity to the virus. Another risk of virus vaccination is that the virus is grown in tissue culture cells of a foreign species, such as chick embryo fibroblasts or monkey or dog kidney. The virus can never be completely purified free of the foreign tissue antigens. In fact, it is believed that certain viruses incorporate foreign tissue antigens into their own structure during replication. These antigens, being tissue antigens, cannot only sensitize the recipient, but theoretically could also induce autoimmune sensitization in the recipient to the tissue of origin, e.g. the kidney. So far no cases of glomerulo-nephritis have been described as being directly attributable to vaccination with viruses grown in foreign kidney cell culture. However, results of experiments in laboratory animals indicates that such a risk, although small, can exist.

A number of viruses can cause non-specific immunodepression, particularly of cell-mediated immunity. Measles can cause a loss of delayed hypersensitivity to tuberculin and tends to aggravate concurrent tuberculosis. It also may aggravate malaria. Similar depressive effects of viruses, such as lymphocytic choriomeningitis virus have been demonstrated in experimental infections in mice. The mechanism for this action has not yet been completely elucidated. However, it is associated with a failure of the lymphocytes of these patients to respond normally *in vitro* by lymphoblastic transformation, in the presence of the non-specific plant mitogen phytohaemagglutinin (PHA).

Bibliography

Books

Developments in Malaria Immunology (1975). Report of a WHO Scientific group. World Health Organization Technical Report Series No. 579. Geneva: WHO.
Immunologic Aspects of Parasitic Infections (1967). Pan-American Health Organisation Scientific Publication No. 150. Washington: Pan-American Health Organisation.
Immunology and Parasitic Diseases (1965). Report of a WHO expert Committee— World Health Organisation Technical Report Series No. 315. Geneva: WHO.
Lurie, M. B. (1964), *Resistance to Tuberculosis: Experimental Studies in Nature and Acquired Defensive Mechanisms*. Cambridge, Mass.: Harvard University Press.
Parasites in the Immunized Host: Mechanisms of Survival (1974). Ciba Foundation Symposium (new series) Associated Scientific Publishers, Amsterdam.
Wilson, G. S. & Miles, A. A. (1964), *The Principles of Bacteriology and Immunity*. 5th edition. London: Arnold.

Articles

D'Arcy Hart, P. (1967), "Efficacy and applicability of mass B.C.G. vaccination in tuberculosis control." *Brit. med. J.*, **i**, 587.
Gray, A. R. (1967), "Some principles of the immunology of trypanosomiasis." *Bull. Wld. Hlth. Org.*, **37**, 177.

Turk, J. L. (1970), "Cell-Mediated Immunological Processes in Leprosy." *Lepr. Rev.*, **41**, 207.

Turk, J. L. & Bryceson, A. D. M. (1971), "Immunological Phenomena in Leprosy and Related Diseases." *Adv. Immunol.*, **13**, 209.

Webb, H. E. & Gordon Smith, C. E. (1966), "Relation of immune response to development of central nervous system lesions in virus infections in man." *Brit. med. J.*, **ii**, 1179.

Chapter V
Immunological Deficiency Diseases: Abnormalities in Immunoglobulin Synthesis

Immunodeficiency as a cause of disease may occur as a direct result of some primary defect in the body's immunological mechanism or secondary to damage to immunological function caused by other disease processes. Whether primary or acquired, immunodeficiency may be non-specific resulting in a defect in phagocyte or complement function or specific affecting immunoglobulin synthesis and cell-mediated immunity either separately or together. Specific immunodeficiency may be due to a defect in immunological stem cells or in the B-lymphocytes or T- lymphocytes derived from them. Stem-cell deficiency will cause a subsequent defect in both B-cells and T-cells. This may or may not be associated with a generalized hypoplasia of haemopoietic tissue. Severe combined immunodeficiency due to a defect in stem-cell development may be genetically inherited and may be X-linked or an autosomal recessive characteristic. Selective deficiency of B-cell function is frequently inherited as an X-linked characteristic. Pure immunoglobulin deficiency may involve all the immunoglobulins or may be selective of IgG and IgA with an increased synthesis of IgM, or for IgA alone. A defect in certain aspects of humoral antibody formation can occur in a pure T-cell deficiency and does not necessarily indicate coexistent B-cell or stem-cell deficiency. As has been discussed previously, reaction between antigen and sensitized T-lymphocytes can cause plasma cells, derived from B-lymphocytes, to give an augmented humoral antibody response to certain antigens. Pure T-lymphocyte deficiency may be due to congenital hypoplasia of the thymus which occurs together with an absence of the parathyroid glands, if there is failure of development of the third bronchial arch in embryonic life, or may occur as a familial isolated developmental defect.

Combined deficiency of T-cell and B-cell function can occur associated with other conditions which may themselves have a hereditary element. These include short-limbed dwarfism, ataxia telangiectasia, Wiskott-Aldrich syndrome and thymoma. Dwarfism in mice due to a deficiency in growth hormone and thyroid function, can be associated with a similar combined immunodeficiency state which can be reversed by hormone replacement therapy. This would appear to indicate that a normal hormonal balance is necessary to have a normal function of both T- and B-lymphocytes and that any fundamental upset of these homeostatic mechanisms can result in immunological deficiencies.

A. Primary Specific Immunodeficiency

1. Combined immunodeficiency syndromes

Severe combined immunodeficiency syndrome can either be found as an autosomal recessive or be sex linked to the X chromosome in which case it is only found in male children. The children become ill within the first few months of life and all die before the end of their second year. There is an absence of all the immunoglobulins from the serum and the peripheral blood lymphocyte count is often less than 1,500 per cu mm. Those lymphocytes which are present do not, however, have the capacity of responding immunologically. There is almost a complete absence of lymphoid tissue in the body. What there is consist of a stroma of reticulum cells, and both lymphocytes and plasma cells are absent. The thymus is underdeveloped and weighs less than 1 gm. The thymic remnant is so small that it can only be found by cutting serial sections of the mediastinum and the tissue is made up almost entirely of epithelial and stromal cells. No true lymphoid cells are seen and Hassall's corpuscles are absent. The lymphoid tissue round the intestines and in the Peyer's patches which possibly control immunoglobulin synthesis is also absent. About a quarter of the children lack adenosine deaminase enzyme activity. In addition their parents may also show low levels. This has suggested a causal relationship. It could be that enzyme deficient lymphocytes are inhibited from dividing by an excess of ADP and ATP.

As evidence of the defect in cell-mediated immunity these children readily accept skin grafts from unrelated persons and cannot be sensitized to produce contact sensitivity with dinitrofluorobenzene. The defect in T-cells is indicated by a failure of the lymphocytes to be stimulated in culture by non-specific mitogens such as phytohaemagglutinin (PHA). These children suffer from repeated and progressive infections both of bacterial, fungal and of viral origin. They are particularly susceptible to Candida and *Pneumocystis carinii* and often have a continuous morbilliform rash possibly due to prolonged measles infection and die from progressive vaccinia when vaccinated. Clinically, these children differ from those with a simple defect in immunoglobulin synthesis in that in the latter condition there is no defect in the ability to deal with virus infections.

Less severe forms of this deficiency are found in which the disease has a later onset and a more gradual downhill course. Occasionally these children have normal levels of one or more immunoglobulins, frequently IgM (Nézelof syndrome).

2. Defect in cell-mediated immunity only

In this condition there is thymic dysplasia and lymphoid tissue depletion similar to that found in the previous condition. There is a marked lymphopenia but normal levels of immunoglobulins are found in the serum. These children are capable of developing normal levels of viral antibodies when stimulated with poliovirus. They cannot, however, reject a skin homograft nor develop contact sensitivity to dinitrofluorobenzene and their lymphocytes fail to respond to PHA *in vitro*. Despite the fact that there is no apparent defect in their ability to produce humoral antibodies they would appear to be unable to cope with virus infections. They are also susceptible to candidiasis and develop *Pneumocystis carinii* pneumonia.

It would therefore appear that humoral antibodies are not sufficient to cope with virus, fungal and certain protozoal infections and cell-mediated immune mechanisms are necessary for survival. An interesting corollary to this, which will be discussed later, is that children with defective immunoglobulin synthesis who cannot produce antibodies can still cope with these infections.

One form of this condition (Di George's syndrome) is due to a defect in the third and fourth branchial arches during embryonic development and is not genetically controlled. As well as thymic dysplasia, there is also an absence of the parathyroid glands and thus hypocalcaemia. Less severe forms of this defect have been described as "partial Di George syndrome". In these children there is a spontaneous return of cell-mediated immunity in later childhood.

The other form is a familial condition in which the thymus tissue is very small and replaced by histiocytes (Nézelof). Both conditions are associated with a complete absence of Hassall's corpuscles from the thymus.

3. *Antibody deficiency syndromes*

(a) *Congenital X-linked hypogammaglobulinaemia.* This condition affects all five immunoglobulin classes and symptoms begin between 4 and 12 months of life. Circulating IgG is generally less than 1 mg/ml (normal 10 mg/ml) and both IgA and IgM are present in concentrations as low as 1% of the normal value. These children fail to develop an immune response when injected with conventional antigens such as diphtheria, pertussis or tetanus toxoid. Anti-A and anti-B isohaemagglutinins are low or absent. On the other hand they are able to reject homografts and develop delayed hypersensitivity to tuberculin, vaccinia and candidin and can be sensitized with dinitrofluorobenzene.

These children are unable to cope with pyogenic infections caused by pneumococci, *Haemophilus influenzae* and staphylococci which cause severe infections in the upper and lower respiratory tract. These may spread giving rise to septicaemia and meningitis. Other complications are brochiectasis and chronic middle ear infection. Chronic diarrhoea may occur due to *Giardia lamblia* or Bacteroides species. A common complication is polyarthritis, which may occur in up to 25% of the patients, affecting mainly the knees.

Histological examination of lymph nodes shows normal proliferation of lymphocytes in the thymus-dependent areas of the lymph nodes associated with the development of cell-mediated immunity. However, they are unable to develop plasma cells in the lymph node medulla, nor germinal centres in the lymphoid tissue of the cortex. The number of circulating lymphocytes is normal. The lymphoid tissue in the appendix and Peyer's patches of the intestine is relatively depleted. However, the thymus does not appear abnormal, with a well preserved cortical and medullary structure. Hassall's corpuscles are normal in most cases.

(b) *Variable forms of hypogammaglobulinaemia*—Hypogammaglobulinaemia may develop spontaneously in either sex or at any age. There is frequently a deficiency of only one or two classes, either IgG or IgA. Deficiences of IgM are rare but may be isolated. These states may be associated with aplastic or haemolytic anaemia, thrombocytopenia, neutropenia and occasionally renal lesions, sometimes developing a lupus like syndrome. Others may present with features of pernicious anaemia, chronic diarrhoea with malnutrition or colitis and may be infected with *Giardia lamblia*. Histologically the lymphoid tissue appears normal or even hyperplastic with germinal centres and plasma cells that can be seen to be making IgM only. Antibodies produced by these patients are generally IgM. Transient hypogammaglobulinaemia may occur as the infant loses maternal immunoglobulins and before it begins to make its own. This might result in transient infections or failure to thrive.

(c) *Selective IgA deficiency*—Isolated absence of IgA can occur in normal people without causing any harmful side effects. However there is frequently a high incidence of respiratory tract infection and some patients with this defect have coeliac disease that responds to a gluten free diet. Examination of the mucous membranes of the intestinal tract shows a marked depletion of IgA producing plasma cells. Occasionally a selective deficiency of IgA is associated with some degree of T-cell deficiency that can be detected by the clinical tests in current use. IgA deficiency is common in patients with ataxia telangiectasia.

One case of ataxia telangiectasia has been described in which IgG was also absent and in which it was also not possible to demonstrate delayed hypersensitivity or a homograft reaction. In another case in which an autopsy was performed the thymus could not be found. It would therefore appear that in some cases of ataxia telangiectasia there is also a defect in cell-mediated immune responses. There may also be a defect in the synthesis of all types of immunoglobulin not just a simple defect in the synthesis of IgA, as other cases of ataxia telangiectasia are also recorded with low levels of IgG. However, it must be remembered that a certain proportion of children with this disease (20% in one series) are described with normal levels of all the immunoglobulins.

4. *Immunodeficiency with eczema and thrombocytopenia—Wiskott-Aldrich syndrome*

This is a sex-linked recessive condition of infants characterized by eczema, thrombocytopenia and recurrent pyogenic infections.patients have a normal level of IgG. However IgA and IgE may be higher than normal. IgM is usually lower than normal. Humoral antibodies appear to be produced normally against typhoid antigens. However, there is a diminished or absent response to diphtheria toxoid and virus antigens. Anti-A and anti-B isoagglutinins are generally absent. Surprisingly these children have a high frequency of precipitins in their serum to milk proteins, present to quite a high titre. They also give positive anaphylactic reactions when skin tested with common antigens including milk. These children seem to be particularly susceptible to virus infections.

Defective cell-mediated immune responses have also been found in these patients, many of whom cannot be sensitized to dinitrofluorobenzene. The thymus in some is smaller than normal, although retaining a normal histological pattern. There is a striking depletion of small lymphocytes from the thymus-dependent paracortical areas of the lymph nodes, while the germinal centres and plasma cells appear to develop normally, consistent with normal levels of IgG and IgA. It has been suggested that this condition results from an inability of the patients to respond to certain polysaccharide antigens, and involves specifically the afferent limb of the immune response. However, this hypothesis does not cover the associated defect in cell-mediated immune reactions where the antigens are invariably proteins and not polysaccharides. Thus the defect in the immune response would appear to be somewhat broader than that originally postulated and involves a more general defect in the recognition or processing of antigens.

The clinical picture of eczema, recurrent infections, multiple skin sensitivities and a high frequency of precipitating antibodies in the serum against milk, indicate that this condition could be a variant of that very common condition among infants—atopic eczema. It is possible that in both these conditions the central immunological mechanisms are geared over to making certain antibodies such as reagins to an excessive degree and are unable to respond with a normal cell-mediated immune response to viral antigens in the same way as unaffected individuals. It may also be that, in the Wiskott-Aldrich syndrome, there is some structural abnormality of some of the IgG molecules so that they are unable to react normally with certain antigens.

B. Acquired Defects

1. *Immunoglobulin synthesis*

(a) *Primary.* Primary acquired hypogammaglobulinaemia may be found in adults, where the levels of circulating IgG is less than 5 mg/ml. This does not appear to be an inherited disease and it can affect both males and females. It can develop either in childhood or in adult life. There is a high incidence of other immunological diseases such as lupus erythematosus, thrombocytopenia and haemolytic anaemia in patients with this disorder. Two conditions which are sometimes found associated with primary acquired hypogammaglobulinaemia are steatorrhoea and non-caseating granulomas of the lungs, spleen, liver or skin. Lymph nodes show an absence of plasma cells as in the congenital form of hypogammaglobulinaemia.

(b) *Secondary.* Low levels of immunoglobulins can occur in a number of other disease states. These include diseases where there is an excessive loss of serum proteins such as exfoliative dermatitis, certain diseases of the kidney, and intestinal disorders.

Secondary hypogammaglobulinaemia can occur in diseases of the reticulo-endothelial system such as Hodgkin's disease, lymphosarcoma and chronic lymphatic leukaemia, and tumours of the thymus. Low levels of IgG are found in multiple myeloma where the neoplastic plasma cells are producing other immunoglobulins and in Waldenström's macroglobulinaemia. A list of the causes of secondary hypogammaglobulinaemia is shown in Table 1.

2. *Cell-mediated immunity*

A non-specific lowering of cell-mediated immunity (CMI) can occur in malnutrition including kwashiorkor a number of other disease states. These changes appear to occur more commonly in granulomatous conditions often involving the reticuloendothelial system. Acquired deficiencies of cell-mediated immunity of these types are generally partial, involving a number of the clinical tests of CMI, but are rarely so complete as to cause a complete failure of host resistance so that the patient develops an overwhelming viral or fungal infection or the development of an increased incidence of tumours. Such complete failure can be acquired as a result of therapy with immunosuppressive agents, drugs and antilymphocytic serum, used to prevent organ allograft rejection.

Partial failure of CMI affecting the regular clinical tests for CMI may be found in patients with Hodgkin's disease, sarcoidosis, Crohn's disease, rheumatoid arthritis, primary biliary cirrhosis and certain acute and chronic infections including virus infections, such as measles and rubella, and chronic bacterial infections such as lepromatous leprosy. The commonest defect found in these diseases is a diminished reactivity to the chemical contact sensitizer 2·4 dinitrochlorobenzene (DNCB). In a number of these conditions, there is also diminished tuberculin reactivity. However, an increased survival time of skin homografts

Classification of the causes of secondary hypogammaglobul naemia
(after Prof. J. R. Hobbs)

(a) *Physiological*
  (i) Premature babies
  (ii) Delayed maturity
  Both these conditions can be distinguished from hereditary hypogammaglobulinaemia as levels of IgA and IgM are normal.

(b) *Catabolic*
    —Increased turnover of protein.
    (i) Nephrotic syndrome
    (ii) Protein losing enteropathy
    (iii) Severe malnutrition
    (iv) Dystrophia myotonica
    (v) Thoracic duct fistula
  Affect IgG but not IgA or IgM.

(c) *Marrow disorders*
    (i) Marrow hypoplasia
    (ii) Extensive bony metastases
    (iii) Myelosclerosis
    (iv) Paroxysmal nocturnal haemoglobinuria
  IgM antibodies present against IgG antigens.

(d) *Toxic factors*
    (i) Renal failure
    (ii) High levels of corticosteroids (50–100 mg prednisone per day)
    (iii) Cytotoxic therapy
    (iv) Diazoxide therapy
    (v) Gluten sensitive enteropathy (IgM deficiency)
    (vi) Thyrotoxicosis
    (vii) Diabetes mellitus without proteinuria
    (viii) Following severe infection
    (ix) Congenital heart disease (? rubella *in utero*)

(e) *Primary reticulo-endothelial neoplasia*
    (i) Reticulosarcoma
    (ii) Mycosis fungoides
    (iii) Hodgkin's disease
    (iv) Lymphosarcoma
    (v) Giant follicular lymphoma
    (vi) Chronic lymphatic leukaemia
    (vii) Thymoma
    (viii) Malignant paraproteinaemia
        —Myelomatosis (low IgM followed by low IgA)
        —Macroglobulinaemia

is rare, as is diminished reactivity to foreign protein antigens injected to produce a primary response. A decreased response of the
lymphocytes to phytohaemagglutinin has also been demonstrated in a
number of these diseases, indicating that a functional decrease of T-
lymphocyte activity is also present. In some diseases, such as secondary syphilis, there may be a serum factor present which depresses such

a lymphocyte response *in vitro*. In Hodgkin's disease, sarcoidosis and lepromatous leprosy, the paracortical or thymus dependent areas of peripheral lymphoid tissue may be replaced by granulomatous infiltration, which might also contribute partially to the observed deficiency.

Similar deficiency of CMI occurs in a proportion of patients with neoplastic diseases, especially those of the reticulo-endothelial system. In the case of Hodgkin's disease it has been reported that non-specific depression of CMI is related to the severity of the disease and the degree of replacement of lymphoid tissue. In other malignant diseases it has not been possible to separate the effect of the malignancy from the effect of the associated debility and wasting. Signs of deficiencies of CMI, however, appear to occur more commonly with some tumours, such as gastric carcinomas than with others such as bronchial cancers. Another situation in which some of the parameters of cell-mediated immunity may show a depression is post-operatively and after a general anaesthetic.

The situation of immunodeficiency states leading to the development of muco-cutaneous candidiasis is somewhat more complicated. Muco-cutaneous candidiasis can occur in patients with non-specific immunodeficiency for cell-mediated immunity as in thymic dysplasia. However, it also occurs in acquired immunodeficiency due to leukaemia or Hodgkin's disease. Another group of secondary immunodeficiencies of CMI associated with muco-cutaneous candidiasis are a hereditary group associated with primary endocrine deficiencies especially hypoparathyroidism, hypoadrenalism, hypothyroidism and diabetes mellitus. In a number of these patients it is difficult to determine the nature of the immunological lesion precisely. In some cases there is a failure of T-lymphocytes to be transformed by phytohaemagglutinin or specific antigen into lymphoblasts. In others, transformation is normal even to specific antigen such as candidin, but there may be a failure of the lymphocytes to produce the chemical mediators of delayed hypersensitivity when stimulated by specific antigen *in vitro*.

Treatment of Immunological Deficiency Diseases

1. *Immunoglobulin deficiency*

Commercial γ-globulin is particularly effective in the prevention of recurrent pyogenic infections in patients where the only defect is one of immunoglobulin synthesis. It has been suggested that raising the level of circulating IgG by 2 mg/ml is sufficient in most cases. This can be achieved by injecting 300 mg/kg body weight monthly. The amount injected can be dropped to 100 mg/kg body weight when the required effect is achieved. In the case of the Wiskott-Aldrich syndrome it has been found that periodic transfusions of whole plasma in a dose of 15 ml/kg body weight kept the patients relatively free from infection. Treatment with commercial γ-globulin alone has not proved effective in this condition.

2. *Severe combined immunodeficiency*

In this condition it is necessary to replace the immunological stem cells, deficiency of which is the basic cause of the condition. In view of the risk of graft versus host reactions, all tissue grafted must be typed for HLA (leucocyte histocompatibility group antigens) compatibility. If only partial compatibility is possible the stem-cell fraction must be grafted under a cover of immunosuppressive therapy or combined with prior administration of enhancing antibody directed against the HLA antigens of the recipient. Graft versus host reactions, if they occur, are fatal and appear one to three weeks after the graft cells are transfused. The transfused cells proliferate and react during this time against host tissues. Such a reaction is manifested as a diffuse rash all over the body associated with marked enlargement of the liver and spleen. There is also fever, haemolytic anaemia and inevitably death. Such reactions, once they occur, are fatal and there is no means of treatment. In severe combined immunodeficiency foetal thymus transplant is not sufficient. The need is for stem cells which can, however, be provided in the form of unfractionated bone marrow from a matched histocompatible donor, usually a sibling. The addition of a thymus graft is not necessary in this condition, nor is the use of foetal liver which was once advocated as a source of stem cells.

3. *Congenital thymic hypoplasia*

Unfortunately, so far it has not been possible to treat this condition successfully. Thymuses from 12–16 week foetuses have temporarily reconstituted cell-mediated immunity in these children so that they can reject skin grafts and develop sensitivity to dinitrofluorobenzene. However, as the immunological defect is partial, involving T-cells only, the grafted thymuses induce an immune response and are eventually rejected despite the absence of cell-mediated immunity. It is likely that those cases which have been reported as recovering following such treatment are examples of "partial Di George syndrome".

4. *Secondary immunodeficiencies*

Secondary immunodeficiency in chronic mucocutaneous candidiasis has been successfully treated with transfer factor. This dialysate from a frozen and thawed extract of human leucocytes (see Chapter III) appears to act as a non-specific T-cell stimulant. Cases of Wiskott-Aldrich syndrome have been described in which depressed levels of circulating T-cells have been restored to near normal levels by treatment with transfer factor. Another substance that appears to have a similar effect is the anti-helminthic drug levamisole. Levamisole has been reported as restoring the ability to show normal delayed hypersensitivity in patients who have become immunologically anergic as a result of cancer. This increased skin reactivity has been found to be associated with a return of the ability of lymphocytes to respond *in vitro*. A similar response to levamisole has been found in patients with Hodgkin's disease. Initial studies with levamisole have been on short term courses of this compound. It will be interesting to see what effect longer term studies will have in increasing host resistance to infection in situations where this has been depressed non-specifically. So far there have been uncontrolled reports of its effectiveness in recurrent herpes infections.

Complement Deficiency States

1. *Hereditary angioneurotic oedema*

This condition is inherited as an autosomal dominant characteristic. Patients lack an α_2 globulin in their serum which acts as an inhibitor of the enzyme (an esterase) which is the first component of complement (C_1). They develop attacks of oedematous swelling of the skin which does not pit on pressure and does not itch. They also have haemorrhages into the gastro-intestinal tract and thus may develop nausea, vomiting and abdominal pains. They can die from asphyxia due to laryngeal oedema. Attacks generally subside within 48–72 hours of onset. During the attack there are low levels of the second component of complement in the blood. After the attack, levels return to normal. This drop is due to the second component being a natural substrate of the uninhibited enzyme. As these patients lack an inhibitor of the first component of complement (an α_2 globulin), the injection of this substance (C_1) intradermally in the purified state can precipitate a severe attack of the angioneurotic oedema. It would appear, therefore, that the first component of complement causes increased vascular permeability which is normally inhibited by the factor which is deficient in these patients.

2. *Deficiency of the second component of complement*

This defect in the complement system is not associated with any untoward acute allergic condition, nor with any increased susceptibility to infection. However about half the cases develop diseases with a possible immunopathological basis. These include systemic lupus erythematosus, glomeurlonephritis and Henoch–Schonlein purpura. It is inherited as an autosomal recessive. The sera of these subjects are partially defective as far as their bactericidal capacity is concerned. However, some bactericidal activity is present indicating that they are not completely deficient in this component. It has been suggested that the association with diseases with a possible immunopathological aetiology is due to inadequate clearing of immune complexes.

The Significance of Raised Levels of Immunoglobulins; Monoclonal Rise in Immunoglobulins

Multiple myeloma may be regarded as a malignant proliferation of a specific group of plasma cells. Such a group has been called a *clone* of cells by analogy with bacterial clones derived from a single bacterial cell. In the disease multiple myeloma, such a malignant clone will produce one particular type of immunoglobulin either IgG or more rarely IgA, IgD or IgE. However, all immunoglobulins form a composite class of proteins of different electrophoretic mobility. The immunoglobulins produced in excess by the malignant proliferating plasma cells of multiple myeloma do not possess a whole spectrum of different electrophoretic mobilities as in normal serum. They always have the same electrophoretic mobility and thus the increased protein in the circulation forms a compact band ("M"-type protein) on electrophoresis. Such an "M"-type band is typical of what is therefore called a "monoclonal gammopathy".

A monoclonal gammopathy is typical of IgG, IgA, IgD or IgE myelomas and also the less malignant Waldenström's macroglobulinaemia where there is a monoclonal rise in the IgM. The actual presence of an M-type protein is not in itself diagnostic of multiple myeloma. For diagnosis to be made there should be either typical X-ray pictures of deposits in bone, plasma cells in excess in a bone marrow biopsy or occasionally in the peripheral blood, or Bence-Jones protein in the urine. It will be remembered that an immunoglobulin molecule of molecular weight 150,000 consists of four polypeptide chains two of molecular weight 25,000 (called light or L chains) and two of molecular weight 50,000 (called heavy or H chains). Bence-Jones proteins are light chains of the myeloma protein which pass into the circulation and out into the urine before the whole immunoglobulin molecule can be assembled.

An increase in "M"-type protein in multiple myeloma is generally associated with a decreased synthesis of normal immunoglobulins. This is associated with a poor immunological response when the patients are immunized against typhoid or other bacterial antigens and an increased incidence of respiratory tract infections in these patients. The poor state of antibody synthesis is often so marked that it has been suggested that such patients be treated by injections of γ-globulin in the same way as patients with hypogammaglobulinaemia.

A monoclonal rise in an immunoglobulin on its own is not however diagnostic of multiple myeloma. It may indicate the proliferation of a clone of cells specifically stimulated to make a particular antibody. Two such cases have been described both making "M"-type macroglobulins, one consisting of antibodies which gave a positive Wasserman reaction and another which contained cold agglutinins. A number of patients with disseminated carcinoma have been described with "M"-type proteins in the serum which have been considered to be antibodies directed against tumour specific antigens. In these cases the antibodies could have been derived from a single colony or clone of plasma cells producing immunoglobulins with the same electrophoretic mobility. These paraproteinaemias associated with disseminated carcinomas are generally IgG. A few have been described which have IgA or IgM. However, recently in a survey of 6,995 normal adult sera in Sweden 64 cases of normal individuals were found containing "M"-type proteins in the serum. The average age of the subjects with these changes was 64. Thus such changes can apparently occur in normal people, though more commonly in the older age groups. Although no disease state could be found to account for these changes, such patients should be followed up frequently to see whether they develop generalized neoplastic disease or multiple myeloma at a later date. In a further study of 7,200 hospital patients observed in London over a period of six months 0·76% were found to have an "M"-type protein in their serum. Of these 53% were diagnosed as being of malignant origin, mainly myelomas. In 40% the finding was considered to be benign. The criteria of benignity were (1) no symptoms related to the presence of the paraproteins (M protein), (2) no palpable enlargement of lymph nodes, liver or spleen, (3) negative radiological survey of the bones, (4) bone marrow normal, (5) followed up for at least three years with no change in their overall clinical picture. If a subnormal level of one of the other immunoglobulin classes was present, the patient was more likely to have a myeloma. 10% of patients in whom a diagnosis could not be made initially were found to develop a malignant condition within three years. In two patients with an "M"-type protein of the IgG type the band disappeared over a period of six months and did not reappear. One such case was followed up over eight years without a recurrence being discovered.

An abnormal globulin which was at one stage thought to be of a myeloma type has been found in patients with the rare skin disease Lichen myxoedematosus (Papular mucinosis). This protein is antigenically an IgG, however it has a much slower electrophoretic mobility than normal IgG. Lichen myxoedematosus is a benign condition and the significance of this IgG with its remarkable slow electrophoretic mobility is not known.

An interesting variant of multiple myeloma is the so-called "Heavy chain disease". In this condition there is a large amount of an abnormal protein both in the serum and in the urine. On analysis this protein is found to consist of the heavy chains of the IgG molecule. The disease appears to be malignant and atypical plasma cells may be found in the bone marrow as well as abnormal aggregates of reticulum cells in the tissues. Atypical granulomas may be seen in the skin consisting of aggregates of reticulum-like cells surrounded by lymphocytes and plasma cells. These patients are unable to produce antibodies normally and thus they are more prone to infection. "Heavy chain disease" is an example of a malignant lymphoma associated with the over production of the heavy polypeptide chains of the IgG molecule, which are secreted unconjugated into the circulation.

Polyclonal Rise in Immunoglobulins

As a result of a strong antigenic stimulus the normal response will be to produce antibodies, generally IgG over a wide electrophoretic range. The response will involve many different clones of plasma cells. Thus the rise in the level of the IgG could be considered to be of a polyclonal type. Such an immune response would be expected to produce only a temporary rise. In certain disease states there is a more prolonged rise of the polyclonal type. These conditions include systemic lupus erythematosus and chronic liver disease. However, sometimes cases exist where there is a prolonged polyclonal rise in IgG. A study of the families of patients with systemic lupus erythematosus (SLE) has shown a high incidence of siblings with so-called "benign essential hypergammaglobulinaemia" who eventually develop SLE. Thus patients with polyclonal hypergammaglobulinaemia must be followed up at very frequent intervals as this would appear to be a precursor of SLE. The condition "purpura hyperglobulinaemia" would also appear to be a precursor of SLE.

The cause of hyperglobulinaemia in chronic liver disease is not known but may be due to a continuous release of antigens from damaged liver causing a prolonged antibody response.

Bibliography

Books
Chini, V., Bonomo, L. & Sirtori, C. (eds.) (1968), *Gammopathies, Infections, Cancer and Immunity*. Milan: Carlo Erba Foundation.
Hayward, A. R. (1977), *Immunodeficiency*. London: Edward Arnold.
Waldenström, J. (1967), *Clinical and Biological Significance of Monoclonal and Polyclonal Hypergammaglobulinemia*. Cambridge University Press.

Articles
Austen, K. F. (1967), "Inborn errors of the complement system in man." *New Eng. J. Med.*, **276**, 1363.
Axelsson, U., Bachman, R. & Hallen, J. (1966), "Frequency of pathological proteins (M-components) in 6,995 sera from an adult population." *Acta med. scand.*, **179**, 235.
Blaese, R. H., Strober, W., Brown, R. S. & Waldman, T. A. (1968), "The Wiskott-Aldrich syndrome. A disorder with a possible defect of antigen processing or recognition." *Lancet*, i; 1056.
Cooper, M. D., Chase, H. P., Lowman, J. T., Krivit, W. & Good, R. A. (1968), "Wiskott-Aldrich syndrome. An immunological deficiency disease involving the afferent limb of immunity." *Amer. J. Med.*, **44**, 499.
Good, R. A., Kelly, W. D., Rotstein, J. & Varco, R. L. (1962), "Immunological deficiency diseases. Agammaglobulinaemia, hypogammaglobulinaemia, Hodgkin's disease and sarcoidosis." *Progr. Allergy*, **6**, 187.
James, K., Fudenberg, H., Epstein, W. L. & Shuster, J. (1967), "Studies on a unique diagnostic serum globulin in papular mucinosis (lichen myxoedematosus)." *Clin. exp. Immunol.*, **2**, 153.
Ruddy, S., Carpenter, C .B., Muller-Eberhard, H. J. & Austen, K. F. A. (1968), "Complement component levels in hereditary angioneurotic oedema and isolated

94 *Immunology in Clinical Medicine*

C_2' deficiency in man." *Immunopathology Vth International Symposium (Mechanisms of Inflammation Induced by Immune Reactions)*. Eds. P. A. Miescher and P. Grabar. Basel: Schwabe.

Soothill, J., Hobbs, J. R., Hitzig, W. H. & Kay, H. E. M. (1968), "Immunological deficiency syndromes." *Proc. roy. Soc. Med.*, **61**, 881.

Waldenström, J. (1962), "Monoclonal and polyclonal gammopathies and the biological system of gamma globulins." *Progr. Allergy*, **6**, 320.

Chapter VI

The Concept of Autoimmunity and its Relation to Disease

In the early days of the study of the subject of immunology, it was thought that an animal was incapable of forming antibodies which would combine with its own tissues. This concept was called "horror autotoxicus" by Erhlich and Morgenroth who in 1900 considered this was the means by which the body protected itself from self-destruction by autoantibodies directed against itself. More recently Burnet introduced the concept of self versus non-self antigens. He postulated that during embryonic life the developing immunological tissues recognized self antigens and developed a state of immunological tolerance to these antigens, as a result of which they were not able to react to these antigens when the animal became immunologically mature. However, one phenomenon which was overlooked for many years was that if a rabbit was injected with bovine lens material, it would develop antibodies which would react with its own lens *in vitro*, but would not cause any disease of the animal's lens *in situ*. To explain this phenomenon, it was suggested that the lens was in a "privileged site" and normally "not immunologically accessible".

This concept was held very strongly until about fifteen years ago when it received a very strong challenge from a number of quarters. The first of these was the demonstration that certain haemolytic anaemias were due to antibodies in the serum which could be demonstrated by the Coombs antiglobulin test to have adhered to the surface of the red cells (Fig. 1). Secondly, there was the demonstration of the LE-cell phenomenon. LE cells develop in the blood or bone marrow, of patients with systemic lupus erythematosus, when incubated *in vitro* and are granulocytes which have ingested nuclear material. Phagocytosis occurs as a result of the reaction between an antibody against nuclear antigens (anti-nuclear factor) present in the circulation. However, the study which caught the imagination of almost the whole of medical science was the demonstration of antibodies in the serum which reacted with thyroglobulin in Hashimoto's thyroiditis. The relationship between these antibodies and the cause of the thyroiditis was brought out by animal experiments carried out at about the same time. When experimental animals were injected with an adjuvant mixture containing an extract of thyroid tissue, they were found to develop a thyroiditis resembling that seen in Hashimoto's disease and at the same time they were found to develop humoral antibodies in their circulation which were capable of reacting with thyroid tissue *in vitro*. However, on no occasion was it found possible to transfer the thyroiditis passively with serum containing these anti-thyroid antibodies. Not long before, it had been found possible to produce orchitis with aspermatogenesis by injection of an extract of testis and in the early 1930's allergic encephalomyelitis had been produced in monkeys by injections of rabbit brain. Another organ in which an autoimmune condition could be produced experimentally was the suprarenal gland. In most of these conditions humoral antibodies could be demonstrated in the circulation. However, the organ disease could never be transferred with serum. It was therefore postulated that these conditions were all cell-mediated and that

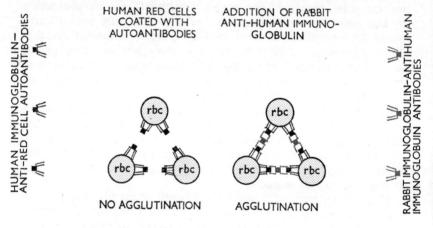

Fig. 1. The direct antiglobulin reaction for detecting non-agglutinating antibody on the surface of red cells (Coombs' test).

the presence of humoral antibodies in the circulation was an associated phenomenon rather than cause of the disease. Moreover, in one condition, experimental allergic encephalomyelitis, it was possible to transfer the disease passively with lymphocytes, apparently confirming the cell-mediated mechanism of the disease. Neither thyroiditis nor orchitis could be transferred with cells alone in outbred animals, although recently it has been possible to transfer orchitis passively with cells injected into animals already making humoral antibody. This would indicate that there needs to be collaboration between cell-mediated immune processes and humoral autoantibodies in the development of organ specific autoimmune lesions. The ability to transfer thyroiditis adoptively with cells from lymphoid organs containing plasma cells and plasma cell precursors is also consistent with this concept.

The significance of autoantibodies in relation to disease can be further assessed by experiments in rabbits injected with homologous liver in an adjuvant mixture. Such rabbits produce autoantibodies which react *in vitro* with extracts of rabbit liver. However, no significant damage to the liver could be found. It would thus appear that the production of autoantibodies to a particular organ need not signify the presence of disease within that organ.

It is probable that there are very few analogies in clinical medicine to the production of autoimmune disease or autoantibodies in experimental animals. There is, however, one well documented condition where there is a direct analogy. This is the encephalomyelitis which develops following the injection of rabies vaccine. Attenuated rabies virus is injected into the patient in rabbit spinal cord. It has been shown that the encephalomyelitis is not due to the rabies virus itself and is therefore directly analogous to the encephalomyelitis produced in experimental animals by the injection of heterologous spinal cord.

Thus in experimental animals and under certain rare conditions in the human an autoimmune disease process can be induced by injection of an extract of the particular organs derived from a different animal. In experimental animals this process can be induced more readily by injection of an extract of the same organ derived from another animal of the same species, especially if emulsified in "Freund's adjuvant". In this way it is possible to overcome the "horror autotoxicus" postulated by Ehrlich and Morgenroth and get the body to produce an immunological response against antigens which would normally be regarded as "self".

In most cases, however, disease which could be regarded as autoimmune or associated with autoimmune phenomena arises apparently spontaneously. In these cases, one needs to ask the question how has the body been induced to react against its own tissue components.

Two possibilities have been considered. In the first, changes could perhaps occur in the central immunological mechanisms, whereby suddenly there appears an inability to recognize "self" from "not self" antigens. This could occur in a number of different ways. It has been suggested by Burnet that under normal conditions clones or colonies of cells do develop with an ability to react against "self" antigens. However, these clones are unable to proliferate, due to some inborn defensive mechanism. It is thought that the precursor lymphocytes which have an ability to react with "self" antigens and thus be stimulated to proliferate, are eliminated as soon as they develop. If, however, these cells are allowed to come into contact with "self" antigens and allowed to proliferate, they will cause the formation of autoimmune humoral antibodies or the development of a cell-mediated immune response. The condition which would then develop would be expected to affect many different organs and tissues at the same time. Systemic lupus erythematosus (SLE) was considered by the protagonists of this hypothesis to be such a disease as many different tissues are

involved in this condition. Moreover the thymus has been thought by
many to have an important physiological role in deleting "aberrant" or
"forbidden" clones of lymphocytes which might develop, possibly by
somatic mutation, and react against constituents of the body's own
tissues. In such a disease as SLE it was thought that the condition could
originate as some defect in the functioning of the thymus gland.
Abnormalities of the thymus have in fact been found in a wide range of
diseases associated with autoimmune phenomena. In SLE and rheumatoid arthritis there is loss of differentiation between cortex and medulla,
the presence of germinal centres and an increased number of plasma
cells as well as changes in Hassall's corpuscles. Germinal centres, not
normally found in the thymus, are seen in patients with thyrotoxicosis
and other diseases of the thyroid associated with autoimmune phenomena. They are also found in a congenital disease of a certain strain of
inbred mice (NZB) associated with haemolytic anaemia and involvement of other organs in a possible generalized autoimmune process.
Germinal centres are also found in the thymus of patients with myasthenia gravis where autoimmune antibodies are found which react both
with skeletal muscle and the myoepithelial elements of the thymus.
However, a certain proportion of patients with myasthenia gravis also
can be found to have a lymphomatous tumour (thymoma) within the
thymus. Thus the association of disease of the thymus and autoimmune processes are well documented.

It has been suggested that germinal centres in the thymus in SLE,
rheumatoid arthritis, myasthenia gravis and in the autoimmune disease
of NZB mice are the actual site of proliferation of the abnormal or
"forbidden clones". However, the disease in the mice still develops even
if the thymus is removed at birth. It is more likely that the presence of
germinal centres and plasma cells in the thymus are the result of direct
antigenic stimulation. Normally antigen does not appear to gain access
to the thymus. However, if antigen is injected into the thymus of experimental animals it will respond as any other lymphoid organ by the
development of plasma cells and germinal centres. Thymectomy is of
value clinically in myasthenia gravis and autoimmune haemolytic
anaemia of infancy. However, it is ineffective in SLE and rheumatoid
arthritis and other diseases with associated autoimmune phenomena.
Moreover both SLE and thyroiditis with associated autoimmune antibodies have been reported as developing even after the thymus had
been removed for myasthenia gravis.

It would thus appear that the relation between the thymus and
autoimmune processes is complex and yet far from resolved. No real
evidence has so far been brought to show either that the function of the
thymus is to destroy "forbidden" clones, or that in diseases with
associated autoimmune processes "forbidden" clones are allowed to
proliferate in the thymus.

Autoimmune phenomena are also found in other diseases of the reticulo-endothelial system where it has also been postulated that they develop as a result of the production of or failure to eliminate "aberrant clones". Examples of these are the haemolytic anaemias and thrombo-cytopenias associated with lymphomas, Hodgkin's disease or lymphatic leukaemias. Again there is no direct evidence of such conditions arising from a secondary defect in the immunological mechanisms. They could arise as easily from a number of other different mechanisms associated with the neoplastic process.

Perhaps the most persuasive argument against the "forbidden clone" hypothesis is the demonstration of lymphocytes in the thymus and blood in healthy individuals that can react with thyroglobulin. These cells have been shown to be B-cells rather than T-cells. Higher levels of these cells are found in patients with Hashimoto's thyroiditis. This leads us to the second possibility which is that a *normal* immunological mechanism is stimulated to develop an immune reaction against the body's own tissues. One of the mechanisms that have been proposed for this suggests that the proliferation of antigen reactive cells is normally controlled by a population of specific T-suppressor cells. Autoimmune phenomena could then occur as a result of a loss of these suppressor cells or from an abnormal stimulus that might overcome the effect of these cells. In experimental animals an immune reaction can be produced against one of the body's own tissues by a single injection of an extract of that organ either derived from an animal of the same species or derived from another species. This can in most cases only be undertaken by combining the antigen in Freund's adjuvant (an oil in water emulsion containing dead tubercle bacilli) which forms a chronic granuloma and gives the central immuno-logical mechanisms an abnormally strong stimulus. Moreover a better response is often produced by injecting heterologous rather than homologous tissue. Thus one might look for a similar situation in the human to produce the development of autoimmune phenomena; that is, an exceptionally powerful stimulus with a modified or cross reacting antigen. To explain this, it is necessary to find out how the human immunological mechanism can receive a stimulus equivalent to or as powerful as that produced by Freund's adjuvant in the experi-mental animal. It is known that Freund's adjuvant produces in the experimental animal sterile granulomata which under certain conditions are metastatic. It may be that an equivalent stimulus is produced by bacterial or viral infections in the human. The incidence of autoimmune phenomena in chronic inflammatory diseases such as the rheumatic group of diseases, leprosy and syphilis is now well documented. IgM antibodies directed against the body's own IgG molecules, the so-called rheumatoid factor, are a diagnostic mark of diseases of the rheumatoid group. In syphilis the antibody which reacts with extracts of heart muscle and is used diagnostically in the Wasserman reaction has been recognized for many years as an autoantibody. However, this is not the only autoimmune phenomenon which occurs in syphilis as the rheumatoid factor can also be demonstrated in 10% of patients with this disease. Another interesting autoimmune phenomenon which can be demonstrated in syphilis is the presence of cryoglobulins which in some cases can be shown to be complexes of IgG and IgM which have been found to occur in 15% of cases in one survey. This is probably just another example of the presence of an IgM or IgG autoantibody complexing with the body's own IgG. However, it appears that the antibody that forms the cryoglobulin is different from that which can be identified in the same disease as the rheumatoid factor. Autoantibodies against thyroglobulin, rheumatoid factor, Wasserman antibody against heart muscle and antinuclear factor have been demonstrated in the sera of patients with lepromatous leprosy. The concentration of antinuclear factor has been so high that granulocytes were found in the peripheral blood which had ingested nuclear material (LE cells), similar to those found in the peripheral blood of patients with systemic lupus erythematosus. As patients with lepromatous leprosy have massive infiltration of their tissues with mycobacteria, they could be considered to be in a state analogous to that of an experimental animal injected with Freund's adjuvant. Rabbits injected with *Mycobacterium tuberculosis* have been shown to develop autoantibodies against a wide range of organs including liver, kidney, spleen, lung and heart homogenates within twelve weeks of infection. Similar autoantibodies against a wide range of organs including, liver, kidney, thyroid gland, spleen, adrenal gland and cardiac and skeletal muscle have been found in the sera of patients with actinomycosis, syphilis and chronic tuberculosis. In time it may well be shown that the commonest cause of autoimmune phenomena are chronic infections and chronic granulomatous diseases.

The stimulation of such an activated immunological system by modified or cross reacting antigens is more easy to understand and a number of examples have now been described of the induction of autoimmune phenomena, with or without actual disease, by cross reacting bacterial antigens or by drugs which bind either directly or in the form of a metabolic by-product to the body's own tissues. The association of autoimmune phenomena with infection with microorganisms some of which contain antigens that cross react with human tissue, will be the first to be discussed. For many years now it has been recognized that the group A streptococcus plays a considerable role in the pathogenesis of rheumatic fever. It has recently been found that streptococci isolated from a patient with acute rheumatic fever have antigens associated with their cell wall which cross react with antigens in the human heart, which could be localized to the sarcolemma or the outer edge of the cardiac myofibrils and also to smooth muscle elements of the vessels and endocardium of the heart. Such an antibody has been found present in the serum of 55% of patients with acute rheumatic fever or inactive rheumatic carditis.

Similarly infection with a particular strain of streptococcus has for many years been associated with the development of acute nephritis. This strain the type 12 or nephritogenic strain has also been found to have antigens on its surface similar to those found in human glomeruli.

A further example of the relationship between a specific infection and the production of autoantibodies occurs in the disease which used to be known as "primary atypical pneumonia". This disease is due to infection with the organism *Mycoplasma pneumoniae* and is associated with the presence of cold agglutinins in the serum which react with the patient's own red cells. Such antibodies are macroglobulins of the class IgM and produce a low grade of haemolytic anaemia sufficient to produce a mild reticulocytosis. They are directed against the I antigen on the red cell. There is no correlation between the presence of antibody to the mycoplasma and these autoantibodies. There is also no cross reaction between the cold agglutinins and antibodies against the mycoplasma. It may be that in some way the infective organism modifies the I antigen on the red cell surface and together with the presence of an infection the body's central immunological mechanisms are stimulated to produce these autoantibodies.

A fourth example of the relation between infection and autoimmune phenomena can be found in the so-called "autoimmune disease" which develops in New Zealand Black (NZB) mice. These mice develop a haemolytic anaemia associated with a positive Coombs' test (demonstrating the presence of immunoglobulin on the surface of their red cells (Fig. 1)), antibodies against cell nuclei (similar to those found in human systemic lupus erythematosus) and renal disease (similar to chronic glomerulonephritis or that found in systemic lupus erythematosus), when four to six months of age. It has recently been found that these mice are infected with a virus which can be demonstrated in lymph nodes, thymus, spleen and pancreas. Similar virus particles have been found in embryos of this strain suggesting that the infective agent could pass across the placenta. Infection with this virus could cause the release of the DNA into the circulation which stimulates anti-DNA antibodies. These then form immune complexes which deposit in the renal glomeruli as in serum sickness, causing nephritis. It is interesting that the nephritis is alleviated by treatment with cyclophosphamide which also reduces the complexes deposited in the glomeruli. It is possible that cyclophosphamide acts in this case as an antiviral agent, killing the virus and reducing the amount of DNA in the circulation, rather than, as has been suggested, as an immunosuppressive agent, directly reducing the amount of antibody.

Whether the disease in these four examples is related to the auto-immune phenomena or to the infective agent is an interesting problem. In the case of rheumatic carditis, although antibodies against heart muscle are present in the circulation, no immunoglobulin can be demonstrated bound to the actual Aschoff lesions which are the areas of inflammation associated with the disease. This might suggest that the disease state could either be a cell-mediated hypersensitivity reaction induced by the streptococcus to cross reacting antigens in the heart muscle or could be a direct toxic action of the organism. In both cases the autoantibodies against heart muscle present in the serum would be related phenomena and not the cause of the actual disease process. In the case of primary atypical pneumonia due to *Mycoplasma pneumoniae* the mild haemolytic anaemia is probably due to the direct action of the autoantibody. However, the pneumonia probably results from a hypersensitivity reaction to the organism itself in the lungs. Fever and pneumonia develop on second contact with the mycoplasma, if the subject has been previously vaccinated with the organism and thus sensitized, but do not develop on first contact even with live organisms.

The relation between the presence of virus particles in many tissues and the development of a multi-organ disease associated with autoimmune phenomena in NZB mice has yet to be worked out. However, this would appear to be a very hopeful model in which it may be possible to determine how certain infections can induce the production of antibodies against the patient's own tissues. In the human the association of what could be an autoimmune encephalomyelitis has been known for many years as an uncommon complication of virus infections such as mumps and measles. This could also result from the modification of the body's own antigens as a result of the infection possibly by direct enzyme action on the tissues concerned. However another possibility is that demyelination in these diseases could be due to reaction between virus and cell-mediated immune processes in the vicinity of the affected tissues.

Diseases resembling so-called autoimmune diseases of unknown aetiology can be induced by a number of drugs. Although in the majority of cases the agent inducing systemic lupus erythematosus is not known, this syndrome has been demonstrated as a side-effect of treatment with a number of drugs. Moreover in many cases this disease which is often fatal can be reversed if the drug is identified and treatment is stopped. The drugs which have been found to induce this condition are hydralazine, penicillin, phenylbutazone, methyl-phenyl-ethyl-hydantoin, trimethadine, sulphamethoxypyridazine, sulphadiazine, procaineamide, isoniazid and tetracycline. The commonest reports are following the use of the drug hydralazine (Apresoline). This drug can induce the typical LE phenomenon. The phenomenon, as mentioned above, is due to an autoantibody present in the serum directed against nuclei of the body's own cells and is often called the "anti-nuclear factor" or ANF. The development of LE cells in the bone marrow, after incubation *in vitro*, or ANF in the serum occurs in all cases of systemic lupus erythematosus. ANF is an immunoglobulin which can be IgG, IgA or IgM. ANF can be detected in the laboratory either by agglutination of latex particles coated with DNA or by labelling the immunoglobulin with fluorescein and detecting the fluorescence produced when the serum reacts with nuclei, under the miscroscope using ultraviolet light. In one recent study 14 out of 32 patients treated with hydralazine for hypertension developed a clinical disease identical in every way with systemic lupus erythematosus and another 4 out of the 15 which did not have clinical symptoms had antinuclear factor in their serum.

The clinical picture of SLE is consistent with a disease developing as a result of the chronic circulation of immune complexes. Many of the conditions found in this disease are also found in serum sickness. The two most important are arthritis and nephritis. In studies of the nephritis of SLE it has been found that there are immune complexes and complement localized as lumpy deposits in the glomeruli. These antibodies have been eluted and have been found to be antibodies against DNA and nuclear histones. It may be therefore that in SLE the body's own nuclear antigens are modified by the action of drugs. This may be a direct chemical effect or the drug might actually bind onto the nucleoprotein as a hapten. The modified nuclear antigens or complexes of drug and nucleoprotein then stimulate the formation of antinuclear antibodies. These antibodies combine with nuclear antigen and as a result immune complexes are formed which cause a disease which would appear to be a modified form of serum sickness. The drug initiating the disease can only be identified in a few cases but some of those which have been identified are compounds which can bind to protein and are known to act as haptens both in man and in experimental animals. Where no identifiable chemical agent can be incriminated in this disease, it is possible that the disease has been caused by an unknown chemical agent acting as a hapten which has bound onto the nucleoprotein or nuclear histones not only making them antigenic, but also converting them to such a form that the body fails to recognize its own antigens as "self" and produces antibodies which react with DNA and nuclear histones.

Another autoimmune phenomenon which is caused by a drug is the haemolytic anaemia produced by the drug α methyldopa which like hydralazine is also used in the treatment of hypertension. DOPA (dihydroxyphenylalanine) is broken down in the body to DOPA-quinone. It is possible, therefore, that α methyldopa is also broken down to a quinone. Quinones are very reactive, bind to proteins and form haptens. One might think that the haemolytic anaemia was caused by the production of antibodies which might react with the quinone bound to the surface of the red cells and thus cause the haemolysis. However, this is not the complete story because the patients treated with α methyldopa have been found to develop autoantibodies directed against Rhesus antigens normally present on the surface of their own erythrocytes, similar to those which develop in autoimmune haemolytic anaemias of unknown aetiology. So far antibodies have not been found against α methyldopa or its metabolic products. Thus it may be that the drug is in some way unmasking antigens present on the erythrocyte surface which do not under normal conditions stimulate antibody production. Possibly this might be by producing antibodies against the carrier protein to which this hapten is linked. Haemolytic anaemia has also been described as a result of penicillin therapy. The red cells have been found to be coated with immunoglobulin which would appear to have bound with haptenic groups on the surface of the red cells. If the immunoglobulin is eluted it can be shown that it is an antibody which will react with metabolic breakdown products of penicillin which were capable of binding as a hapten to any protein. In this case the hapten had bound to the patient's red cells. The patient had then pro-duced antibodies directed against this chemical grouping, and thus the red cells had been lysed by the reaction of the antibody with the penicillin grouping on its surface. If the antibodies against the red cells had not been identified as reacting with the penicillin group, it might have been thought the penicillin had induced an "auto-immune" haemolytic anaemia. There may be many other examples where phenomena are thought to be autoimmune, but are in fact due to antibodies produced against chemical substances which bind as haptens to the body's own proteins and thus make them antigenic. The action of physical as opposed to chemical agents in modifying the antigenicity of the body's own tissues must also be considered. An example of this is cold. Application of an ice-cube to the skin for a relatively short period of time can modify the antigenic nature of certain proteins in the skin. This could be due to a change in the tertiary structure of the molecule. There would then be a failure of recognition of a "self" antigen as such and an immune response would be set up. Next time the person comes in contact with cold an urticarial weal might develop within 15–30 minutes in the skin, if the antibodies produced were reagins of the class IgE. However, if the response was a "cell-mediated" one, the application of cold would produce a reaction in the skin more like a tuberculin reaction taking 24–48 hours to develop. Other physical agents which might modify the proteins of the skin in this way are pressure and ultra-violet light.

A further factor which can predispose to the development of auto-immune phenomena appears to be age. A progressive increase in the level of circulating immunoglobulins has been described with age. There is also an increased frequency of positive serological reactions for syphilis in non-syphilitic elderly people. These reactions, as mentioned above, indicate the presence of macroglobulin autoantibodies directed against an extract of heart. Similarly there is an increase in the incidence of anti-IgG antibodies usually associated with rheumatoid arthritis, in normal elderly subjects over the age of 65 without any history of rheumatoid arthritis and also an increased incidence of antinuclear factor in the serum of a similar group of elderly subjects without any obvious disease process. No correlation has been found between the presence of anti-immunoglobulin antibodies and antinuclear factor in old age, indicating that these two autoantibodies are produced independently. It would therefore appear that the central immunological mechanisms are more easily stimulated to produce autoantibodies in older people than in young subjects. It is interesting that the autoantibodies that have so far been described in old people do not cause actual disease. They are some of those which occur together with diseases either of known infective origin or with diseases that have been considered by some to be of autoimmune aetiology, because of the associated autoimmune phenomena, but which could as easily be due to an infective agent or the result of the toxic effect of some chemical substance.

Autoantibodies are known to occur at low concentration in the circulation of normal animals and people against a wide range of antigens, without causing any harmful side-effects. These range from antibodies against components of tissues such as the lens of the eye to antibodies against determinants on the immunoglobulin molecule. Antibodies are present in normal rabbit serum which react with an extract of homologous skin. Antinuclear antibodies are also present in the sera of normal people, and the incidence of these antibodies in the population increases as a function of age. Over the age of 60, more than 50% of normal subjects have one or more of the following autoantibodies in the serum: antinuclear antibody, rheumatoid factor, antibody against smooth muscle, anti-mitochondrial or anti-microsomal antibody, or antibody to adrenal, thyroid or gastric cells. Many of these naturally occurring antibodies are macroglobulins (IgM) rather than IgG and are not tissue or species specific. It is thought that these antibodies arise as a result of antigenic stimulation, possibly as a result of immunization with crossreacting antigens derived from microorganisms or even from ingested foodstuffs. Although anti-tissue autoantibodies of this type can be found in normal people, there is a marked increase in their incidence in certain disease states, particularly liver and kidney diseases and especially systemic lupus erythematous and paraproteinaemias or infections with trypanosomes.

The increased incidence of natural autoantibodies as a function of age appears to be inversely related to the presence of natural antibodies to certain extrinsic antigens of bacterial origin, which decreases with age.

The reason for this is somewhat obscure at present. Superficially, these results appear to dissociate the presence of anti-tissue antibodies from natural antibodies derived from microorganisms. However, until there has been an investigation of the incidence of a wider range of antibodies to both extrinsic and intrinsic antigens as a function of age, the dissociation of these two types of antibody cannot be accepted as a general phenomenon. If it is shown that the development of antibodies to newly encountered extrinsic antigens generally decreases as a function of age whereas those to intrinsic antigens increase, this could be an important contributory factor in the ageing process. Such a process has been considered to be related to the failure of immunological surveillance mechanisms which is thought to be a vital aspect of ageing. Failure to eliminate clones of immunocompetent cells capable of making autoantibodies could be related to a failure to eliminate abnormal clones of neoplastic cells. It has moreover been suggested that such a failure is related to the depletion of thymus cells which occurs increasingly with age. The fundamental lesion in such an ageing process would be a failure of function of the T-lymphocytes involved in cell-mediated immune processes.

Another way in which infective or toxic agents could cause the production of antibodies against the body's own tissues is thought to be by exposure of antigens which would normally be protected from the immune system. Such antigens would not have been recognized as "self" in embryonic life and the central immunological tissues would not have developed a state of "normal" immunological tolerance to them. Some of these antigens such as those present in the testis probably do not develop until after birth. If these antigens then get exposed to immune processes in adult life an immune reaction will be mounted against the tissue and the body will attempt to reject it as though it was foreign.

In summary two main hypotheses have been put forward to explain the development of autoimmune phenomena. In the first it has been postulated that there was some defect in the central immunological mechanisms as a result of which either abnormal clones of immunologically active cells were produced possibly by somatic mutation or else there was some defect in a regulator mechanism, which caused the elimination of such abnormal clones which might be produced continuously. The supporters of this hypothesis have sited the frequent occurrence of changes in the thymus associated with certain autoimmune disease in support of their views. Although changes can be found in the thymus, it is not possible to link the actual changes found with the function postulated. Moreover removal of the thymus in acute systemic lupus erythematosus and rheumatoid arthritis does not affect the course of these diseases. In myasthenia gravis where thymectomy does appear to help, the disease is probably directed more against the myoepithelial structures of the thymus than against its immunological function.

A second approach to the cause of autoimmune phenomena is to consider that there is no fundamental defect in the central immunological mechanisms. However, immune reaction against the body's own tissues are either the result of these central mechanisms receiving an abnormal stimulus or as a result of the release of these normal mechanisms from the action of suppressor cells. In the case of experimental animals the use of Freund's adjuvant seems to have such an effect and cross reacting heterologous tissues are more effective than homologous tissues. In man there is the frequent association of autoimmune phenomena with infections which are often granulomatous such as syphilis, or with a modification of the body's own antigens by possible combination with highly reactive drugs such as hydralazine.

Many of the autoimmune phenomena found associated with so-called "autoimmune diseases" cannot themselves cause pathological changes and are probably phenomena associated with a disease of which the actual aetiology is not itself "autoimmune" but infective or toxic. However, in many cases a hypersensitivity reaction against an infective or toxic agent is involved in the pathogenesis of the "autoimmune disease", and the disease though not primarily "autoimmune" is caused by immunological processes.

Bibliography

Books

Anderson, J. R., Buchanan, W. W. & Goudie, R. B. (1967), *Autoimmunity: Clinical and Experimental*. Springfield, Ill.: Charles C. Thomas.
Buchanan, W. W. & Irvine, W. J. (eds.) (1967), *Symposium on Autoimmunity and Genetics. Clin. exp. Immunol.*, **2**, Suppl.
Glynn, L. E. & Holborow, E. J. (1974), *Autoimmunity and Disease*. Oxford: Blackwell. Second edition.
Mackay, I. R. & Burnet, F. M. (1963), *Autoimmune Diseases, Pathogenesis, Chemistry and Therapy*. Springfield, Ill.: Charles C. Thomas.

Articles

Asherson, G. L. (1968), "The role of microorganisms in autoimmune response." *Progr. Allergy*, **12**, 192.
Burnet, F. M. (1970), "An immunological approach to ageing". *Lancet*, **ii**, 358.
Isacson, E. P. (1967), "Myxoviruses and autoimmunity." *Progr. Allergy*, **10**, 256.
Roberts, I. M., Whittingham, S. and Mackay, I. R. (1973), "Tolerance to an auto-antigen: antigen binding lymphocytes in thymus and blood in health and auto-immune disease." *Lancet*, **ii**, 937.

Chapter VII
Immunosuppressive Agents

Over the last two decades there has been a considerable amount of research into agents which could modify the immune response. This has been stimulated to a large extent by the need of such agents to suppress the immune response so as to obtain a successful transplantation of organs, especially the kidney. As both cell-mediated immunity and the induction of humoral antibody production involve considerable cellular proliferation, it is not surprising that the agents which were found to have some success in suppressing immune responses were those designed initially to suppress cellular proliferation. Many of these agents had already been found to modify or suppress the proliferation of neoplastic cells, before they were examined for an immunosuppressive effect.

A. The Effects of Irradiation

Much of the initial work was done on the effect of irradiation on the immune response, although this has turned out to be the least effective of all the immunosuppressive agents used now in clinical practice. However, this chapter will begin with a discussion of the effect of irradiation as more is known about the way in which this agent works than any of the other agents in current use. Moreover irradiation is used considerably in clinical practice. In many cases it is used in the treatment of neoplasia without any account being taken of its effect on the immune response. Thus, although irradiation has little clinical application, at the present time, in affecting the rejection of organ transplants or in the treatment of immune complex disease, the immunological status of patients being irradiated for the treatment of cancer must be considered most seriously. Very little work has been done on the effect of irradiation on the immune response in man, but much can be learnt from its effect on experimental animals.

Whole body irradiation of sufficient intensity strongly inhibits the immune response if given before immunization or just after exposure to antigen. X-irradiation probably acts by causing breakages in the nucleic-acid chains and causing cross linkages across the double helix spiral. This will inhibit further nucleic acid and protein synthesis and inhibit cell division. The most effective dose of radiation that will completely suppress an immune response without killing all the animals appears to be in the range of 500–700 r. Maximum inhibition is found if immunization is two days after irradiation. The capacity to respond to antigen recovers gradually between one to four weeks after irradiation. Some experimental animals were found to produce a subnormal immune response, if given antigen as long as eight weeks after irradiation. An interesting effect of irradiation is that it can, under certain circumstances, produce a stimulating effect if given before exposure to antigen. This has been explained as a rebound phenomenon, immunization taking place at a time when there was increased proliferation of cells to compensate for the depression caused by the effect of irradiation. However it might also result from a differential effect on the proliferation of precursors of suppressor lymphocytes. Irradiation does not appear to affect the formation of other serum proteins and thus does not have a direct effect on protein synthesis. Its effect is mainly to suppress the proliferation of cells which is the main process taking place during the inductive phase of the immune response, whether cell-mediated or for the production of humoral antibody. Such a suppression has been found to be associated with damage to the mechanism of nucleic-acid synthesis. This can be reversed to a certain extent by providing the animal with extracts of cells which can provide substitutes for those substances, involved in the early stages of nucleic-acid synthesis, which have been damaged. The substances which can restore immunological activity after irradiation are highly polymerized degradation products of nucleic acids. These can be provided in the form of extracts of cells, or nucleic acids incubated with enzymes which can degrade them. Another way of providing such products is by causing their release from the irradiated animal itself. This can be done by an injection of colchicine or bacterial endotoxin, or surprisingly by local irradiation of the animal's own tissues with doses as high as 5,000–10,000 r. The immune response can also be restored by the transfusion of unirradiated cells. However, if these are not genetically identical to the irradiated recipient they will react against the recipient and produce a graft versus host reaction. Such reactions have been observed in patients with leukaemia treated with whole body irradiation to destroy their leukaemic cells, and transfused with bone marrow cells from an unrelated donor to restore both erythropoietic tissue and immunologically active tissue. Such a graft versus host reaction is an immune reaction of the donor cells against the recipient in which the patient becomes very ill and among other conditions may develop an exfoliative dermatitis.

Certain chemical substances are known to have a protective effect against the action of irradiation on the immune response under experimental conditions. One of these substances is cysteamine, which is believed to protect some biochemical mechanism essential for the proliferation and differentiation of immunologically active cells after antigenic stimulation. This action may be associated in some way with the metabolism of nucleic acids in the irradiated lymphoid tissue.

It is interesting that the secondary response to an antigen is much less sensitive to irradiation than the primary response. Another effect that has been observed is that if an animal is irradiated after a primary response the anamnestic ability of the animal is destroyed. On second exposure to the same antigen it will not produce a rapid rise in the level of circulating antibody, typical of a secondary response, but will produce a slow rise with a final low concentration of antibody more typical of a primary response. It appears that in this case the effect of irradiation given after a primary response is to modify what might be called the "immunological memory" which is produced by a primary response in the central immunological tissues. This might be due to the inhibition of division of long-lived T-lymphocytes which form the memory cells in an immune response.

One of the more recent discoveries concerning the effect of irradiation on antibody production is the finding of an effect on macrophages during the earliest stage of the reaction of the humoral antibody producing mechanism to antigen. It appears that antigen needs to be processed by macrophages before it can stimulate plasma cell proliferation and antibody production. It has been found that macrophages lose the property of processing some antigens into an immunogenic form, as a result of irradiation. They do not however lose their property of being able to phagocytose antigenic material, only the property of being able to process it.

Humoral antibody production is much more radiosensitive than cell-mediated immunity. Delayed hypersensitivity can be demonstrated to be unaffected by a dose of irradiation sufficient to suppress the humoral antibody response completely. However, with higher doses of irradiation both delayed hypersensitivity and the humoral antibody response are eliminated.

The role of irradiation in increasing susceptibility to infection is of great clinical importance. Microorganisms and other parasites are much more resistant to the effects of irradiation than the human or mammalian body. It has been found that an overwhelming bacteraemia with bacteria derived from the gastro-intestinal tract develops during the second week after a dose of irradiation sufficient to kill a proportion of animals. That this is often the cause of death, can be shown by the effect of antibiotic treatment in protecting animals from the lethal effect of radiation at this level. The effect of radiation has been found to be mainly the one on macrophages described above in relation to the effect on antibody production. Macrophages do not lose their ability to phagocytose organisms but once phagocytosed the organisms are not killed and digested in the normal way. Microorganisms phagocytosed by macrophages from irradiated animals remain viable and can still multiply. Another factor involved in the reaction of the body to microorganisms after irradiation is that there is also a reduction in the number of available macrophages.

In some infective conditions, as discussed above, harmful effects are due not to the direct toxic action of the organism, but to the hypersensitivity reaction on the part of the body against the organism. Under these conditions irradiation far from making the body more susceptible to the harmful effects of the organism, actually protects it. This aspect of the effects of irradiation has not been fully studied, but is obviously a subject of much interest.

B. Immunosuppressive Drugs

The search for an effective immunosuppressive agent or combination of agents, which would allow the successful retention of an organ transplant or treatment of immune complex disease, is far from complete. A number of agents have been used either alone or in combination and so far the ideal system has not been obtained.

One might suggest the following criteria for successful immunosuppression.

1. There should be a wide margin of safety between the toxic dose and the therapeutic dose.
2. The drugs should have a selective effect on the lymphoid cells of the reticulo-endothelial system, and not cause damage to the rest of the body. Specifically they should not block erythropoiesis.
3. If possible this effect should only be on those cells which are specifically involved in immunological processes.
4. The drugs of choice should only need to be administered for a limited period, until such a time as the immunological processes become familiar with the foreign antigen and begin to recognize it as part of "self". After this time it should be possible to reduce the dosage and finally to dispense with the drugs so that the animal can maintain its own immunological defences against microbial infections.
5. The drugs should be effective against the immune processes once they have already developed.

At the present time none of the available immunosuppressive drugs attain these ideal conditions.

Although the initial impetus to find a suitable drug or combination of drugs which would suppress an immune response came from the need of these agents in allowing the successful retention of an organ transplant, more recently much interest has been shown in the possible use of these agents in suppressing pathological states arising from other immunological processes. The effects of these compounds is currently being assessed in three main groups of conditions which have previously shown little response to a more conventional therapeutic approach. The diseases on which most work is being done at the moment are systemic lupus erythematosus, nephritis and plasma cell hepatitis, all three of which show many features consistent with their development as a result of some form of hypersensitivity mechanisms. Although many other diseases develop primarily from hypersensitivity states or have associated immunological phenomena, these three conditions are diseases with an overall poor prognosis.

Most of the compounds have been chosen because they are able to suppress a primary immunological response in experimental animals. However, there has been an increasing awareness that their therapeutic effects may not be limited to this. The majority of compounds now in use have been chosen or synthesized specially for their ability to interfere with the proliferation of rapidly dividing cells. Thus in many cases they were in use as cancer chemotherapeutic agents some years before their immunosuppressive action was discovered. It is logical that a substance that will reduce the rate of neoplastic growth will also inhibit the proliferation of lymphocytes or plasma cell precursors which is such a vital part of the latent inductive phase of the immune response. Compounds have been synthesized on a very rational basis, either to affect the further synthesis of DNA or interfere with the transmission of the message from DNA to the RNA involved in protein synthesis. The drugs acting on DNA have been designed either to block enzyme action necessary for DNA synthesis or to introduce foreign groups into the DNA molecule, affecting the structure or the composition of the molecule. The known action of each of the drugs used will be discussed at greater length later. However, although the drugs have been designed for a specific action, it appears to be a principal of pharmacology that no compound can in fact have a single simple action. Although designed for a specific purpose, when the drug is given to a living animal, many other effects can be discovered that had not been considered by the chemists who originally synthesized the compound for a particular purpose. Surprisingly it has been shown in a number of different ways that a chemical compound designed to block a particular pathway to inhibit cellular proliferation, may have the desired effect of inhibiting cellular proliferation by blocking a completely different pathway from that which it was designed to block. Another interesting effect is that almost all drugs, designed to inhibit the cellular proliferative phase of the induction of an immune response can be shown also to have a further effect of blocking the immune response in the periphery. In some cases the compounds will have a beneficial effect on diseases due to an immunological mechanism, purely by an anti-inflammatory effect often without having much effect on the central immunological mechanisms. Most compounds discovered so far have little effect on an immune response once it has already developed. The phase of the immune response which is most sensitive to the drug is the phase of cellular proliferation which precedes the circulation of immunologically active lymphocytes in the cell-mediated immune response or the secretion of humoral antibody. However, many of these drugs, designed as immunosuppressive, have a marked effect in suppressing immunological diseases once they have been fully developed at a time when the central immunological mechanisms are at their least sensitive. The therapeutic effect can in these cases only be explained as one directly on the inflammatory process which occurs as a result of the interaction of immunologically active cell or humoral antibody with the target antigen. This is particularly brought out in the finding that cyclophosphamide is to some extent effective in the treatment of "lipoid nephrosis" which is one of the conditions of the kidney where so far no evidence has been found for the disease being due to an immunological disturbance. Another example of the anti-inflammatory effect of a primarily immunosuppressive drug is the finding that 6-mercapto-purine can affect the capacity of experimental animals to manifest the Arthus phenomenon without producing a drop in circulating antibodies. More recently much evidence has been produced to show that anti-lymphocyte serum which is particularly active in allowing the retention of organ transplants also has a marked non-specific anti-inflammatory effect as well as its more well known immunosuppressive action.

Another possibility that should be considered is that immunosuppressive drugs, being powerful antimetabolites, are also acting as antibacterial or viricidal agents. It is possible that cyclophosphamide could act in suppressing the nephritis of NZB mice by killing a virus that could cause the release of DNA antigen which results in the autoimmune processes leading to the nephritis.

At this stage it is profitable to list these compounds which are at the present time used for their immunosuppressive action. Those used in experimental work only, will be discussed as well as those used in current therapy as some of these compounds or related compounds may come to be used in future therapeutic trials.

Drugs which are either in use now or in the experimental stage may be listed under six main headings—

(i) Adreno-cortical hormones

(ii) Alkylating agents

(iii) Purine and pyrimidine analogues

(iv) Drugs affecting specific enzyme pathways especially that involving folic acid

(v) Antibiotics which inhibit either the synthesis of RNA or the synthesis of proteins

(vi) Anti-lymphocyte sera

(i) *Adreno-cortical hormones*

The effect of adreno-cortical hormones in suppressing immunological reactions followed very soon after the demonstration by Hench and his co-workers that rheumatoid arthritis could be strikingly modified by the use of adreno-corticotrophic hormones or cortisone. The earliest work on these compounds showed that the effect was mainly an anti-inflammatory effect on the peripheral manifestations of these reactions and over subsequent years there has been little to indicate that these compounds have a significant effect in suppressing the response of the central immunological mechanisms to antigenic stimulation in man. Even when such an effect has been suspected this has been shown to be due to a mechanical failure in access of antigen to the draining lymph node as a result of a primary anti-inflammatory effect of the steroid hormone. In certain experimental animals large doses of these hormones cause a lymphopenia and can thus suppress the central immunological mechanisms, but such an effect cannot be found in other animals nor in man. Extensive studies on the effect of steroid hormones on the tuberculin reaction in experimental animals has shown that the inhibition of the peripheral manifestation of this reaction was due to an effect on carbohydrate metabolism by causing an excess of a particular product which was found to inhibit the allergic reaction. It is possible that the anti-inflammatory effects of steroid hormones can be partially explained in the same way.

Another way that cortisone can affect the peripheral effect of immuno-logical reactions is by its action on lysosomes. Lysosomes are packets of hydrolytic enzymes surrounded by a phospholipid membrane. The granules of polymorphonuclear leucocytes are lysosomes and it is con-sidered that as part of their reaction in inflammation they can release hydrolytic enzymes into the tissues. The Arthus phenomenon is one type of immunological reaction in which polymorphonuclear leucocytes play a considerable part, possibly by the release of hydrolytic enzymes from their granules. Cortisone and its analogues have been found to exert an effect in stabilizing the phospholipid membrane of lysosomes. It is believed that part of its anti-inflammatory action takes place in this way. It is of particular interest that cortisone is very much more effective on the Arthus reaction in the human than on the tuberculin reaction. It is thought that this may be through its particular action on stabilizing the phospholipid membrane of the lysosomes of polymorphonuclear leucocytes which form the major cell type infiltrating the tissues in the Arthus reaction. Polymorphonuclear leucocytes appear to play little part in delayed hypersensitivity reactions in the human.

Cortisone or related steroid compounds are now used extensively in the treatment of a wide range of diseases where there is an immuno-logical background. These include rheumatoid arthritis, systemic lupus erythematosus, autoimmune haemolytic anaemia, idiopathic thrombo-cytopenic purpura, various types of nephritis and nephrosis and ulcera-tive colitis. They are also used, together with other compounds, in inhibiting the immunological reaction, directed against the rejection of organ transplants. However, the toxic side-effects of these compounds are considerable and certain patients are unable to tolerate these compounds in the dosage necessary to relieve symptoms caused by the immunological reactions in these conditions. The side-effects which particularly contribute against the use of these compounds are osteoporosis, pathological fractures of bone, gastro-intestinal haemorrhage and psychotic disorders. A number of patients can be found who never respond to steroids whatever the dose.

(ii) *Alkylating agents—cyclophosphamide*

This group of drugs acts in a similar kind of way to X-irradiation. They are sometimes called "radiomimetic agents". The principle of action of both these compounds and of X-rays is that they modify both DNA and protein. X-rays are thought to act by modifying the tertiary structure of these molecules, the alkylating agents however probably act by substituting chemical groups within these biologically active molecules. The first of these alkylating agents to be used in clinical practice was nitrogen mustard, a very simple but highly reactive organic compound, capable of combining irreversibly with proteins and especially nucleoproteins. The simplicity of this compound is illustrated by its chemical structure.

$$
\begin{array}{c}
Cl-CH_2-CH_2 \\
\diagdown \\
NH \\
\diagup \\
Cl-CH_2-CH_2
\end{array}
$$

Other alkylating agents which have also been used in cancer chemotherapy and have also been found to be powerful immunosuppressive agents are Busulphan (Myleran), Chlorambucil, and Melphalan. A simple molecule such as nitrogen mustard shown above has two reactive side chains attached to chloride atoms. It is thought to act as an antimitotic agent by its action on nucleic acids. The molecule can act by disrupting the orderly arrangement of bases on the DNA molecule by forming a bridge across different parts of the DNA spiral or actually rupturing the DNA molecule. In this way it would destroy the template for DNA replication and messenger RNA formation. At the present time the alkylating agent used most frequently in clinical medicine is cyclophosphamide. This compound is itself an ineffective transport form of nitrogen mustard. However, once taken up by the body it is converted into at least two cytostatic alkylating agents, one of which is nitrogen mustard. These agents then tend to accumulate in rapidly dividing tissues such as tumours or antigenically stimulated lymphoid tissue and inhibit the process of cell division.

However, alkylating agents are not only active on nucleic acids involved in cell division but can also have an inhibitory and disruptive effect on other proteins such as enzymes and this effect probably accounts for the marked anti-inflammatory effect that can be demonstrated with these compounds on immune reactions in the periphery.

Cyclophosphamide is one of the drugs which has been used in the prevention of the rejection of organ and tissue transplants. In this case its effect has probably been mainly as a cytostatic drug in the prevention or impairment of the immune response of the host against the graft. In fact, marked impairment of differentiation and proliferation of antigenically stimulated lymphoid tissue can be demonstrated in animals treated with this compound. Under experimental conditions it has been found that cyclophosphamide is most effective against the more rapidly turning over populations of lymphocytes. As a result it appears to have a preferential effect on B-lymphocytes more than T-lymphocytes, although it is equally effective on both populations once they have been stimulated by antigen to rapid cell proliferation. In situations where B-lymphocytes are modulating a T-lymphocyte response, cyclophosphamide can effectively be used to increase cell-mediated immunity. This action may be particularly relevant to its use in the treatment of Burkitt's lymphoma.

Cyclophosphamide has been shown to be particularly effective in suppressing certain diseases of an immunological nature when started some time after the disease has reached its maximum severity and often after other drugs such as corticosteroids have failed. Diseases in which this drug has been effective have been autoimmune haemolytic anaemia and systemic lupus erythematosus, glomerulonephritis and nephrosis. In the case of systemic lupus erythematosus the improvement was associated with a slight drop in objective immunological phenomena. However, this was not sufficient to account for the marked improvement, which could be the result of the marked anti-inflammatory effect of the drug. In the case of the autoimmune haemolytic anaemia, although there might be some effect on the circulating antibody level, a considerable part of the effect of this compound could be due to some inhibition of the removal of antibody coated red cells by the phagocytic cells of reticulo-endothelial system. Cyclophosphamide is well known to suppress the immune response to bacteria as a complication of its therapeutic action against diseases of an immunological nature.

(iii) *Purine and pyrimidine analogues—6 MP and imuran*

Nucleic acids are formed of a series of purine and pyrimidine bases linked together in strands which in the case of DNA forms the well known double helix. Analogues of these purine and pyrimidine bases have been synthesized so that they can be used in the place of the natural bases and thus form an abnormal DNA or RNA template, thus disorganizing cell replication and protein synthesis.

The commonest compound of this type used in clinical practice is an analogue of the purine guanine, 6-mercaptopurine

GUANINE   6-MERCAPTOPURINE

An example of a pyrimidine analogue is 5-fluorouracil and another 5-bromodeoxuridine

URACIL   5-FLUOROURACIL

Many such compounds have been synthesized and are being used to inhibit the immune response in experimental animals. However, in clinical practice it is the compound 6-mercaptopurine and its analogue Azathioprine (Imuran) which have been used the most. Imuran is split *in vivo* to 6-mercaptopurine (6-MP), although it is more readily absorbed than 6-MP. 6-MP itself is converted into another compound 6-thioguanine which is probably the compound incorporated into the DNA molecule as a "fraudulent base".

6-MP and Imuran are the two immunosuppressive agents used most commonly in clinical medicine. They have been shown to be particularly effective in combination with other compounds in suppressing the immune response against organ transplants. They are used more frequently than cyclophosphamide because they appear to have a slightly better therapeutic/toxic index. Although these compounds were synthesized specifically to act as "fraudulent bases" to be incorporated into DNA molecule and in this way to suppress the immune response, they have been also shown to have a marked non-specific anti-inflammatory effect *in vivo*. It is not difficult to conceive how alkylating agents which can denature proteins as well as nucleic acids can have a peripheral anti-inflammatory effect. However, it is more difficult to conceive how 6-MP and Imuran have such effect, but there is no doubt now that such an effect does exist. This has been demonstrated quite convincingly in experimental animals and it is thought that this effect might explain a considerable part of the therapeutic action of these drugs on such diseases as systemic lupus erythematosus, glomerulonephritis and nephrosis. 6-MP has been shown to produce a marked depression of the normal mononuclear response which occurs in the skin during inflammation.

6-MP or Imuran have been tried together with reduced doses of corticosteroids in those patients with systemic lupus erythematosus who show marked steroid side-effects. Reduction of the steroid dosage allows resolution of the toxic side-effects and the main disease can be kept well under control by the combination of the steroids with the immuno-suppressive drug.

(iv) *Inhibition of enzyme action—methotrexate*

Methotrexate (Amethopterin) was originally synthesized as a folic acid inhibitor. *In vitro* it can be shown to bind the enzyme folic reductase and prevent the conversion of dihydrofolinic acid to tetrahydrofolinic acid, which acts as a coenzyme in the conversion of uracil desoxyriboside into thymidine which is necessary for DNA synthesis. Again although synthesized to have a specific effect on a single enzyme pathway, this compound as all other immunosuppressive agents, can be shown to have multiple effects. *In vivo* it has been shown to have some effect on RNA and protein synthesis, but specially to be able to block enzymes with such diverse actions as dehydrogenases and alkaline phosphatase. It has been suggested that this effect may be due to this compound also being a chelating agent capable of binding the metal ion zinc which is necessary for the action of certain enzymes such as dehydrogenases.

Methotrexate has not been so widely used as an immunosuppressive agent in clinical medicine as 6-MP, Imuran or cyclophosphamide. This is due to the fact that as an antifolic acid agent it is capable of inducing megaloblastic anaemia as a toxic side-effect. There is a suggestion, however, that its immunosuppressive effect might be separate from its antifolic acid effect and in some experimental animals marked immuno-suppressive action can be demonstrated in the absence of toxic side-effects. In experimental animals it has been shown that the immunosuppressive action persists when given in a potentially toxic dose, if the animal receives at the same time high doses of folinic acid, capable of suppressing the toxic side-effects of the drug. If such an effect could be demonstrated in man a combination of methotrexate and folinic acid might possibly turn out to be a far less toxic immuno-suppressive combination than any produced so far. Another advantage of methotrexate over other immunosuppressive drugs is that it appears to act at a lower level in the proliferation of immunologically active cells than the alkylating agents or the purine analogues. Both cyclo-phosphamide and 6-MP block the differentiation of lymphocytes into immunoblasts, the precursors of the immunologically active cells, whereas methotrexate does not prevent the stage of differentiation into immunoblasts but prevents the division of these cells. If an immunosuppressive drug acts at a late stage in the development of immunologically active cells, its action on the immune response could be expected to be more specific.

(v) *Antibiotics*
Antibiotics derived from fungal or bacterial sources act as antibacterial agents, often because of their effect in inhibiting either nucleic acid or protein synthesis of bacteria. Such an effect is often not specific to micro-organisms but is a general biological phenomenon also affecting higher organisms. If the effect on the host is too great this often accounts for the toxicity of the compound. A number of antibiotics which are very powerful bacteriostatic agents have been rejected as therapeutic agents because of this so-called toxicity. However, these agents are often more active on rapidly dividing tissues such as those involved in cancerous proliferation, haemopoietic tissues or lymphoid tissue rapidly proli-ferating in response to antigenic stimulation. Some of these antibiotics have been on occasion used to supplement the immunosuppressive action of other compounds in preventing the immune response occur-ring as a result of an organ transplant. Although the immunosuppressive effects of these agents has been studied in isolation on experimental animals, in transplantation surgery they are more often used in con-junction with other more conventional immunosuppressive agents. Three antibiotics are known from experimental work to have a powerful immunosuppressive action. Actinomycin C, Mitomycin C and Chlor-amphenicol.

(a) *Actinomycin C.* The actinomycins have been found to have the highest activity of all the antibiotics against proliferating tissues in man. Actinomycins are derived from cultures of *Streptomyces antibioticus.* They are designated A, B, C, D, etc., originally according to their chemical composition. In fact all except for Actinomycin D are mixtures of related compounds. Actinomycin D is the purest of the various mixtures and contains the active principle in highest concentra-tion. Actinomycin D is thought to act by complexing selectively with DNA thus inhibiting RNA and protein synthesis. Pure Actinomycin D is in very short supply. Thus the compound or mixture of compounds used mostly for their immunosuppressive action is Actinomycin C, which contains a certain amount of Actinomycin D. Actinomycin C in combination with Imuran has been found to be more effective than Imuran alone in preventing the rejection of renal homografts in dogs. In some cases it was found to reverse a rejection process which had already begun in animals treated originally with Imuran alone. It has also been found of value as a supplementary treatment in the human in whom graft rejection was starting, despite the use of the maximum dose of Imuran that the patient could tolerate.

(b) *Mitomycin C.* Mitomycin C is another antibiotic derived in this case from a *Streptomyces caespitosus*. It acts by suppressing DNA dependent RNA synthesis and has also been used clinically in the treatment of malignant disease. It has however so far only been used as an immunosuppressive agent under experimental conditions where it has been shown to block the ability of immunologically active lymphocytes to react in cell-mediated immune reactions.

(c) *Chloramphenicol.* This antibiotic was originally obtained from *Streptomyces venezuelae*, but is now generally synthesized. It is probably one of the antibiotics most commonly used as a bacteriostatic agent on a world-wide scale, although for a large number of years it has been known to have a number of severe side-effects, the commonest of which are blood dyscrasias such as aplastic anaemia. It has been shown to stop protein synthesis in mammalian cells by blocking the formation of peptide chains from amino acids on the ribosomes, by stopping the attachment of the RNA template to the ribosomes. It has also been found to be immunosuppressive in experimental animals. It acts by blocking the synthesis of messenger RNA in proliferating cells such as lymph node cells, making a new protein such as antibody.

In experimental animals chloramphenicol in very large doses has been found to block the primary response of antibody production. However, it does not stop immunologically-active cells from receiving an antigenic message, so that when the animals receive a second contact with antigen while off the drug they are able to respond with a secondary increased response, as though they had produced a normal primary response. Chloramphenicol also blocks a secondary response in an animal which has shown a primary response before it was on the drug. In addition, it is a powerful immunosuppressive agent in preventing the rejection of skin transplants in experimental animals. However, the doses used are far greater than those used normally in clinical medicine.

In clinical medicine chloramphenicol has been shown to have a beneficial effect on nephritis associated with systemic lupus erythematosus. Owing to its combined bacteriostatic and immunosuppressive action, this drug could have much wider use in transplantation surgery, where other immunosuppressive drugs act incidentally to suppress the immune response against bacterial infection.

(vi) *Anti-lymphocyte serum (ALS)*
Anti-lymphocyte serum has occasionally been used as an immunosuppressive agent. The antiserum is prepared generally in the horse

by the injection of human lymphocytes, derived from thoracic-duct lymphocytes, lymph nodes or thymuses. The serum produced is often purified partially so that only the IgG fraction is used and adsorbed with packed red cells as it contains antibodies directed against erythrocytes as well as lymphocytes. Such a serum can produce a marked depletion in the circulating lymphocytes. The factor which makes this preparation so useful is that its action appears to be directed preferentially against cell-mediated immune reactions, although under certain conditions lesser effects can be demonstrated on the production of some humoral antibodies. As cell-mediated immune reactions are more important than humoral antibodies in the rejection of tissue and organ transplants, the first condition in which this serum was used clinically was on the immune response associated with the rejection of renal homografts. The course of injections was usually started some days before transplantation. In many cases it was found that patients treated with ALS needed far less Imuran or corticosteroids to suppress the graft rejection mechanism. This is important as it has been assessed that much of the mortality following renal transplantation is especially due to the toxic side-effects of corticosteroid therapy. There is an indication that, by including ALS in the therapeutic mixture and reducing the dose of corticosteroids, the morbidity and mortality following renal transplantation can be reduced

ALS is however far from being an ideal therapeutic agent, as treatment can be associated with a number of toxic side-effects. The first is due to the fact that even in its purest form ALS is a foreign serum protein and patients on this compound can develop many of the well known side-effects of sero-therapy. Anaphylactic side-effects such as urticaria, collapse and low blood pressure have been recorded in these patients. However, the organs, which are mostly at risk whenever there are circulating immune complexes, are the kidneys. Side-effects can be expected in the kidneys as there are antigens common to lymph nodes and the kidney. To minimize anaphylactic reaction ALS is given subcutaneously and not intravenously, and in the form of the purified immunoglobulins. The risks of chronic serum sickness are lessened by the fact that ALS is never used alone in clinical practice but together with other immunosuppressive agents such as Imuran. However, patients develop a very painful tended swelling at the site of injection starting after 12 hours and lasting for two to six days. This is generally associated with fever. It has also been suggested that ALS should be given only during the first few post-operative months as after this the risks of serum sickness become greater.

Owing to its greater effect on cell-mediated reactions as opposed to humoral antibody production, ALS does not appear to make the person more susceptible to bacterial infection. However, it can produce an increased susceptibility to infection with viruses, fungi and protozoa.

Little is known about the action of ALS as its immunosuppressive action does not parallel the drop in circulating lymphocytes. It does not act simply by reducing the circulating lymphocytes, but its effect seems to be specifically on the mobile pool of small lymphocytes which are under the influence of the thymus. Examination of lymph nodes from experimental animals shows that it appears to have a markedly specific effect in eliminating the T-lymphocytes from the thymus-dependent paracortical area of the lymph nodes without affecting the germinal centres or the plasma cells at the cortico-medullary junction. It also has a very strong non-specific anti-inflammatory effect on all types of reaction both immune and otherwise in the periphery. A number of theories have been put forward for the action of ALS. Probably its final action is the resultant of a number of different effects.

ALS has been shown to reduce auto-allergic encephalitis and thyroiditis in experimental animals. So far it has not been tried out extensively in clinical practice apart from its action in preventing the rejection of tissue and organ homografts.

One of the main problems with the use of ALS at the present is that it has not been possible to standardize the preparations used in different centres. This is due to the difficulty in correlating its activity *in vitro* with its activity *in vivo*. Moreover there has been no agreement even as to the method by which the horses should be immunized. Thus although results are comparable within one clinic using one batch of serum, these results are not comparable with those from another clinic using another batch of serum, probably from horses immunized in a different way. Another point, which makes it even more difficult to assess the results of ALS, is that there is apparently no correlation between its immuno-suppressive action and its ability to decrease the number of lymphocytes in the circulation.

Sera prepared against polymorphs have been found to suppress the Arthus reaction and non-specific inflammatory reactions, but have no effect on cell-mediated immune reactions. So far this reagent has not been used in clinical medicine.

Specific Immunological Tolerance Induced by an Immunosuppressive Agent

As mentioned at the beginning of this section, one of the attributes that one would consider desirable, is that once the drugs had been stopped the patient should remain unresponsive to the particular antigen to which unresponsiveness existed during the period of drug therapy. Work has been done on experimental animals to find out whether this is possible and, under certain conditions, results are promising. Initial work with 6-MP showed that if a moderate dose of antigen was given during a course of 6-MP, the animal would remain specifically unresponsive to that particular antigen once the drug had been stopped.

Other experiments show that cyclophosphamide can have a similar effect. Both the cell-mediated immune response and humoral antibody production have been specifically inhibited by these means. Similar results have been found in transplantation immunity. One report has been made of a dog which had had a kidney transplant while receiving 6-MP. Thirteen months after transplantation, the drugs were stopped and the animal retained the transplanted kidney, which was from an unrelated dog, for a further seven months. This is an isolated report as, in all other cases, humans and dogs have begun to reject their transplanted kidneys very soon after drug treatment has ceased, when the foreign kidney is recognized again as "not self".

However, drug-induced tolerance has been demonstrated on frequent occasions, using simple antigens in experimental animals. It is probably only a matter of time before these results can be applied to transplantation in man.

Bibliography

Books

Bach, J.-F. (1975), *The mode of action of immunosuppressive agents.* North-Holland Publishing, Amsterdam.

Bertelli, A. and Monaco, A. P. (eds.) (1970), *"Pharmacological treatment in organ and tissue transplantation."* Excerpta Medica Foundation, Amsterdam.

Longmire, W. P. (ed.) (1967), *Conference on Transplantation. Transplantation,* **5,** 775.

Porter, K. A. (ed.) (1967), *Symposium on Tissue and Organ Transplantation. Suppl. J. clin. Path.,* **20,** 415.

Rapaport, F. T. & Dausset, J. (eds.) (1968), *Human Transplantation.* New York: Grune and Stratton.

Taliaferro, W. H., Taliaferro, L. G. & Jaroslow, B. N. (1964), *Radiation and Immune Mechanisms.* New York: Academic Press.

Articles

Amos, D. B., Billingham, R. E., Lawrence, H. S. & Russell, P. S. (eds.) (1970), "Proceedings of the Conference on Antilymphocyte Serum". *Fed. Proc.* **29,** 97–229.

Gabrielson, A. E. & Good, R. A. (1967), "Chemical suppression of adaptive immunity." *Adv. Immunol.,* **6,** 91.

Michael, A. F., Vernier, R. L., Drummond, K. N., Levitt, J. I., Herdman, R. C., Fish, A. J. & Good, R. A. (1967), "Immunosuppressive therapy of chronic renal disease." *New Engl. J. Med.,* **276,** 817.

Miescher, P. A. & Grabar, P. (eds.) (1968), "WHO Conference on use of antimetabolites in disease associated with abnormal immune responses." *Immunopathology Vth International Symposium. Mechanisms of Inflammation Induced by Immune Reactions.* Basel: Schwabe.

Schwartz, R. S. (1965), "Immunosuppressive drugs." *Progr. Allergy,* **9,** 246.

Swanson, M. & Schwartz, R. S. (1967), "Immunosuppressive therapy. Relation between immunological competence and clinical responsiveness." *New Engl. J. Med.,* **277,** 163.

Chapter VIII
Transplantation of Tissues and Organs

The immunological basis for the rejection of allogeneic (homologous) transplants of organs and tissues has only been generally accepted for the past twenty-five years. For much of this time most of the experimental work has been done on the mechanism of the rejection of skin allografts (homografts). The initial stimulus for this work was provided by plastic surgeons who wished to replace large areas of skin damaged by burns and, as many major advances in science, this came as a direct result of needs engendered during World War II. Later the emphasis in interest has shifted from the skin to the kidney and so much work has been done in this field that it has recently been stated that "a patient receiving a transplant from a living related donor should have at least a 65% likelihood of survival for two years or more". With the prospect of consistent survival of renal transplants in sight, experimental work is now being directed to a study of the problems that might be encountered in transplantation of the liver, pancreas, heart and lungs. So much work is now being done by surgeons in the field of experimental organ and tissue transplantation that it must be considered only a matter of time before organ transplantation becomes a regular part of modern surgical procedure. Before discussing the problems inherent in the transplantation of different organs and tissues, it will be profitable to discuss the immunological mechanism lying behind graft rejection both in man and in experimental animals. The techniques at present used to suppress these immunological mechanisms especially in relation to the allograft (homograft) reaction will then be described, emphasis being made on the techniques used at present to prevent renal allograft rejection in clinical practice. Finally reference will be made to the immunological problems special to the transplantation of other organs and tissues.

The Immunological Background of Allogeneic (Homologous) Graft Rejection

1. *The cell-mediated immune reaction*

The suggestion that there was an immunological basis for the breakdown of skin allografts (homografts) came from the observation that a second graft placed on a recipient animal would be rejected more rapidly if the recipient had already rejected a first graft from the same donor. An analogy was therefore drawn between the more rapid "second set rejection" and a more rapid secondary immune response of an animal to the injection of a foreign soluble antigen such as for instance diphtheria toxoid. The slower "first set graft rejection" was considered to be analogous to the slower primary immune response to diphtheria toxoid. However, the immunological basis of allograft rejection differed in one major respect from the immune response to diphtheria toxoid. Immunity to the toxoid could be transferred passively from animal to animal by means of serum and thus would be shown to involve serum antibodies. However, the ability to immunize an animal passively so that it would reject a first set graft more rapidly as though it was a second set graft could not be undertaken by the injection of serum from an animal which had already rejected a first set graft from the same donor. In this way graft rejection appeared to be more analogous to bacterial allergy such as the tuberculin reaction and to chemical contact sensitivity. This was further emphasized by histological examination of the skin grafts during the rejection process. The cellular infiltrate in a graft during rejection was found to be mainly mononuclear like that found in the tuberculin reaction and contact sensitivity, whereas the infiltrate in an Arthus reaction caused by the reaction between antigen and soluble antibody consists mainly of polymorphonuclear leucocytes.

Soon after it was demonstrated that tuberculin sensitivity and contact sensitivity could be transferred passively with lymphocytes, it was shown that transplantation immunity could also be transferred passively with these cells. It thus became obvious that transplantation immunity, just as the tuberculin reaction and chemical contact sensitivity, was another example of a cell-mediated immune response. Although later on it was shown that humoral antibodies could play quite a significant role in allograft rejection, this role has always been found in practice to be an auxiliary role. It does appear that humoral antibodies cannot initiate allograft rejection, and that allograft rejection needs to be initiated in the first place by a cell-mediated immunological reaction.

This is because the transplanted graft acts as a fixed antigen, in the same way as in chemical contact sensitivity the antigen is fixed in the tissues, because the low molecular weight foreign chemical substance is bound firmly to the skin. Only a small proportion of the antigen diffuses down to the medulla of the lymph node where it is taken up by macrophages to stimulate plasma cell proliferation and humoral antibody production. Most of the antigen remains fixed in the periphery where it stimulates T-lymphocytes passing through the tissues. These cells migrate down through the peripheral lymphatics to the draining lymph nodes and pass from the peripheral sinus down into the paracortical area of the cortex of the lymph node between the lymph follicles where they find the right milieu to differentiate into immunoblasts and divide into immunologically competent small lymphocytes. These lymphocytes carry membrane receptors analogous to the antigen reactive site of an antibody, that allows them to react specifically with a target tissue, in this case the initial graft itself or a second set graft placed subsequently on the animal. This reaction will initiate an inflammatory process as a result of which the graft will be rejected. Similar T-lymphocytes are cytotoxic for target cells in tissue culture *in vitro*. However, it is unlikely that this is the mechanism of graft rejection *in vivo*. *In vivo* it can be shown that macrophages form a significant proportion of the infiltrate and would appear to be stimulated by a factor released by the lymphocytes after reaction with antigen. This factor may be a lymphokine similar to that released after reaction between specifically sensitized T-lymphocytes and soluble antigen.

The cell-mediated immune response in the allograft reaction can be regarded in some way analogous to a reflex arc with an afferent limb in which lymphocytes get sensitized in the periphery and pass down to the local lymph node which is analogous to a nerve ganglion. The lymph node is the site of proliferation of these lymphocytes in that it provides the correct milieu for this process. The immunologically competent lymphocytes passing out to the periphery are then analogous to the efferent limb of the reflex arc passing coded messages out to the peripheral tissues to cause the rejection of the tissue or organ which can now be recognized as "not self" and initiate the process of graft rejection. The lymphocytes on the afferent side of the arc which respond immunologically to the presence of an allograft are normal T-lymphocytes and do not develop if the thymus gland is removed during neonatal life. In the same way they appear to be more susceptible to the action of anti-lymphocyte serum than the B-cells which are the precursors of plasma cells involved in antibody production.

2. *The role of humoral antibodies in organ graft rejection*

Whereas allograft rejection cannot in most cases be initiated by humoral antibodies except under highly artificial conditions in the laboratory, evidence has recently been accumulating that antibodies can play an ancillary role especially in the rejection of organ allografts. Most of the transplantation antigen resides in a fixed state in the tissues, a small amount is released and travels in a soluble form to the medulla of the lymph node or to the spleen where it initiates the production of circulating antibody. There is one tissue however in which it is thought by some that graft rejection is initiated almost completely by humoral antibodies and this is the cornea of the eye. The cornea, however, holds a privileged site as far as graft rejection is concerned and this will be considered as a separate subject. Very few lymphocytes pass through the cornea to stimulate a cell-mediated immune reaction and thus in many cases a corneal allograft is never rejected. However, soluble antigen can diffuse from this transplanted tissue and occasionally could stimulate sufficient circulating antibody to cause the rejection of the graft.

Much of the evidence for the role of circulating antibody in organ graft rejection comes from a study of the rejection of renal allografts during late rejection that has been delayed by immunosuppressive therapy which has, however, been insufficient to abolish the immune response completely. Evidence for the involvement of humoral antibody can be found by examining the rejected graft histologically and histochemically. In the first place as well as infiltration of the graft with immunoblasts and lymphocytes, plasma cells can be seen, recognized under the electron microscope by the presence of the typical rough endoplasmic reticulum, which indicates that these cells are involved in the secretion of protein (antibody). Furthermore these cells can actually be shown to contain the immunoglobulins G and M (IgG and IgM). Evidence can also be found that there is a substantial antigen–antibody reaction going on in the body as the level of serum complement can be shown to be falling during the phase of acute graft rejection, rather as it does during the acute phase of a disease caused by the circulation of immune complexes, such as systemic lupus erythematosus or acute glomerulonephritis. Histologically the blood vessels in the rejected kidney show many of the features found in the Arthus phenomenon. There is fibrinoid necrosis of the walls of many of the afferent and efferent glomerular arterioles and IgG, IgM and complement can be shown in these lesions. Some of the smaller arteries in the kidney can be found to have developed fibroblastic thickening of the intima and rupture of the internal elastic lamina. Finally platelets can be seen aggregating in the lumen of the capillary loops and it is known that platelet aggregation can be induced by contact with antigen–antibody complexes. Another indication of the involvement of platelets in the intravascular thrombosis which occurs with this form of graft rejection is that it is associated with a fall in the number of circulating platelets. This fall parallels the sequestration of platelets within the rejected transplant. It has been suggested that part of the effect of corticosteroids in reversing renal graft rejection is that it reverses platelet aggregation caused by antigen–antibody interaction.

If rejection occurs several months or years after transplantation there may be no evidence at all of cell-mediated immune rejection. It appears that the cell-mediated response can still be suppressed by therapy but that humoral antibody production can break away from immunosuppression independently. Under these conditions there is virtually no evidence of cellular infiltration of the renal graft. The histological appearance resembles that seen in glomerulonephritis and a fine deposit of IgM and IgG or complement can be demonstrated outlining the glomerular capillary wall and mesangial cells. The deposits of immunoglobulin and complement form a continuous smooth layer outlining the glomerular capillary tuft rather like that seen in Goodpasture's syndrome rather than the lumpy deposits of immune complexes seen in serum sickness, acute glomerulonephritis or systemic lupus erythematosus (see Chapter X). Experimentally this can be reproduced by the injection of nephrotoxic antiserum induced in a foreign species or in allergic glomerulonephritis induced by immunization with glomerular capillary basement membranes. Antibodies against the kidney can rarely be demonstrated in the serum during the rejection process as they are taken up by the kidney as soon as they are formed, but if the rejected kidney is removed antibodies will begin to appear in the serum and can be detected with ease. It appears that the synthesis of IgM antibodies are the least affected by immunosuppression with 6-MP, the drug most commonly used in the treatment of renal allografts. Thus it appears that the synthesis of IgM antibodies is more readily able to break away from immunosuppression with 6-MP as late as many months or even years after the transplantation, and cause acute rejection of the graft.

Thus the way in which humoral antibody can cause renal graft rejection is by the production of an acute glomerulonephritis and allergic obliterating vasculitis in the kidney transplant. There is often no evidence of direct target cell damage by infiltrating lymphocytes and macrophages, similar to that which occurs in cell-mediated graft rejection.

Tissue Typing for Organ Transplantation in Man—The HLA System

As mentioned in Chapter I the HLA system present on chromosome 6 forms the major histocompatibility system equivalent to the H-2 system in the mouse. Four loci controlling a number of antigenic specificities have been defined. Three of these loci, A, B and C control three groups of antigens that can be defined serologically. The fourth or D locus controls antigenic determinants that are defined by lymphocyte activation in the mixed lymphocyte reaction. Each individual will therefore inherit the potential to manifest two sets of antigens, one set derived from each parent.

The antigens controlled by the A, B and C loci have been defined serologically on the surface of circulating leucocytes. Sera specific for these antigens are cytotoxic for leucocytes and have been produced in multiparous women, transplant patients and those that have received multiple transfusions, as well as by immunizing volunteers with a skin graft from a single donor or by the subcutaneous injection of peripheral white cells. Identification of the HLA antigens carried by an individual is generally by means of a microcytotoxicity test, using these sera in the presence of complement. Incubation is generally for one hour at 37°C and cell death determined by the use of trypan blue or eosin, which are taken up by dead cells. Most of these antigens so far discovered segregate into the A and B groups. Studies on the alleles at the C locus have only just started. As the loci are so close together the frequency of recombination between them is low. For practical purposes the antigens have in the past been considered to belong to two segregational groups controlled by the A and B loci. The individual thus inherits the potential to manifest two antigens from those controlled by the A locus and two from those controlled by the B locus. In practice as the loci are so closely linked the two A and B antigens are frequently inherited together.

HLA antigens are surface glycoproteins of about 44,000 molecular weight and are associated with another 12,000 molecular weight glycoprotein which is structurally related to the immunoglobulin molecule and is electrophoretically a β-microglobulin. Differences in HLA specificity are due to the amino-acid composition of the larger molecule.

It is generally accepted that the ABO compatibility is necessary for successful transplantation in man. The value of HLA compatibility is far from being completely accepted. There is no doubt that grafts matched for three or four antigens survive significantly better than grafts matched for one or two antigens. However very few grafts have been performed in which there was identity of all four serologically defined antigens. Even if there is identity at the A and B loci, rejection can still occur as a result of non-identity at the C or D locus. Non-identity at the D locus can be determined by mixed lymphocyte culture as the antigens controlled by this locus are all lymphocyte activating determinants. In mixed lymphocyte culture, lymphocytes from the two individuals are mixed and incubated *in vitro*. Incompatibility at the D locus is demonstrated by the cells transforming in culture into lymphoblasts. This can be demonstrated by adding a radioactive precursor of DNA (^{3}H-thymidine) which is then taken up by these cells during DNA synthesis. The problem of HLA matching is that in practice it may not be possible to match much more than 5% of individuals for three or all four of these HLA antigens: in most cases surgeons have to be content with a match for one or two antigens Another problem with potential transplant recipients is that certain patients develop lymphocytotoxic antibodies as a result of multiple blood transfusions. However it has been found that patients who have received multiple transfusions without developing antibodies have a significantly better survival.

The frequency of serologically defined HLA antigens of the A and B groups varies in different ethnic groups. Thus HLA-A1 is relatively absent and HLA-B8 has a very low frequency in Japanese as compared with Caucasians. A1 and B8 are found together in Caucasians with a greater degree of frequency than would be expected, as also are A2 and B12. As has been mentioned earlier Hodgkin's disease occurs more frequently in those with the A1,B8 haplotype, whereas acute lymphatie leukaemia occurs with greater frequency in those with A2,B12. The strongest disease association is however the association between B27 and ankylosing spondylitis, acute anterior uveitis, Reiter's syndrome and psoriasis. B8 shows an association with coeliac disease, dermatitis herpetiformis, thyrotoxicosis, myasthenia gravis and chronic active hepatitis.

Bone marrow Transplantation—Graft versus Host Disease

Bone-marrow transplants are used in the treatment of severe combined immuno-deficiency disease to replace the absent stem cells in this congenital disorder. They are also used to replace haematopoietic and immunologically-active tissue in patients who have received massive doses of irradiation or chemotherapy in the treatment of leukaemia, Hodgkin's disease and other neoplastic conditions of the haematopoietic and reticulo-endothelial systems. It is also indicated in the treatment of aplastic anaemia and severe leucopenia. Patients with transplanted bone marrow are generally referred to as haematopoietic chimeras, in that they have circulating erythrocytes and leucocytes with antigens of donor origin. The establishment of chimaerism is the most reliable proof of the take of a graft. This can be done by chromosome studies, transplanting male into female and vice versa. Allogeneic bone marrow transplanted into patients who have never had or have lost a functioning immunological system will not be rejected in the same way as it would be in normal subjects. However, it is capable of being stimulated immunologically by the host's tissues to react against the host. This will result in the grafted lymphoid cells mounting a rejection process against the host's tissues. "Graft versus host" disease is severe and relentless. The spleen and liver, being the sites at which the graft lymphocytes are proliferating, become massively enlarged. The symptoms of "secondary" or "graft versus host" disease are rapidly progressive loss of weight, diarrhoea, nausea and vomiting, desquamative erthrodermia (exfoliative dermatitis) (with infiltration of the dermis with mononuclear cells). If the disease progresses it is inevitably fatal. "Graft versus host" disease can be avoided by close HLA matching, and good survival of patients transplanted with bone marrow can now be obtained if the graft is obtained from a closely HLA matched sibling donor.

Normally, bone marrow transplants are performed in patients with leukaemia and Hodgkin's disease whose own immunologically-active tissue has been suppressed by the use of X-irradiation or cyclophosphamide. However, if recipients are pre-treated with anti-lymphocyte serum as an immunosuppressive agent, there is evidence that "graft versus host" disease does not develop in such an acute or subacute form. This could be because residual antilymphocytic serum in the circulation at the time of the transplant makes the graft lymphocytes to some degree tolerant of the host.

Immunosuppression and Transplantation

(a) *X-irradiation*

The original concept was to irradiate the patient with a supralethal dose of X-rays as this would completely abolish the immune response. As this process is inevitably associated with complete bone marrow destruction, the patient has to be transfused with bone marrow, preferably from the donor of the transplanted organ. However, the transfused cells will react immunologically against the recipient producing a "graft versus host" disease, causing death of the recipient. Sublethal total body irradiation was then introduced and long term renal graft survival was occasionally encountered using this technique especially in grafts from non-identical twins or siblings, but this procedure has now been discontinued.

Local irradiation of the transplant before actual transplantation does not appear to affect graft survival. Another technique is local irradiation of the graft *in situ* on the 1st, 3rd, 5th and 7th days after transplantation. This does not produce any damage to the function of the kidney but does appear to have a certain beneficial effect on renal graft survival. The effect of irradiation would appear to inhibit graft rejection by interfering with the afferent arc of the immune response, although a non-specific effect in preventing sensitizing lymphocytes from destroying the graft cannot be excluded.

Attempts have also been made to irradiate the circulating blood in isolation from the rest of the body. This has been attempted either by irradiating the afferent artery to the transplant or by implanting Yttrium[90] pellets into the centre of the abdominal aorta in the case of renal transplants. Both these techniques have produced prolonged survivial of renal transplants in experimental animals.

Irradiation has also been used in patients receiving organ transplants by passing the blood through an extracorporeal shunt in a box containing Strontium[90] as a source of irradiation. This procedure has not been used as a sole source of immunosuppression, but has been used in patients undergoing episodes of graft rejection while on more conventional immunosuppressive therapy. The equipment necessary is very light and can be strapped to the patient so that he remains ambulatory. As Strontium[90] is a pure β ray emitter only light lead shielding is necessary. The technique has been used in a series of patients undergoing vigorous rejection despite azathioprine and prednisone therapy and succeeded in reversing the rejection process in at least one patient. The effect of this treatment is to produce a marked lymphopenia and the surviving lymphocytes showed definite signs of radiation damage. Extracorporeal irradiation of thoracic duct lymph has been attempted experimentally but would not be considered to be applicable to use in transplantation of organs such as the kidney where the afferent arc of sensitization is by way of the blood stream rather than the lymphatics.

(b) *Immunosuppressive drugs*

The standard treatment of patients who receive renal allografts has been for a number of years now a combination of the drugs azathioprine (imuran) and prednisone. The timing and dosage of these two drugs has been varied from centre to centre. Until recently there has been little use of donor recipient selection by tissue-typing techniques as these have only recently been fully developed. Thus it can reasonably be stated that these drugs have not yet been used consistently under ideal conditions.

Initially toxic effects were due to too high a dose of azathioprine being used. Often this was used alone and was only supplemented by prednisone and actinomycin C when the patient showed signs of rejection. Subsequently patients have been treated with half the dose of azathioprine used initially but prednisone has been given continuously from the beginning of therapy. Under these conditions there was a reduction in the incidence of severe early rejection. The onset of early signs of graft rejection are indicated by an increased blood urea and decreased creatinine clearance. Rejection crises can be controlled by two or three intravenous injections of 1 gram methylprednisolone, which is far less toxic than the high doses of oral steroids previously used. This, however, brings the risk of increased susceptibility to infection. In patients transplanted with kidneys from live donors, death in unsuccessfully treated cases was due almost solely to infection with uncommon fungi, protozoa or viruses which could not be controlled by conventional antibiotic therapy, rather than by uraemia resulting on graft rejection. These are the organisms controlled normally by cell-mediated immunity which has been suppressed non-specifically by the drugs used to suppress graft rejection. Many of the series of patients described have been transplanted with cadaver kidneys and these appear to have a higher rejection rate than kidneys from live donors; rejection in these cases may frequently be non-immunological.

Where patients die, often the sequence of events is that there is an impending rejection which leads to more intensive immunosuppressive therapy which in turn leads to irreversible bone marrow failure, followed by a fulminating infection which cannot be controlled. Much better effects of renal transplantation have been seen over the past few years since experience has been gained in individual centres. There has been an increased experience in both operative technique and in the use of immunosuppressive therapy. The use of haemodialysis both before operation and during a rejection has reduced the incidence of drug toxicity. There is no doubt that immunosuppressive drugs are more toxic in a patient with renal failure and to a certain extent drug toxicity can be reduced by haemodialysis. The most critical phase appears to be in the third week after transplantation during the first rejection crisis. It is surprising that if this can be overcome most patients adapt themselves to both the graft and immunosuppressive therapy so that they can be discharged on maintenance levels of azathioprine and prednisone lower than that used initially and become free from further rejection crises.

One disturbing feature has recently been described in patients treated for long periods with immunosuppressive drugs for renal transplants and this is that a few but significant number of these patients have developed reticulosarcomata, which could be the result of the prolonged immunosuppressive therapy.

(c) *Antilymphocyte serum (ALS)*

Recently in a number of centres antilymphocyte serum has been used as an adjuvant to azathioprine and prednisone therapy in the prevention of the rejection of renal allografts. In one series daily injections are started 5 days before operation and continued daily for 10–17 days afterwards, then every other day for 2 weeks, followed by twice a week for one month and then once a week for one month. In other centres it is only used during rejection crises. Injections have been of 1–5 ml of purified globulin. However, the level of antibody given cannot be assessed as there are no means of assaying and standardizing the immunosuppressive effect of the serum especially as the immunosuppressive effect appears to be independent of the lymphopenia produced. The serum generally used in the human is prepared in horses by injection of human lymphocytes and the globulin fraction of the serum containing the antilymphocyte antibodies is generally purified. The amount of protein injected is usually between 100 and 500 mg/kg/week. By covering the early critical phase of transplantation with antilymphocyte serum the total dose of azathioprine can be somewhat reduced. However, the most important claim is that the dose of prednisone used can be reduced by as much as a half. It has also been claimed that there is a marked reduction in the incidence of acute rejection episodes during the first three months after transplantation, and a reduction in mortality. This is possibly due to a reduction in the amounts of prednisone and azathioprine used and thus a marked reduction in the susceptibility of the patient to infection.

However, toxic side-effects of ALS do occur. The patients all have pain and tenderness at the site of injection and run a fever when on ALS. In some cases therapy has to be stopped due to the development of anaphylactic reactions, since ALS is itself a foreign protein. One of the risks of ALS that has been poorly emphasized is that as a foreign protein it induces a state of chronic serum sickness in the patient since ALS does not suppress humoral antibody production to the same extent as it suppresses the cell-mediated immune reaction. Immune complexes containing ALS, recipient IgG and recipient complement are deposited in the renal glomeruli which can potentially cause glomerular damage in the transplant and thus defeat ultimately the aim of the whole procedure, transplantation and immunosuppression.

The Use of "Immunological Enhancement" in avoiding Graft Rejection or "Graft versus Host" Disease

The phenomenon of "immunological enhancement" was first described in relation to tumour allografts in mice. Tumour allografts which have had contact with specific antisera have enhanced growth and are protected from the host's immunological reaction directed against them. Skin grafts in experimental animals can similarly be protected from rejection by specific antisera. It is considered that specific antibody has a dual effect in affecting the cell-mediated immune response. Antibody can protect the graft itself by modifying it so that it is no longer susceptible to the cell-mediated immune reaction, once the response has already developed. It is also believed to inhibit the cell-mediated immune response centrally.

The principle of "immunological enhancement" has been used to prevent a "graft versus host" reaction in bone marrow transplantation. In this situation an antiserum is prepared against HLA antigens absent in the donor but present in the recipient. The serum is injected at the same time as the marrow is transplanted. In two cases treated in this way there has been prolonged survival of a bone marrow graft without the development of "graft versus host" disease.

Immunological enhancement has also been shown to allow the indefinite survival and functioning of renal allografts in experimental animals. An attempt has been made to use this approach to induce the increased survival of a renal allograft in man. The subject was transplanted with a maternal kidney and at the same time given an antiserum prepared in the father against maternal leucocytes. The antiserum was absorbed so as to be against those HLA antigens in the donor that were not common with the recipient. Partial immunological enhancement was obtained as the renal graft was able to survive for 3 months without immunosuppressive therapy from the 8th to the 20th week after grafting. It is likely that the kidney has organ specific transplantation antigens as well as HLA antigens. Therefore immunological enhancement cannot be expected to be complete using only antibodies against HLA antigens. However, these results are encouraging enough to suggest that immunological enhancement, which could become a regular technique in bone marrow transplantation, may be used in the future more frequently to supplement immunosuppressive therapy in renal transplantation.

Transplantation of the Liver and other Organs

There is no doubt that it is easier to get a patient to accept a transplant of a kidney from another individual using modern techniques of immunosuppression, than it is to get a patient to accept a skin graft. It would therefore appear that the strength of immune response and the subsequent rejection will vary from tissue to tissue and organ to organ. It has been suggested that certain sites in the body are privileged in that a transplant at this site will initiate an immune response to a lesser extent than at another site. This is undoubtedly true of the cornea which will be discussed later on in this chapter. The liver, however, provides a very interesting example of this. Spurred on by successes in the field of renal transplantation, surgeons have recently been approaching the problems of liver transplantation. Perhaps the most interesting finding is that liver allografts in outbred pigs can survive for many weeks, in some cases longer than 15 months without any immunosuppressive therapy, under conditions where the animals would be expected to reject skin grafts within 9–10 days. It appears that the transplanted liver, if completely healthy, apparently does not stimulate a cell-mediated immune response. Moreover, it also appears to protect skin and kidney grafts transplanted from the same donor at the same time. Such skin grafts are rejected six times more slowly than a skin graft transplanted on its own. Injected soluble-liver antigen extracts have also been shown to prolong the survival of skin and renal grafts from the same donor. It has therefore been suggested that the liver releases histocompatibility antigens in a tolerogenic form which induces a state of partial immunological tolerance to these antigens. However, if the liver is damaged in any way, antigen is released and an immune response is stimulated resulting in immunological rejection. In the experiments on pigs, the donor's liver was attached to the recipient's vasculature immediately after removal. If the liver was allowed to undergo even slight ischaemia during operation the damage would be sufficient to release antigen and stimulate an immune reaction in the recipient.

Liver transplantation has been attempted in the human. As the liver is not a paired organ cadaveric transplants have to be used in which some degree of ischaemia has already occurred. Moreover, most of the recipients have been extremely ill, in hepatic coma. Immunosuppression has been provided with azathioprine, prednisone and ALS. However, these patients are extremely sensitive to the toxic effects of azathioprine and prednisone which are also primary hepatoxic agents. Many non-immunological problems have to be overcome before liver transplantation becomes a regular procedure in the human, but the experimental results in pigs are most promising.

Experiments are under way on the transplantation of the heart, lungs, pancreas and stomach in experimental animals and man. At the present many of the problems are technical as well as immunological. But as the technical problems are overcome, it is becoming more and more apparent that the problems of immunosuppression in man are greater for some organs than others. It is often extremely difficult to suppress graft rejection without weakening the patient's defence mechanisms against microorganisms to such an extent that they develop severe overwhelming and fatal infections. This risk is especially strong during episodes of so-called "rejection crises" when the dose of immuno-suppressants has to be increased to continue graft survival. Survival and function of lung allografts have been described in experimental animals using conventional immunosuppressive therapy. However, in man immunosuppressive therapy has not so far been able completely and successfully to prevent immunological rejection. Similarly, although immunological rejection has been delayed in some cases of heart transplantation in man and in one series 50% of patients have survived for at least one year. The problems of immunosuppression appear to be far more difficult for this organ than for the kidney.

Corneal Transplantation

The cornea provides a very special case in clinical transplantation. It is estimated that 80% of corneal allografts will remain permanently *in situ* without being rejected. This has been considered to be possibly due to the transplant consisting of a relatively small amount of tissues and cells containing a low content of transplantation antigens, also because the site is avascular. The reason that a cornea is normally not rejected is known to be due to a failure of sensitization on the afferent side of the immune arc, since if the subject is transplanted simultaneously with skin from the same donor the patient will become sensitized and the graft rejected. Moreover, if the corneal graft is implanted into another tissue such as muscle, it will be rejected in the same time as a skin graft. Thus there is no lack of transplantation antigens and the cornea is easily rejected once the subject is sensitized. The reason that sensitiza-tion does not occur appears to be related to the fact that the tissue is avascular, since the incidence of graft rejection is proportional to the degree of vascularization of the cornea. Also there is a higher incidence of graft rejection if the eye is the site of certain diseases at the time of transplantation. If the recipient cornea is oedematous, there is a higher risk of rejection of a donor graft; also if the cornea is the site of infection with the herpes virus, graft rejection is more likely. Being avascular the cornea is not normally visited by circulating lymphocytes. Thus lymphocytes cannot normally be activated by contact with the foreign antigens of the cornea and initiate a cell-mediated response in the draining lymphoid tissue. If a corneal graft is not vascularized, immunologically activated lymphocytes will not be able to reach the graft and cause a cell-mediated rejection.

Clinically rejection of a corneal graft takes the form of an opacification. This may occur between three weeks and two years after transplantation. The infiltration is mainly polymorphonuclear and although it has been suggested that this is a humoral antibody reaction rather than cell-mediated, so far immunoglobulins have not been demonstrated in the graft during rejection. The injection of corneal material, from a human donor eye, into the skin of the forearm of recipients with corneal grafts which were becoming cloudy due to a rejection process, produces an erythematous hypersensitivity reaction. Corticosteroids alone, administered systemically before the onset, will prevent graft rejection, but once clouding has begun the response is only modified.

The use of azathioprine $5 \cdot 0$–$5 \cdot 6$ mg/kg initially, followed by a maintenance dose of $3 \cdot 3$–$3 \cdot 6$ mg/kg daily for up to two years, together with prednisolone has been found a satisfactory course of treatment to cause retention of corneal grafts in patients who were consistently rejecting corneal grafts despite corticosteroid therapy. This dose of azathioprine was found to be insufficient to block a humoral antibody response to a conventional antigen.

Transplantation of Cartilage and Bone

Cartilage does not provoke an immune response at all when transplanted allogeneically. It appears to be weakly antigenic. However, if the cells normally enclosed in matrix are exposed, antigen will be released and immunization will occur so that accelerated rejection of a skin graft from the same donor will be obtained. Apparently it is not the chondrocytes but other cells which are antigenic.

Bone, on the other hand, is extremely antigenic. If transplanted allogeneically it will stimulate a cell-mediated immune response and be rejected in the same way as any other tissue. The intensity of the immune response is proportional to the number of cells within the graft. Cell survival, however, is not an essential part of the function of a bone graft. The bone graft will be resorbed, but while being resorbed it will be replaced by normal recipient bone. The bone graft acts as a scaffold which supports and guides new bone invasion of the graft. It is said that a bone allograft during rejection and resorption has osteoconductive properties, stimulating new bone formation. Whereas bone from individuals of the same species have these properties, bones from a foreign species excite a particularly violent immune reaction and will not be osteoconductive. Bone grafts even from a different species can be treated chemically and their antigenicity reduced so that they will be accepted by a recipient and not rejected immunologically.

138 *Immunology in Clinical Medicine*

Appendix

TRANSPLANTESE   (The language of the transplanter)

Noun	Adjective	Meaning
Autograft	autochthonous	Graft from individual to himself
Syngeneic homograft	syngeneic	Graft within genetically identical inbred strains of animals or identical twins
Allogeneic homograft or allograft	allogeneic	Graft within same species, however between genetically different individuals
Xenograft	xenogeneic	Graft between animals of different species

Bibliography

Books

Calne R. Y. (1975), *Organ Grafts*. London: Edward Arnold.
Longmire, W. P. (ed.) (1967), "Conference on transplantation." *Transplantation*, 5, 775.
Porter, K. A. (ed.) (1967), "Tissue and organ transplantation." Suppl. *J. clin. Path.*, 20, 415.
Rapaport, F. T. & Dausset, J. (ed.) (1968), *Human Transplantation*. New York: Grune Stratton.
Rycroft, P. V. (ed.) (1969), *Corneo-plastic Surgery*. Oxford: Pergamon.

Articles

Batchelor, J. R. & Hackett, M. (1970), "HL-A matching in treatment of burned patients with skin allografts." *Lancet*, ii, 581.
Batchelor, J. R., Ellis, F., French, M. E., Bewick, M., Cameron, J. S. & Ogg, C. S. (1970), "Immunological enhancement of human kidney graft." *Lancet*, ii, 1007.
Mathé, G., Amiel, J. L., Schwarzenberg, L., Choay, J., Troland, P., Schneider, M., Hayat, M., Schlumberger, J. R. & Jasmin, Cl. (1970), "Bone marrow graft in man after conditioning with antilymphocytic serum." *Br. Med. J.*, 2, 131.
"Nomenclature for factors of the HLA system." *Bull. Wld. Hlth. Org.*, 52, 261 (1975).
Oliver, R. T. D. (1976), "Histocompatibility matching and renal graft survival." *Proc. roy. Soc. Med.*, 69, 531.
Salaman, J. R. (1976), "Current status of organ transplantation." *Proc. roy. Soc. Med.*, 69, 527.

Chapter IX
Connective Tissue Diseases

This group of diseases include rheumatic fever, rheumatoid arthritis and systemic lupus erythematosus (SLE). Clinically these three conditions have a common feature in that arthritis plays an important part in each disease. Immunologically, rheumatoid arthritis and SLE are associated with the presence of auto-antibodies in the serum. The nature of these auto-antibodies will be discussed at length. However, the presence of auto-antibodies in the serum should never conceal the fact that we know very little about the aetiology and pathogenesis of these diseases. The presence of arthritis with other signs of a generalized systemic disease suggests to the immunologist that these diseases could be caused by a continuous circulation of immune complexes, such as occurs in chronic serum sickness. These would localize in different sites depending possibly on the physico-chemical nature of the antigen. In rheumatic fever especially and occasionally in rheumatoid arthritis there is often evidence of involvement of the cardiovascular system, whereas in SLE there is involvement of the kidneys as well as the heart. In SLE and occasionally rheumatoid arthritis the skin may be involved; in the latter there may be a diffuse vasculitis, whereas in SLE patients may occasionally have the typical indolent "lupus" rash on the face or more frequently on other areas of the body. Vasculitis appears to be a regular finding in all three diseases, although it is more common in rheumatoid arthritis, and purpura hyperglobulinaemia is often a precursor of fully developed SLE. In all three diseases, a marked increase in circulating immunoglobulins indicates an increased production of circulating antibodies, although these cannot be identified completely. The increase in IgG is always of the polyclonal variety. Haematological changes occur frequently, and these may take the form of thrombocytopenia, and anaemia with or without leucopenia, in the case of SLE.

Systemic disease due to the circulation of immune complexes may take many forms. In SLE many different tissues and organs are attacked. In glomerulonephritis lesions are mainly limited to the kidney. In rheumatic fever it is the heart and joints which are most affected, whereas in rheumatoid arthritis it is more common to have the joints only affected. In so-called Henoch-Schonlein purpura there is generally a diffuse haemorrhagic vasculitis in the skin associated with glomerulonephritis. Although the pathogenesis of these diseases appears very similar, the reason why a particular organ or tissue is affected would appear to depend upon the nature of the antigen. It may be that the physico-chemical nature of the antigen will influence the particular organ or tissue to be affected. More is becoming known about the nature of the antigens both in SLE and in rheumatic fever. However, many questions have yet to be answered to account for the way in which the body reacts to these antigens.

Systemic Lupus Erythematosus

The demonstration by Hargreaves and his associates of the "LE" cell in the bone marrow of patients with SLE was the first step in unravelling the complex nature of this multiorgan disease. The typical LE cell is usually a polymorphonuclear leucocyte which has engulfed a large weakly basophilic inclusion body. Although originally described only in bone marrow preparations, these cells can be seen in smears of peripheral blood, if careful preparations of the buffy coat are examined after incubation *in vitro*.

It was next found that serum from patients with SLE contained a factor which could produce the LE phenomenon using leucocytes from normal subjects. The process of formation of LE cells could then be observed *in vitro*. It was found that the serum had the effect of lysing the nuclei of certain leucocytes and these lysed nuclei were then phagocytosed by other leucocytes. The LE factor was then isolated from the sera of patients with SLE and found to be an immunoglobulin of type IgG. It was thus found that the LE factor was a circulating autoantibody directed against the patient's own nuclei (Antinuclear factor— ANF). Serum from patients with SLE was also found to have the property of precipitating DNA *in vitro*. The precipitates could then be isolated and the IgG released from the immune complex. This purified antibody against DNA was also found to be capable of inducing the LE phenomenon *in vitro*.

The next stage in the investigation of the pathogenesis of this disease was the demonstration that both immunoglobulin and complement were present in the various visceral lesions of the disease. The technique used to demonstrate this is the fluorescent antibody technique. The principle of this reaction is illustrated in Fig. 1. Human antibody or complement can be demonstrated by preparing antisera in a rabbit against the antigenic determinants of these human proteins. These antisera are then conjugated with fluorescein and can be used as histochemical reagents to demonstrate the presence of specific antigens in tissue sections using microscopy with ultraviolet light to localize the presence of fluorescence on the section. This technique can be called the direct method. An indirect technique can be used in which these antisera themselves are not conjugated directly with the fluorescein but their presence on the section bound to antigens on human immunoglobulin or complement molecules, can be demonstrated by a sandwich technique using a fluorescent antiserum against the rabbit immunoglobulin which has first been bound to the specific antigens in the tissues. Antiserum

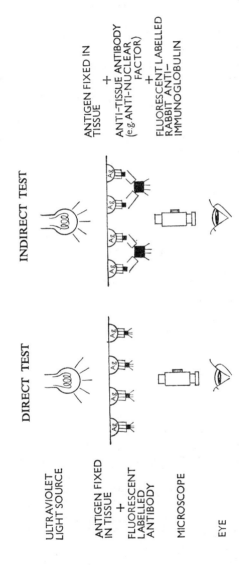

FIG. 1. The fluorescent antibody technique for detecting antigen fixed in tissues (direct) and anti-tissue antibodies in serum, e.g. antinuclear factor (indirect). (Coons.)

against rabbit immunoglobulin is prepared in goats or sheep and conjugated with fluorescein.

Antinuclear factor can also be demonstrated in the serum of patients with SLE and other diseases associated with autoimmune phenomena by the use of the fluorescent antibody technique, described above. Antinuclear factor in human serum will react with the nuclei of a wide range of animal tissues. The patient's serum is allowed to react with a section of rat liver. The section is then washed leaving the human antibody molecules attached to antigens in the nuclei of the rat liver. The section is then incubated with a rabbit anti-human IgG serum which has been conjugated with fluorescein. If antinuclear factor is present in the human serum, the nuclei of the rat liver will be found to fluoresce when examined by the microscope under ultraviolet light. Different sera containing different types of antinuclear factor produce different patterns of nuclear fluorescence and an attempt has been made to correlate these patterns with SLE and other chronic diseases in which antinuclear factor is found in the serum. Antibodies in SLE may be against double stranded (DS) DNA, single stranded (SS) DNA and other polynucleotides including ribonuclear proteins.

In addition to arthritis 60% of patients with SLE have renal disease. In a few this may take the form of "minimal change" nephritis. However in others there may be a membranous or focal glomerulonephritis and eventually a diffuse glomerulonephritis in which all the glomeruli are involved. In the minimal change disease IgG and C3 may be found in the mesangium, and in the membranous type the entire glomerular basement membrane is thickened. In active glomerulonephritis there will be granular and "lumpy bumpy" deposits. Activation of complement may be by DNA—antiDNA complexes or other polynucleotide—antibody complexes through the classical pathway as indicated by the presence of Clq or by the alternative pathway as indicated by the presence of properdin.

Direct evidence also exists for the presence of immune complexes in the circulation. Free DNA has been demonstrated in the circulation of some patients with SLE. Study of patients over a period of time show that either free DNA is present or antiDNA antibodies. However, neither are present together. This would appear to indicate that at some stages during the disease immune complexes are being formed and deposited in the tissues in antibody excess, whereas in other stages of the disease the complexes are formed in antigen excess. Free DNA has also been observed in the joint fluid from inflamed joints and immune complexes containing DNA have been observed in the skin lesions. Evidence for circulating complexes in SLE is derived not only from the deposits in the glomeruli from which DNA and antiDNA can be eluted but also from the finding of low levels of circulating complement. In addition the presence of nuclear antigen in the circulation alternates frequently with that of antinuclear antibodies, suggesting that the immune complexes are formed in antigen equivalence or excess. A test for circulating immune complexes has been devised involving the precipitation of Clq which is frequently positive in SLE. However this test is liable to produce false positives for a number of reasons including the fact that Clq is precipitated non-specifically by a wide range of biological polyanions. Finally indirect evidence for circulating immune complexes is provided by the observation that treatment of serum with DNAase increases the titre of antiDNA antibodies, presumably by releasing antibody from the complexes.

As well as the presence of immune complexes containing DNA, there are other phenomena which have to be accounted for. There is no doubt that in this disease there is an abnormal increased sensitivity of the antibody-forming system. Thus autoimmune antibodies are produced reacting with erythrocytes, platelets and probably also leucocytes. There is also a high incidence of drug allergy and blood group iso-immunization. This increased activity of the immunological mechanisms could arise as a result of the chronic inflammatory disease produced in the first place by the circulation of immune complexes. It is known that auto-antibodies such as rheumatoid factor and thyroid auto-antibodies can be produced as a result of a chronic inflammatory disease due to a known infective agent, such as in syphilis, or in leprosy. It may be that chronic inflammatory diseases cause an increased activity of the central immunological mechanisms in the same way as Freund's adjuvant in experimental animals. Both rheumatoid factor and organ specific auto-antibodies directed against the thyroid and stomach are found in SLE just as in syphilis and leprosy.

Of more interest in the aetiology of the disease is the high incidence of its occurrence following treatment of patients with a number of different drugs. The most common of these is hydralazine (Apresoline) used for hypertension. However, a wide selection of other drugs have been associated with the production of a lupus-like syndrome. These include anticonvulsants of the phenytoin group and troxidone, phenylbutazone, and antibiotics such as penicillin, streptomycin, tetracycline and isoniazid, as well as procaineamide used to treat cardiac arrhythmias. The wide distribution of these different chemical compounds makes it very difficult to suggest a common pathway by which these substances could act in initiating SLE. Indeed some authors believe that drugs themselves do not initiate the disease but unmask a predisposition to the disease which already exists. It has been suggested that certain patients have a "lupus" diathesis and treatment with these different compounds or perhaps an infection will uncover a latent process. If the drug which initiates the process is stopped the disease may become dormant again. However, in some cases reported, the disease has continued at the same level despite discontinuing the drugs.

Many of the drugs which instigate SLE such as hydralazine or penicillin are capable of reacting with proteins or nucleoproteins and acting as haptens. It may be that combination of the drug with nucleoprotein and sensitization to the carrier as well as to the hapten starts off the whole process by which the patient eventually produces antibody which can combine with his own unconjugated nucleoprotein. Hydralazine, however, has another property in that it is a strong enzyme inhibitor and it may be that it acts by inhibiting circulating DNAase and allowing free DNA to appear in the circulation and thus in the environment of the antibody stimulating mechanisms. At the moment the mechanism by which the body becomes sensitized to its own nuclear products is conjectural. However, once sensitized, immune complexes containing DNA and other nuclear components as antigens circulate and cause a disease similar to that of chronic serum sickness.

Mention should be made of the relationship between SLE and discoid lupus erythematosus which may have similar skin manifestations but is not associated with systemic disease. Despite the presence of antinuclear factor in the serum of up to 35% of patients with discoid LE, overt SLE develops in less than 5% of these patients. It is therefore considered by most authorities that discoid LE and SLE are separate disease entities with different ratios of sex and age-onset and thus probably occur in two different genetic groups.

Many people consider that SLE has an infective aetiology. Evidence for this is mainly from observations on the autoimmune disease of New Zealand black (NZB) mice. These mice develop a Coombs positive haemolytic anaemia and antinuclear factor in the serum. They also have nephritis with the deposition of immune complexes containing DNA in the glomeruli, and germinal centres and plasma cells in the thymus. This lupus-like disease has been shown to be associated with infection by an RNA virus. In addition an SLE-like syndrome has been described in dogs. In man electron microscopic evidence has been produced showing the presence of tubular structures, that could be of viral origin, in the cytoplasm of renal glomerular endothelial cells. Both antinuclear factor and LE cells are found as a result of a chronic infective disease process in leprosy where there is marked tissue damage. It may be therefore that in some cases SLE itself could have an infective origin due to a virus or another tissue destroying microorganism.

Most patients with SLE are treated with corticosteroids, the dose used being the minimum that will keep the disease under control. Imuran (Azathioprine) is now used in a number of centres in addition to the steroids. The dose used varies from centre to centre but is in the range of 1·5–3·0 mg/kg/day (in children 0·75 mg/kg/day). Those who use this drug state that it might take 6 weeks or more for the full effectiveness of this drug to be felt and after this, it is possible to lower the dose of steroids. 5 mg/kg/day has been found much too toxic a dose.

The margin between the therapeutic and toxic level of this drug is thus very slight. Some people feel that Imuran is more toxic than 6-MP. Imuran might be acting in SLE as an antiviral or anti-inflammatory agent, rather than by its immunosuppressive properties.

Rheumatoid Arthritis

This disease is much more widespread and much more chronic than SLE, but also has many features which suggest that it might also be another manifestation of the chronic circulation of immune complexes over a long period of time. As in SLE, germinal centres and plasma cells are found in the thymus indicating the possibility of similar aetiology. Apart from the arthritis there is the frequent occurrence of subcu-taneous nodules which develop as granulomata particularly around blood vessels. Granulomatous lesions are also found in the myocardium and lungs. The heart valves may also be involved in a rheumatoid granuloma or in a non-specific chronic endocarditis. Histologically the lesions of rheumatoid arthritis differ from those of SLE by the relative absence of fibrinoid deposits that are found in SLE. ˙

(a) *Rheumatoid factor*

The immunological nature of rheumatoid arthritis has been highlighted by the presence of "rheumatoid factor" in the serum of patients with rheumatoid arthritis. The original observation embodied in the Rose-Waaler test was that sera from patients with rheumatoid arthritis would agglutinate sheep erythrocytes coated with a subagglutinating dose of rabbit anti-sheep cell antiserum. It was later found that cells coated with γ-globulin from any species would be agglutinated by rheumatoid sera. Finally it was shown that rheumatoid sera would also agglutinate human red cells which had reacted with incomplete anti-Rhesus (D) antibodies. Latex particles coated with human γ-globulin are the particles generally used now to detect the presence of rheumatoid factor in patients' serum. Heat denatured γ-globulin can also be precipitated by rheumatoid sera. It appears that some alteration has to occur to the γ-globulin before it will react with rheumatoid sera. It either has to have reacted with antigen, be fixed non-specifically to particles or be denatured by heat. Thus rheumatoid factor appears to be an antibody directed against γ-globulin molecules which have had their tertiary structure modified either by reaction with antigen or by heat denaturation, so that certain antigenic groups, normally inacces-sible to reaction with a specific antibody, become unmasked.

Rheumatoid factor has a molecular weight of approximately 900,000 and is an immunoglobulin of the type IgM. By immunohistochemical techniques it can be shown to be made by plasma cells not only in the lymph nodes but also in the granulation tissue in the synovial mem-branes and the subcutaneous nodules. The same cells can be shown to be making IgM. Recently lower molecular weight theumatoid factors, IgG, IgD and IgA have also been found.

The antigen in human IgG which reacts with rheumatoid factor is not present in the IgG of all people. By the use of rheumatoid factor it is possible to divide people into two groups, one with IgG which reacts with rheumatoid factor and the other with IgG which does not react with rheumatoid factor. These antigens on the IgG molecule are analogous to bloodgroups and are called Gm groups or allotypes of human γ-globulin. Those sera, which contain IgG which reacts with rheumatoid factor, are designated as being of serum group Gm (a+), whereas those lacking it are of serum groups Gm (a−). This characteristic of IgG molecules is genetically determined by a dominant autosomal gene. Other similar genetically controlled antigens have been discovered on the IgG molecule by the use of other antisera and have been designated Gm (b) and Gm (x). Although rheumatoid sera only react with IgG molecules which are Gm (a+), when bound to antigen, they will however react with all IgG molecules whether Gm (a+) or Gm (a−) if they are denatured by heat. Thus the rheumatoid factor appears to consist of antibodies which react with other antigens than the Gm (a+) antigen on the IgG molecule as well as the Gm (a+) antigen, but these are only revealed when the molecule is unfolded to a greater degree by heat denaturation than by reaction with antigen.

There has been considerable speculation as to the role of the rheumatoid factor in the pathogenesis of rheumatoid arthritis. As with the antinuclear factor, it can be found in the serum of a small proportion of patients with a wide range of other diseases, especially granulomatous diseases such as leprosy and syphilis in the absence of any clinical signs of arthritis. However, IgG-rheumatoid factor and IgG-β_{1c} globulin complexes have been demonstrated in the synovial membrane of patients with rheumatoid arthritis. Moreover, the injection of autologous IgG into the quiescent joints of patients with rheumatoid arthritis results in acute synovitis, if rheumatoid factor can be demonstrated in either the serum or joint fluid. Synovitis also occurs if the IgG is obtained from another rheumatoid patient but not with that from normal subjects. Despite these findings, it is likely that the rheumatoid factor is an autoantibody which develops as a result of the disease and is not involved in the pathogenesis of rheumatoid arthritis.

(b) *The possible pathogenesis of rheumatoid arthritis*

It is generally accepted that rheumatoid arthritis is a disease in which immunological mechanisms play a considerable role in the pathogenesis. However, as yet no clue has been given to the nature of the antigenic stimulus. Two possible causes have been considered. In the first it is suggested that the disease might have an infective origin. The other possibility that has been investigated is that the disease could be an autoimmune process, possibly to fibrin which has been altered antigenically. A number of models exist for the production of arthritis in experimental animals. A condition more akin to rheumatoid arthritis is the polyarthritis caused by *Mycoplasma hyorhinis* in pigs, where the disease can be transferred from animal to animal by the organism under controlled conditions. This disease resembles rheumatoid arthritis in man, in a number of ways. The histological picture of the inflammatory process is very similar. The disease is chronic and non-suppurating. The infiltrating cells are lymphocytes, macrophages and plasma cells, and lymphoid follicles can be seen in the granulation tissue round the joints. Other mycoplasmas have been isolated from cases of spontaneous arthritis arising in cattle, goat, sheep, rats and mice. However, the disease process in these cases is more acute and the infiltrate contains more polymorphonuclear leucocytes than the disease in man or pigs.

The possibility that rheumatoid arthritis in man could be caused by infection with mycoplasma is only a suggestion at the present time. This is partly based on the frequent association of arthritis in other animals with these organisms. There have recently been reports of increased delayed hypersensitivity to *Mycoplasma fermentans* in patients with rheumatoid arthritis using *in vitro* techniques. *Mycoplasma fermentans* has also been isolated with an increased frequency from the joints of patients with rheumatoid arthritis. However, it is not known whether under these circumstances the organism is acting as a pathogenic agent or whether it is merely present as a commensal. Moreover the positive *in vitro* delayed hypersensitivity tests have been shown to be directed against IgG bound tᵣ the Mycoplasma rather than to the organism itself.

Another possibility that has been considered seriously is that the disease is a hypersensitivity reaction to the patient's own fibrin which has been altered antigenically in some way. The subcutaneous implantation of heterologous fibrin in an experimental animal is followed after several weeks by a reaction which resembles very closely that found in a rheumatoid nodule. If an animal is sensitized to a foreign fibrin and then that fibrin is injected into a joint, the joint will develop typical hyperplasia of the synovial lining cells, pannus formation with erosion of the articular cartilage and adjacent bone, and chronic inflammation of the synovial membrane. Lymphoid follicles with germinal centres and many plasma cells can also be seen in the granulation tissue round the affected joint, just as in rheumatoid arthritis in man.

Another experimental model which should be mentioned is the so-called "adjuvant arthritis" in rats. If rats are injected intradermally in the footpad with an oil in water emulsion containing dead tubercle bacilli (Freund's complete adjuvant) they develop a disease which has many parallels with Reiter's syndrome, Behçet's disease, Stevens-

Johnson syndrome, and post-gonococcal arthritis as well as rheumatoid arthritis. As well as polyarthritis with a mononuclear infiltration and typical pannus formation, skin lesions are seen at other sites of frequent trauma—these are eyes, ears, skin, penis, and the surface of the tail.

Opinion is divided as to whether rheumatoid arthritis is fundamentally caused by cell-mediated immunity or humoral antibodies. At the present time it would appear more likely that the disease could be initiated by circulating immune complexes, which localize at the sites of maximum trauma, in this case the joints, or to antigen–antibody interaction across blood vessel walls. However, the relative parts played by humoral antibody and cell-mediated immunity has yet to be determined. The association of plasma cell proliferation and germinal centre formation in areas of chronic inflammation and in the thymus as well as in the lymph nodes and spleen would be consistent with humoral antibodies playing a considerable role in this disease.

(c) *Treatment*

In very severe cases corticosteroids have to be used and occasionally a combination of Imuran and the steroid has been used as in SLE, when the dose of steroids necessary to control the patient becomes too great.

Rheumatic Fever

This again could be a disease caused by the circulation of immune complexes and their localization in areas of trauma. The polyarthritis associated with the acute myocardial and valvular disease are consistent with this concept. Acute rheumatic fever has been shown to occur consistently following streptococcal infection, usually of the throat. The illness generally begins at a time when antibodies are beginning to be produced against the organism. Thus if there was absorption of streptococcal antigen into the blood stream, there is every reason why there should be the circulation of immune complexes. However, one of the main problems in this interpretation is that only approximately 2-3% of patients with streptococcal infection develop the signs and symptoms of rheumatic fever. The low incidence of the disease following streptococcal infection could be related to the type of immune response produced by the patient against the streptococcal antigens and the avidity of the antibody produced, as immune complex disease appears to develop only when complexes are formed in antigen excess. The incidence of rheumatic fever has been shown to be proportional to the magnitude of the antibody response to the streptococcal antigens. The type of immune response occurring can be judged by following the levels of antibodies in the serum against streptolysin O.

The reason why the heart is so frequently involved in rheumatic fever is that there is a cross reaction between streptococcal antigens and organ specific antigens in heart muscle. This cross reaction also exists with skeletal muscle and with blood vessels. Antibodies reacting with both human heart muscle and streptococci can be found in the serum of patients with rheumatic fever. Both can be absorbed out with either streptococci or heart muscle and the antibody can be shown to be the same. This antibody reacts with the sarcolemma of cardiac myofibrils. The antibodies persist after the streptococcal infection is over and are present in patients with chronic rheumatic carditis. In rheumatic fever γ-globulin and complement may be found deposited in cardiac muscle and in the smooth muscle of vessel walls as well as in altered connective tissue. These are the sites which have been shown to be reactive with streptococcal antiserum that cross-reacts with heart muscle. Scattered deposits are found in chronic rheumatic heart disease. However, in fatal cases of acute rheumatic fever associated with cardiac failure the deposits may be quite massive. Although the cross-reacting antibodies which react with both streptococcal M antigens and heart muscle may be found in uncomplicated streptococcal infections, there is an increased frequency of the occurrence of these antibodies in rheumatic fever and rheumatic heart disease. It is probable that cell-mediated reactions could also play a considerable role in the mechanism of rheumatic carditis, as little or no immunoglobulin can be found in the typical granulomatous lesions of the disease, the Aschoff lesions in the heart muscle. This cell-mediated reaction could be directed against the same sarcolemmal antigens as the circulating antibodies. Immunoglobulins can, however, be demonstrated on the sarcolemmal surface of the cardiac muscle fibres. Arthritis of probable immune complex aetiology may also be associated with infectious diseases due to a wide range of organisms. These include gonococci, meningococci, Shigella, *Yersinia enterocolitica*, viruses such as rubella and measles, and chlamydia.

Polyarteritis Nodosa

The necrosis and fibrinoid changes found in the media of small arterioles in the disease polyarteritis nodosa in man are very similar to the change in blood vessels found in the Arthus reaction produced in experimental animals. Similar lesions have also been found in experimental serum sickness and after repeated streptococcal infections in experimental animals. In man polyarteritis nodosa has been associated with chronic bacterial infections but there is also a marked association with drug therapy. In some cases the development of the lesions has actually occurred during a serum sickness type of disease known to be caused by a particular drug. In other cases an attack of polyarteritis nodosa has been precipitated in the same patient on different occasions by the use of a drug. The drugs which have been incriminated in this way are thiourea, thiouracil and neoarsphenamine.

Polyarteritis nodosa is one form in which a vasculitis can cause disease. Sometimes the vasculitis is limited to the skin. The actual nature of the lesion will depend on the level at which the antigen–antibody reaction occurs in the peripheral circulation and whether the lesion is due to the deposit of immune complexes in the vessel wall or whether there is antigen–antibody interaction across the vessel wall as in the Arthus phenomenon. Lesions may be haemorrhagic, infarcts or form nodular granulomata. A severe form of polyarteritis is that known as Wegener's granulomatosis in which ulcerating lesions of the upper respiratory tract may be accompanied by widespread vasculitis and glomerulonephritis. Vascular lesions in the skin in various types of allergic vasculitis have been examined by immuno-histochemical methods using the fluorescent antibody technique, described above. In a number of cases deposits of immunoglobulin and complement have been demonstrated in the inflamed vessel wall with the same distribution as that found in the Arthus reaction in experimental animals. Strepto-coccal, staphylococcal, mycobacterial, Hepatitis B and Candida anti-gens have been demonstrated in the lesions in the skin of patients with different forms of allergic vasculitis diagnosed variously as polyarteritis nodosa or nodular vasculitis, sometimes associated with IgG or IgM and complement. The evidence that these complexes have caused the lesions in which they can be demonstrated is so far circumstantial, as similar lesions can be induced experimentally with bacterial antigens alone and these can then predispose to the localization in the lesion of immune complexes containing other non-cross-reacting antigens. These complexes which may be deposited in a secondary fashion may not even exacerbate the existing lesion in the tissues. Despite these findings, the resemblance between these lesions and Arthus reactions associated with the time relation between their development and infection in a number of cases suggests that an immunological basis should not yet be too readily discarded.

Dermatomyositis

This is a diffuse erythematous rash often with thickening of the skin and muscle weakness, which sometimes occurs as a dermatological complication of neoplastic disease. In some of these cases antibodies have been found in the serum which react with extracts of the tumour. At the same time immunoglobulin can be demonstrated on the surface of striated muscle and on the surface of collagen bundles in the skin. It is possible that antibody could be reacting with tumour antigens released into the circulation, on the surface of muscle bundles and collagen fibres.

Diffuse Scleroderma

The thickening of the collagen in the skin typical of scleroderma can be associated in some cases with features of a diffuse disease in which there is fibrosis not only of the skin but also around joints, in the lungs and in the myocardium. There may also be fibrinoid necrosis of blood vessels in the kidney, involving the glomeruli. A picture similar to this disease has been produced in rats by the injection of homologous lymphocytes into a recipient which had previously been made tolerant to these cells. This graft versus host disease, sometimes called "homologous disease" is associated with the development over a period of three weeks by listlessness, weight loss, purpura and arthritis. The arthritis is associated with a mononuclear cell infiltration involving the synovial membrane and adjacent connective tissue. The cell types seen are histiocytes, lymphocytes and plasma cells. The skin lesions are characterized microscopically by an increase in the collagen of the dermis with some atrophy of the epidermis and skin appendages. There is little cellular infiltration, as in scleroderma in the human. These changes in the skin can progress ultimately to extreme atrophy of the epidermis with marked hyperkeratosis and thickening of the dermis due mainly to the large increase in the content of collagen.

The fact that scleroderma can be produced in experimental animals by the injection of immunologically active cells which react against the recipient but cannot be rejected, suggests an immunological mechanism in this disease in the human. Moreover antinuclear factor occurs in the serum of up to 80% of patients with this disease. At present there have been no suggestions as to the actual mechanism of the immunological reaction that might cause this disease, especially as there is often very little cellular infiltration in the thickened dermis.

Sjögren's Disease

This disease in which there is chronic inflammation of the salivary and lachrymal glands is often associated with rheumatoid arthritis. Precipitating antibodies exist in the serum which react with extracts of salivary and lachrymal glands. However, antibodies also exist which react with thyroglobulin. There is also a high incidence of LE cells and antinuclear factor in the serum as well as rheumatoid factor. It may be that the disease is basically one due to chronic infection in which the autoimmune phenomena are secondary to a primary infective process, with associated circulation of immune complexes causing the arthritis. However, at the present time little is known about the aetiology of this disease and many workers seem satisfied with just calling this an "autoimmune disease" without looking any further for the cause of the associated autoimmune phenomena. As in SLE and rheumatoid arthritis germinal centres and plasma cells may be found in the thymus, indicating the possibility of a related aetiology.

Bibliography

Books

Dubois, E. L. (ed.) (1966), *Lupus Erythematosus*. New York: McGraw-Hill.
Dumonde, D. C. (ed.) (1976), *Infection and Immunology in the Rheumatic Diseases*. Oxford: Blackwell.
Glynn, L. E. & Holborow, E. J. (1974), *Autoimmunity and Disease*. Oxford: Blackwell. Second edition.
Maini, R. N., Glass, D. N. and Scott, J. T. (1977), *Immunology of the Rheumatic Diseases*. London: Edward Arnold.
Rotstein, J. (ed.) (1966), *Rheumatology. An Annual Review*. Vol. 1. Basel: Karger.
Samter, M. (ed.) (1971), *Immunological Diseases*. 2nd edition. Boston: Little Brown and Co.

Articles

Alarçon-Segovia, D., Worthington, J. W., Ward, L. E. & Wakin, K. (1965), "Lupus diathesis and the hydralazine syndrome." *New Engl. J. Med.*, 272, 462.
Beck, J. S. & Rowell, N. R., "Discoid Lupus Erythematosus." *Quart. J. Med.*, 35, 119.
Parish, W. E. (1971), "Studies on Vasculitis I., Immunoglobulins, β_1c, C-reactive protein and bacterial antigens in cutaneous vasculitis lesions." *Clinical Allergy*, 1, 97.
Stastny, P., Stembridge, V. A. & Ziff, M. (1963), "Homologous disease in the adult rat, a model for autoimmune disease. I. General features and cutaneous lesions." *J. exp. Med.*, 118, 635.
Stastny, P., Stembridge, V. A., Vischer, T. & Ziff, M. (1965), "Homologous disease in the adult rat, a model for auto-immune disease. II. Findings in the joints, heart and other tissues." *J. exp. Med.*, 122, 681.

Chapter X
Immunological Processes in Diseases of the Kidney

As has been mentioned frequently in previous chapters the "serum sickness" syndrome due to circulation of soluble immune complexes is commonly associated with clinical features attributable to involvement of the kidney in this disease complex. Study of serum sickness in its various forms, both acute and chronic, in experimental animals has reproduced many of the histological features associated with glomerulonephritis in the human. This has stimulated considerable study of the various ways renal damage can be produced by immunological means in experimental animals. Attempts are also being made to correlate further the changes produced in the kidney under controlled experimental conditions in animals, with those observed in human renal disease, so that more information can be gained about both the aetiology and pathogenesis of these conditions. As a direct result of the realization that much renal disease can involve immunological processes, successful steps have already been made in the treatment of these diseases with immunosuppressive drugs. It is therefore logical to start a chapter on the immunological basis of renal disease with a description of the methods used to produce renal disease as a result of immunological processes in experimental animals and compare the different renal lesions thus produced. This will be followed by a comparison of these lesions with those found in human disease and finally there will be a discussion of the present status of the immunosuppressive treatment of both acute and chronic renal disease.

The Experimental Production of Renal Disease

A. *Experimental serum sickness*

Glomerulonephritis can be readily produced in experimental animals by circulating antigen–antibody complexes. Soluble immune complexes are localized in the glomeruli for purely mechanical and non-immunological reasons and thus induce renal damage.

Acute glomerulonephritis can be demonstrated as a feature of the serum sickness produced by a single large injection of a foreign protein and develops at the time that the animal begins to make circulating antibody which can complex with the circulating foreign antigen. This occurs about one week after the injection of the antigen and is associated with the presence of protein and casts in the urine and a raised blood urea which may last for several days or weeks. The disease begins to subside as soon as circulating immune complexes are eliminated from the circulation.

Histologically there is proliferation of the endothelial cells of the glomeruli and occasionally epithelial crescents are seen. However, in this acute condition little change is seen in the glomerular basement membrane. Using immuno-histochemical methods (the fluorescent antibody technique, see p. 122) antigen, antibody and complement can be seen as fine granular ("lumpy bumpy") deposits along the glomerular capillary wall (Fig. 1).

The disease is thus due to the immune complexes being trapped in the glomerular filter. A similar form of glomerulonephritis can be produced readily by the intravenous injection of prepared immune complexes. Evidence exists that nephritis occurs under experimental conditions when complexes are formed in antigen excess, rather than

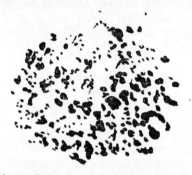

FIG. 1. "Lumpy bumpy" distribution of immunoglobulin and complement in the glomerulus in "serum sickness" type nephritis.

in antibody excess. Dissociated immune complexes will not localize in the glomeruli and the size of the immune complex formed is important in its localization. The larger the complexes formed, the more readily they are localized in the glomeruli and eliminated from the circulation. Light weight complexes are not held up by the glomerular filter. The immune complexes are not phagocytosed by the endothelial cells nor have they any affinity for the vascular membrane cells, but they appear to be held up at the vascular basement membrane which acts as a filtering device preventing their passage. Release of histamine and other vasoactive amines by immune complexes favours the localization of these complexes at the glomerular basement membrane, and this localization can be inhibited by antihistamine drugs and inhibitors of serotonin, which reduce the intensity of experimentally produced glomerulonephritis. The complexes held up at the glomerular basement membrane activate complement which attracts polymorphonuclear leucocytes chemotactically and thus sets in motion the chain of events leading to disease.

There are probably two phases in the glomerular vasculitis caused by the deposition of immune complexes, the first is the attraction of polymorphonuclear leucocytes to the site and this is then followed by the release of enzymes, which damage tissues, and substances which cause an increased vascular permeability. Polymorphs contain a number of such substances in their granules. Among these are proteolytic enzymes which can degrade the vascular basement membrane. These proteolytic enzymes can also cause the release of the vasoactive substance bradykinin from serum proteins. Bradykinin causes further attraction of polymorphs, increased vascular permeability and capillary dilatation. Other permeability increasing substances are released as well as fibrinolytic enzymes.

It has been known for many years that repeated injections of foreign proteins into experimental animals caused the development of chronic glomerulonephritis. Animals may respond in three ways to such injections: (1) no antibody response—thus no immune complex formation and no disease; (2) massive antibody response and thus rapid elimination of circulating antigen by phagocytosis; (3) small to moderate antibody response allowing formation of immune complexes in antigen excess. Animals producing massive antibody response will develop an acute glomerulonephritis at the onset of the antibody response but this will be a self-limiting disease and will resolve as soon as enough antibody is produced for the complexes to be formed in antibody excess and phagocytosed. Almost all animals which develop a mild or moderate antibody response will have circulating immune complexes formed in antigen excess due to the repeated injection of foreign antigen. These animals will gradually develop proteinuria over a number of weeks. Histologically the disease is different from that seen in acute serum sickness as there is thickening of the glomerular basement membrane as well as proliferation of the endothelial cells. This leads to the formation of epithelial crescents and scarring of the glomeruli. Antigen, γ-globulin and complement can be found localized as dense "lumpy bumpy" deposits. The more intense the deposit of immune complexes, the more severe is the disease seen. Once the disease is established, it can be only partially reversed when antigen injection is stopped.

B. *Nephrotoxic serum nephritis*
In this experimental model the donor is immunized with renal tissue from an animal of a different species. A serum is produced and injected back into an animal of the species from which the renal tissue was originally taken to immunize the donor. This serum contains antibodies directed mainly against the glomeruli. However, the recipient also produces antibodies against the foreign serum thus two processes occur, one following the other. During the first week the disease is due purely to the effect of the foreign antiserum on the glomeruli,

but as soon as the recipient starts making antibody against the foreign serum, immune complexes are formed in which host antibody reacts with the foreign antibody deposited on the renal glomeruli, causing a more severe immune reaction. Heterologous nephrotoxic antibodies are directed mainly against the glomerular basement membrane and the foreign antibody can be demonstrated by the fluorescent antibody technique to form a uniform linear deposit (Fig. 2) along the glomerular capillary wall. When the host antibody is formed against the foreign serum, this also can be shown to have the same uniform linear distribution. This uniform linear distribution of immunoglobulin and complement seen in "nephrotoxic serum nephritis" contrasts strongly with the "lumpy bumpy" deposits seen in serum sickness nephritis.

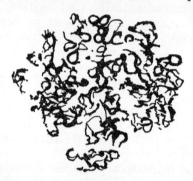

FIG. 2. Uniform distribution of immunoglobulins and complement along the glomerular capillary walls. Appearance found in nephrotoxic serum nephritis in experimental animals and Goodpasture's syndrome in the human.

The histological lesion seen in "nephrotoxic serum nephritis" also differs from that seen in "serum sickness nephritis". In "serum sickness nephritis" the lesion is on the epithelial side of the basement membrane, whereas in "nephrotoxic serum nephritis" the lesion is on the luminar side of the basement membrane. A mixed pattern of proliferative and membranous glomerulonephritis is seen in "nephrotoxic serum nephritis". Although immunoglobulin and complement deposits are localized to the glomeruli, changes are also found histologically in the convoluted tubules. These consist of cellular proliferation and a loss of enzyme activity, followed by some atrophy of the tubules.

It is considered that the process by which antiglomerular antibodies injure the kidney is by fixing complement. This then attracts polymorphonuclear leucocytes which release the proteolytic enzymes and pharmacological mediators which cause the damage. However, it has been found that the antiglomerular antibodies can also damage the glomeruli directly in the absence of complement.

Another factor causing damage to the glomeruli is that deposits of antibody in the glomerular capillary wall can cause deposition of fibrin and thus thrombosis. The importance of this in the pathogenesis of the disease is emphasized by the fact that the disease is not so severe in animals treated with anticoagulants. Anticoagulants can also prevent fibrin deposition and thus crescent formation in Bowman's capsule.

In conclusion it must be emphasized that nephrotoxic serum nephritis forms an experimental model for the presence of foreign antigen deposited in a linear uniform manner along the glomerular basement membrane in such a way that host antibody reacts with it directly and thus sets in motion a train of events leading to renal damage. It is therefore forming one experimental model of what would happen if autoantibodies were produced against antigens in the glomerulus in the human.

C. *Autoimmune nephritis*

A further experimental model for the type of nephritis which could be produced by autoimmune process in man, can be produced by immunizing animals either with homologous or heterologous renal antigens. Nephritis can be induced reproducibly in experimental animals by the intraperitoneal injection of kidney extract in adjuvant mixture at biweekly intervals for 3–5 months. This type of nephritis is a chronic membranous disease with very little proliferation or exudation. The glomerular basement membrane is thickened, but there are also prominent interstitial and tubular lesions. As in nephrotoxic serum nephritis the tubular lesions may sometimes appear to be secondary to the glomerular changes. Immunoglobulin and complement can be seen deposited in the glomerular capillary wall in a uniform but fine granular pattern. The distribution is different from that seen in nephrotoxic serum nephritis and more like that seen in serum sickness nephritis. Immunoglobulin can also be seen in some species localized on the tubular basement membrane.

The antigen involved in the immunization is not organ specific as similar renal disease can be produced by injections of liver. In the kidney the effective antigen is derived from the tubules and not from the glomeruli as might be expected. This, together with the granular deposition of immune complexes in the glomeruli suggests that the renal disease is actually produced by the circulation of immune complexes and not by the direct effect of the antiglomerular antibodies.

Nephritis in Animals Caused by Virus Infections

(a) *NZB mice*. Mice of this strain have been found spontaneously to develop "autoimmune" haemolytic anaemia, hepatomegaly, splenomegaly and antinuclear factor in their serum. Some of these mice also develop a chronic membranous glomerulonephritis. Immunoglobulins are detected in the glomeruli with a "lumpy bumpy" distribution reminiscent of "serum sickness" nephritis due to the deposition of circulating immune complexes. In fact the mice have antibodies which react with an antigen also present in the serum of these mice which deposits in the glomerular capillaries.

Further studies have shown that these mice are infected from birth with a virus which has been identified within the kidney and that the renal disease has been transferred to uninfected mice of a different strain by filtrates of tissues from NZB mice. The antigen causing the "serum sickness"-like lesions in the renal glomeruli appears to be DNA which could have been released by the action of the infectious agent. This complexes with anti-DNA antibodies and is deposited in the renal glomeruli. Treatment of the mice with cyclophosphamide causes improvement in the nephritis and a reduction in the amount of immune complexes deposited. It is possible that this is not an immunosuppressive effect and could be the result of a viricidal action of the drug. Decrease in the amount of virus present would result in a decrease in the amount of DNA released into the circulation and a decrease in the amount of immune complexes deposited in the glomeruli.

(b) *Other virus diseases of animals.* Glomerulonephritis can occur in induced or natural infections in which immune complexes containing viral antigen occur in the circulation. These include lymphocytic choriomeningitis (LCM) of mice, Aleutian disease of mink and lactic dehydrogenase virus infections of mice. In LCM infection the virus in the circulation is present complexed with host immunoglobulin and complement in 2–3 month old mice. There is a progressive accumulation of IgG, complement and viral antigen in irregular deposits along the capillary wall and mesangia from the first 3 weeks of life. Moreover, IgG can be eluted from the kidneys and can be shown to be antibody which reacts specifically with LCM virus antigen.

In Aleutian disease of mink there is also a progressive renal disease which has been shown to be caused by a filterable virus. In severely affected animals, the glomerulus shows thickening and distortion due to the accumulation of large amounts of abnormal eosinophilic material. There is marked increase in the number of mesangial and endothelial cells. The appearance of the glomeruli is very similar to that seen in the disease of NZB mice described above. Other changes are due to the presence of fine thrombi in the glomerular capillaries. Immunoglobulins are found in the glomeruli of affected animals but the distribution is different to that seen in "serum sickness" nephritis or nephrotoxic serum nephritis, and has been described to have a mesangial pattern. Although it has been suggested that renal damage may probably be due to intravascular coagulation, there is no doubt that this condition is also an immune complex nephritis.

Human Renal Disease

A. *Immune complex nephritis due to infectious agents*

The immunological origin of post-streptococcal glomerulonephritis has been suspected for many years. The delay between streptococcal infection and the appearance of the nephritis is similar to that between the injection of foreign serum and the development of serum sickness.

Examination of glomeruli during this disease has shown deposits of IgG and complement in discrete nodules similar to that seen in serum sickness nephritis in the experimental animal. Streptococcal antigen can also be demonstrated in the glomeruli of some patients with this disease. It has been suggested that this form of nephritis was due to cross reaction between glomerular antigens and streptococcal antigens. If this was so the distribution of immunoglobulin and complement would have been of the smooth linear type seen in experimental nephrotoxic serum nephritis.

Immune complex nephritis may also be found in infections with *Plasmodium malariae, Schistosoma mansoni, Treponema pallidum,* hepatitis B, measles and EB virus. In all these conditions either antigen or specific antibody have been demonstrated or eluted from the kidney. Immune complex nephritis has been conceived of as a relative "immunodeficiency" disease, in which the immune response is insufficient to eradicate the antigen, allowing its persistence, while at the same time sufficient antibody is produced to allow immune complex formation.

B. *Chronic renal disease*

Steroid sensitive minimal change nephritis (lipoid nephrosis) accounts for 20–30% of patients with nephrotic syndrome. In this condition there is no microscopic evidence of immune complex deposition, although evidence is accumulating for the presence of immune complexes in the circulation.

IgG and complement are generally distributed as nodular deposits in a linear pattern along the glomerular capillary wall in the proliferative or membranous types of nephritis, or where both these patterns coexist. In the more severe nephrotic syndrome, the glomeruli may show thickening of the mesangium and glomerular stalk region due to an increased number of mesangial cells and focal areas of proliferation. In these patients immunoglobulins and complement can be demonstrated in a focal and local pattern at the base of some glomeruli in the stem or mesangial region. This pattern of deposition of IgG and complement may be unassociated with the basement membrane.

The uniform linear distribution of immunoglobulin within the basement membrane without extramembranous deposits seen typically in experimental nephrotoxic serum nephritis is seen in some patients with chronic nephritis associated with purpura in the lungs (Goodpasture's syndrome). In Goodpasture's syndrome anti-glomerular antibodies are present in the circulation. Passive transfer of serum from a patient with Goodpasture's syndrome to a monkey has been found to produce a glomerulonephritis in which immunoglobulin could be demonstrated with the same typical linear distribution as that found in the human disease.

C. *Nephritis associated with systemic lupus erythematosus (SLE)*

In SLE, nephritis is associated with presence of deposits of immuno-globulins (IgG and IgM) and complement in the discrete nodular form typical of "experimental serum sickness nephritis". This is also the same distribution as that found in the glomeruli of NZB mice with nephritis which also have circulating antinuclear antibodies in their plasma. The glomeruli have also been shown to contain nucleo-protein antigen which can be eluted. Thus it appears that the nephritis may be a serum sickness type in which circulating immune complexes containing DNA or nucleoprotein as antigen are held up by the glomerular basement membrane and thus initiate the well-known disease process.

D. *Different types of glomerular deposits found in human disease*

Glomerular lesions in human renal disease may contain IgG, IgA, IgM, C3, C1q, C4, properdin and fibrinogen. This would indicate activation of both the classical and alternative pathways of complement. Apart from the lesions of Goodpasture's syndrome, the appearance of the deposits have the so-called "lumpy bumpy" appearance typical of "immune complex disease". These deposits may be extramembranous lying on the Bowman's capsule side of the basement membrane of the glomerular tuft, or else may be subendothelial lying on the capillary side. In some cases the deposition may have a mesangial distribution, the deposits being located between the mesangial cells and the basement membrane. The relationship between the different forms of deposit and the type of glomerular damage found is very obscure. These extramembranous deposits are found both in acute post-streptococcal nephritis and in the nephrotic syndrome following infection with *Plasmodium malariae* and subendothelial deposits occur mainly in membranoproliferative glomerulonephritis. Mesangial deposits may be found particularly associated with focal glomerular lesions. The extramembranous deposits of acute glomerulonephritis usually con-tain IgG and C3, whereas those of membranous glomerulonephritis contain IgG only. The subendothelial deposits of membranopro-liferative nephritis contain IgG and IgM as well as C3 but in the later stage of the disease may contain C3 only. The mesangial deposits of focal glomerulonephritis may contain IgA as well as IgG and C3. In the nephritis of systemic lupus erythematosus the deposits may be extramembranous, mesangial or subendothelial and contain IgA as well as IgG, IgM and C3. In Henoch Schonlein purpura there may be mesangial or subendothelial deposits. These can contain IgA, IgG and C3. The pathophysiological processes, that underly whether deposits in the glomeruli are immunoglobulin, complement or fibrin, are little understood. At the present time there is no direct evidence that mesangial deposits are produced by immunological processes. Moreover, focal subendothelial deposits of these proteins can be found in the glomeruli in hypertensive and diabetic nephropathies indicating the possibility that these could also be deposited secondary to non-specific damage.

Complement Changes in Glomerulonephritis

The level of circulating complement has been found to be depressed in up to 75% of cases of acute glomerulonephritis. If the patient recovers the levels return to normal. However, if the disease progresses to sub-acute nephritis levels generally remain low. Depression may be of total haemolytic complement (CH50), C3, C4 and C3PA (C3 proactivator or Factor B, a participant in the alternative pathway). Simultaneous depression of C4 and C3PA means activation of both the classical and alternative pathways. Immune complexes activating complement by the classical pathway could result in a release of C3b which itself could cause alternative pathway activation. Low complement levels are found particularly in membrano-proliferative glomerulonephritis. These patients may initially appear to have acute nephritis or recurrent haematuria, but the majority have persistent proteinuria or a nephrotic syndrome with hypertension and haematuria. Levels of total haemolytic complement and C3 are variable in chronic nephritis and have no diagnostic or prognostic value. Clq, C4 and properdin levels may also be low, indicating involvement of both the classical and alternative pathways. In membrano-proliferative glomerulonephritis the serum often contains a factor known as C3 nephritic factor (C3Nef) which causes C3 conversion when added to normal human serum. As a result of this, C3d, one of the breakdown products of C3 is frequently found in the serum of these patients. C3Nef has been found to contain IgG and may be a low molecular weight circulating immune complex.

The Use of Immunosuppressive Drugs in the Treatment of Chronic Renal Disease

Cyclophosphamide has been shown experimentally to inhibit the lupus-like nephritis of NZB mice, and encouraging results have been found with this drug in man. However, the best treatment of steroid resistant nephritis has been found to be a combination of high doses of prednisone with azathioprine. In one series significant improvement was found in between 50–70% of cases treated. The best results have been found in lupus nephritis or those with proliferative, membranous or mixed proliferative and membranous lesions. Poor results were obtained in one series in the nephrotic group of patients where there were minimal or no glomerular changes seen histologically, whereas in another study however, some improvement was seen in patients in this group.

Signs of improvement, that have been found, are a decrease in proteinuria, increase in creatinine clearance (glomerular filtration rate) and an increase in the level of circulating complement. In a number of cases there was a marked decrease in the amount of immunoglobulin and complement deposited in the glomerulus. There was also a marked improvement in the histological appearance of the glomeruli seen on renal biopsy. The reduction in the deposition of immune complexes in the glomeruli or deposition of antibody in Goodpasture's syndrome, associated with evidence of a reduction in circulating immune complexes, as shown by a rise in serum complement activity, would indicate that treatment with combined azathioprine and prednisone was producing an actual reduction in antibody and that this was true immunosuppression rather than an anti-inflammatory effect.

The dosage used in one trial was azathioprine 10 mg/kg body weight for one to two days, followed by 6–8 mg/kg for one to two days and then 4 mg/kg daily. Prednisone was given in a dosage of 60 mg per square metre body surface per 24 hours. This was then reduced after a month to a better tolerated level. Treatment was continued for up to a year and after stopping treatment a number of the patients maintained their improvement. Anti-lymphocyte serum has been used in the treatment of glomerulonephritis. Results are, however, difficult to interpret and at the best equivocal.

Bibliography

Books

Germuth, F. G. & Rodriguez, E. (1973), *Immunopathology of the Renal Glomerulus.* Boston: Little Brown.

Articles

Dixon, F. J., Edgington, T. S. & Lambert, P. H. (1968), "Non-glomerular antigen-antibody complex nephritis." *Immunopathology Vth International Symposium. Mechanisms of Inflammation Induced by Immune Reactions*, p. 17. Éds. P. A. Miescher & P. Grabar. Basel: Schwabe and Co.

Drummond, N., Michael, A. F., Good, R. A. & Vernier, R. L. (1966), "The nephrotic syndrome of childhood: Immunologic, clinical and pathological considerations." *J. clin. Invest.*, **45**, 620.

Markowitz, A. S., Battifora, H. A., Schwartz, F. & Aseron, C. (1968), "Immunological aspects of Goodpasture's syndrome." *Clin. exp. Immunol.*, **3**, 585.

Michael, A. F., Vernier, R. L., Drummond, K. N., Levitt, J. I., Herdman, R. C., Fish, A. J. & Good, R. A. (1967), "Immunosuppressive therapy of chronic renal disease." *New Engl. J. Med.*, **276**, 817.

Miescher, P. A. & Grabar, P. (eds.) (1968), "WHO Conference on use of antimetabolites in disease associated with abnormal immune responses." *Immunopathology Vth International Symposium. Mechanisms of Inflammation Induced by Immune Responses*, p. 359. Basel: Schwabe and Co.

Morel-Maroger, L. (1976), "Histopathological analysis of glomerular disease." In *Advances in Medicine* 12. Ed. D. K. Peters. London: Pitman Medical.

Unanue, E. R. & Dixon, F. J. (1967), "Experimental glomerulonephritis: immunological events and pathogenetic mechanisms." *Adv. Immunol.*, **6**, 1.

Chapter XI
Skin Diseases

It is surprising that, although diseases of the skin can be observed morphologically with ease throughout various phases, little is known about the aetiological mechanisms behind the majority of these conditions. More is known about diseases of the internal organs which cannot be readily visualized than about diseases of the skin. Possibly the cause for this is that a single pathogenetic mechanism can produce a number of superficially dissimilar lesions in the skin, although the mechanism behind the disease process is identical. Being on the surface and exposed to the outside world a lesion in the skin is often the result of combined internal and external influences. Thus it has become extremely difficult to analyse the multiplicity of pathological conditions of the skin seen in the human. In order to determine to what extent the various clinical conditions of the skin which are seen in the human have an immunological component, it is necessary to recapitulate the type of lesions which can be produced in the skin by immunological processes under controlled conditions in experimental animals and compare the reactions in experimental animals with those seen in the human. It will then be possible to look for counterparts to these experimental lesions among the various clinical syndromes seen in man.

Comparison of the Lesions of the Skin Produced by Immunological Means in Experimental Animals and Those Developing in Man

In experimental animals three types of immunological lesions have been fully characterized in the skin (1) Anaphylactic; (2) mediated by immune complexes—the Arthus reaction; (3) cell-mediated immune reactions—delayed hypersensitivity.

1. *Cutaneous anaphylaxis*

This reaction takes 15–30 minutes to develop and is associated with marked increased vascular permeability. The antibody (γ_1 globulin) involved is different from and electrophoretically faster than that involved in the Arthus reaction (γ_2 globulin). It also has a higher affinity for tissue and is thus analogous in many ways to the reagins or skin sensitizing antibodies in the human (IgE). Histologically there is little cellular infiltration. This reaction is associated with the release of pharmacological agents, such as histamine, serotonin and bradykinin.

Many cases of urticaria in the human are directly analogous to this reaction, especially those where there is obvious weal and flare formation which can be attributed to the local release of histamine, serotonin or bradykinin and which can often be blocked clinically by antihistamine drugs. Urticarial reactions due to drugs, such as penicillin, which can act as haptens forming chemical linkages with the patient's own proteins making them antigenic, fall into this group, as do the urticarial reactions found in serum sickness. Other forms of true urticaria are found which appear to be mediated directly by pharmacological agents without an immunological stimulus. Urticarial reactions to insect bites are true anaphylactic reactions due to antigens present in the saliva of the insects rather than to any toxic substance which might be injected.

2. *Cutaneous reactions due to the formation of immune complexes*

These reactions are due either to the interaction between antigen and antibody across the vessel wall causing an Arthus reaction, or due to the deposition of preformed immune complexes, probably in antigen excess, as in renal disease, in the capillaries of the skin. The antibody has no special affinity for sticking to tissues as does the antibody in anaphylactic reactions and is electrophoretically slower (γ_2 globulin—IgG). These reactions also differ from anaphylactic reactions in that the complement system is activated causing the release of factors which are chemotactic for polymorphonuclear leucocytes. There is also marked vascular damage due to the immune reaction taking place often within the vessel wall and thus the blood vessels are damaged often with much extravasation of fluid and erythrocytes. Necrosis of the vascular wall leads to thrombosis and the area of the skin at the centre of the reaction in the more severe forms becomes the site of infarction and necrosis. Under experimental conditions these reactions take between four and eight hours to develop.

So-called "anaphylactoid" purpura (Henoch-Schlonlein) in the human is in fact not a true anaphylactic reaction but due to the deposition of immune complexes in the skin and is often associated with the deposition of similar immune complexes in the kidneys causing the simultaneous development of glomerulonephritis. Allergic vasculitis whether haemorrhagic or nodular is caused by the same mechanism. The presence of haemorrhage or necrosis is not a necessary concomitant of these reactions in the human which in their milder forms may present as an area of erythema and oedema. Histologically, in the less severe form, immune complex formation may not even elicit a considerable infiltration with polymorphonuclear leucocytes, previously considered to be a necessary concomitant of these reactions. Thus if the time course of the reaction cannot be determined, the minor forms of this condition may be clinically grouped among the urticarias.

Erythema nodosum leprosum presents many of the features of an Arthus reaction as seen in the experimental animal. Lesions may surround a local area of vasculitis often with fibrinoid necrosis and there is generally an intense local polymorphonuclear leucocyte infiltration. Immune complexes containing immunoglobulin, complement and occasionally mycobacterial antigen can be demonstrated in the lesions. Other forms of vasculitis can be found associated with cryoglobulins in the serum. In some cases there may be similar immunoglobulins to those present in the cryoglobulins, deposited in the tissues. Such deposits usually also contain β_{1C} globulin. Cryoglobulins are generally only found in the serum of patients with recurrent vasculitis-type lesions occurring over a period of 2 years. Cryoglobulins are not generally a feature of patients with short-time attacks of cutaneous vasculitis. As mentioned above (Chapter IX) microbial antigens have been demonstrated in the lesions of patients with cutaneous vasculitis. However, the evidence that immune complexes containing these antigens cause the lesions is purely circumstantial, although the time relation between their development and infection in a number of cases suggests an immunological basis for the lesions.

The placing of erythema nodosum on the immunological spectrum causes a considerable amount of difficulty. Erythema nodosum, which is associated histologically with a mononuclear rather than a polymorphonuclear perivascular infiltrate in the skin, is associated clinically with infection, drug allergy or sarcoidosis. In some cases it occurs between 1 and 2 weeks after a streptococcal infection at a time when antibody production would have been expected to have begun to develop and immune complexes would be circulating possibly in antigen excess, the conditions known to be ripe for immune complex deposition. The absence of demonstrable immune complexes in the lesions and the presence of a mononuclear rather than polymorphonuclear infiltrate are features of an Arthus-type reaction more than 12 hours old, when the immune complexes are no longer demonstrable and the histological pattern changes to a mononuclear one. However, these are also features of a cell-mediated immune reaction. Thus erythema nodosum could either represent a late form of reaction involving humoral antibody in which a mononuclear cell infiltration predominates or a condition involving cell-mediated immunity. The complexes formed with humoral antibody would presumably be small, diffusing through and damaging vessel walls. This would account for the bruising. As the antigenic stimulus diminishes the complexes would disappear and complete restitution would occur without infarct or scarring. This distinguishes erythema nodosum from nodular vasculitis where vascular damage is more severe. In certain situations such as in tuberculosis or drug allergy, erythema nodosum may appear and disappear irregularly. This could be due to the condition only developing when there are critical proportions of antigen to antibody in the circulating immune complexes. The different clinical pictures produced by vasculitis in the skin could be due to the depth of the vessels in the skin affected by the immune reaction and to different physico-chemical characteristics of the immune complexes causing the lesions.

The lesions of erythema multiforme whether due to drug allergy or to immunological reaction with an infecting organism such as a mycoplasma, are also consistent with being caused by a circulation of immune complexes at a time when the levels of antigen and antibody combine in the right proportion to produce soluble complexes of the right size. The molecular size of the complex formed is probably critical in determining the form of the lesion seen in the skin in all these reactions, as this will determine the size of the blood vessel and thus the level in the dermis in which the reaction occurs. The typical target form of lesion often seen in erythema multiforme can be seen occasionally during the development of Arthus reactions in experimental animals. Reactions in the skin due to the deposition of immune complexes do not respond to treatment with antihistamine drugs, but are more responsive to treatment with corticosteroid drugs than cell-mediated immunological reactions. The mechanism of action of these drugs in these reactions is not known, but is probably on their peripheral manifestations rather than on the production of antibodies in the central lymphoid tissue. Immunosuppressive drugs such as azathioprine have not been used in the treatment of uncomplicated skin conditions due to immune complexes. However, a mixture of prednisone and azathioprine has been used successfully in the treatment of "anaphylactoid" purpura associated with proliferative glomerulonephritis. Naturally more emphasis has been placed on the improvement in glomerular function in this condition than on the effects of these drugs in suppressing the appearance of cutaneous lesions.

3. *Cutaneous reactions due to cell-mediated immunological reactions.*

Contact sensitivity to simple chemical groupings, whether organic or inorganic, which bind irreversibly to epidermal proteins, is the commonest manifestation of cell-mediated immunity in the skin. Sensitivity of this type can be induced with ease in guinea pigs, often to the same degree that it can be induced in man. Contact sensitizers may be to organic compounds such as picryl chloride or p. phenylenediamine. A wide range of common organic dyes are sensitizers because of the one property that makes them of such use in industry; this is their ability to bind irreversibly to proteins. Other organic compounds which are becoming increasingly known as sensitizers are the epoxyresins used specially in the electronics industry. Sensitizers may also be present in modern lubricants. Thus contact sensitivity must run high in the causes of industrial morbidity in a modern highly technological society. Another group of organic compounds which cause contact sensitivity are drugs, such as penicillin, which can bind to proteins *in vivo*.

Among the inorganic compounds which bind to epidermal proteins *in vivo* and are the cause of contact sensitivity are potassium dichromate, the cause of cement dermatitis, and metals such as nickel, mercury and beryllium. The ability to be sensitized to simple organic and inorganic compounds appears to be controlled genetically in both man and in experimental animals.

The lesions of contact sensitivity, being cell-mediated, take 24–48 hours to develop and are associated with marked erythema and induration, this is associated with thickening of the epidermis (acanthosis), intraepidermal cell oedema (spongiosis) and vesicle formation. The lesions may take a week or more to subside leaving the epidermis thickened and with hair follicles, sweat and sebaceous glands permanently damaged. This condition, if aggravated by trauma, may result in prolonged damage to the skin. Histologically these lesions are associated with an infiltration of the dermis with lymphocytes and macrophages both round blood vessels in the dermis and forming a band of infiltrate at the dermo-epidermal junction just below the basal layer. This is the position in the skin where the antigen (composed of the foreign chemical bound to the epidermal protein) is found at its highest concentration. The cellular infiltrate may persist in the skin for many weeks or months after the actual erythema has subsided. After some time a few of the B-lymphocytes in this infiltrate being in continuous contact with antigen are stimulated to transform into plasma cells and can secrete humoral antibody locally into the skin, which may account for the chronicity of some of the lesions.

In both man and experimental animals, a cell-mediated immunological response rarely occurs in complete isolation. At the same time as T-lymphocytes are passing through the site of fixed antigen in the periphery and passing down to the paracortical area of the lymph node to proliferate and initiate cell-mediated sensitivity, some of the antigen is being released in a soluble form and is passing down to the medulla of the lymph nodes. This soluble antigen will initiate the development of a humoral antibody response at the same time. Thus the patient will have antibodies in his serum, at the same time as he is able to develop a cell-mediated immune response to further contact with the chemical sensitizer. As well as antibodies in the serum, there will be the local production of humoral antibodies at the site of a previous cell-mediated immune reaction in the skin.

If the patient is then exposed to a heavy contact with sensitizer at a later date, as well as there being fixed antigen in the skin, a small amount of antigen will be absorbed systemically. This will react with antibody produced locally at the site of a previous cell-mediated reaction, causing a flare-up of the old reaction site. Immune complexes will also be formed with antibody in the circulation and be deposited in the skin at a number of different sites. This causes the well known phenomenon of "secondary rash" which occurs so frequently in highly sensitive individuals, when in contact with a chemical sensitizer to which they show contact sensitivity. Whereas the contact reaction itself is a cell-mediated phenomenon, the flare-up of old contact sites and more important the secondary rash are probably both mediated by humoral antibodies. If patients are exposed to a heavy contact with the sensitizer, they may become permanently desensitized. This desensitization is an example of immunological tolerance developing subsequent to sensitization and may be permanent.

The role of the systemic absorption of bacterial antigens in the production of cutaneous conditions of "unknown aetiology". In the same way as it is known that the systemic absorption of antigen from the site of heavy contact with a chemical sensitizing agent will cause a "secondary rash" at distant sites in the body, it has been known for a long time that the systemic absorption of fungal antigens in a patient who is highly sensitive will cause a rash at a site distant from the site of actual fungal infection.

It is also known that patients with varicose ulcers, which are the site of heavy bacterial contamination, are frequently liable to develop a "secondary rash" all over the body. This can be accounted for by the absorption of bacterial antigens from the site of the ulcer. Such patients can be shown to be exquisitely sensitive to a wide range of bacteria, showing Arthus reactions and delayed hypersensitivity to a wide range of bacterial antigens injected intradermally. In a few cases it has been demonstrated that circulating polymorphonuclear leucocytes or macrophages from patients with varicose ulcers with secondary rash or pyoderma gangrenosum, another condition where there is massive ulceration and infection of the skin, have ingested and carry antigens to which the patient is sensitive. In these patients the intradermal injection of a suspension of polymorphonuclear leucocytes or mononuclear cells, derived from the circulating blood, back into the patient's own skin will elicit a local skin reaction. The antigen is probably of bacterial origin and absorbed from the ulcer. It probably complexes with circulating antibody and is then phagocytosed by circulating leucocytes.

In these cases there is an obvious focus of infection from which bacterial antigens can be absorbed. In other cases cutaneous lesions could develop in patients with a critical level of circulating antibody when bacterial antigens are released from foci of infection in other less obvious sites. Thus repeated attacks of "anaphylactoid" purpura may be associated with the flare-up of a focus of infection in the genito-urinary tract or other sites in the body. The form of the cutaneous lesion whether a simple morbilliform rash, papular, nodular, with or without haemorrhage will depend on the physico-chemical nature of the antigen, the proportion of antigen to antibody in the immune complex and the molecular size of the soluble immune complex. These factors will determine the size of the vessel and the depth in the dermis at which the immune complexes will localize as well as the intensity of the inflammatory reaction evoked and the degree of extravasation of tissue fluid and erythrocytes. Severe damage to vessel walls will result in localized tissue death and nodule formation.

Similar patterns of cutaneous reactivity can be produced by the systemic absorption of drugs from the gastrointestinal tract. The drug acts as a hapten reacting with the patient's own proteins forming an antigen. If the patient produces anaphylactic antibodies (reagins—IgE) the reaction in the skin will be urticarial. However, if the antibodies are IgG or IgM, immune complexes will be deposited in the smaller cutaneous vessels.

Chronic mucocutaneous candidiasis. *Candida albicans* is not a pathogenic organism under normal conditions. Chronic diffuse infection of the skin and mucous membranes occurs, however, in conditions where there is a lowered state of cell-mediated immunity to this organism, as indicated by the finding of a diminished or absent state of delayed hypersensitivity to candidin. Investigation of patients with chronic mucocutaneous candidiasis has indicated a number of ways in which a low resistance form of chronic infection by a relatively non-pathogenic organism can occur. This may in the first place be associated with a well-defined non-specific absence of cellular immunity, as in congenital thymus aplasia with or without associated immunoglobulin deficiency. Another group of patients are those with primary endocrine disorders, especially hypoparathyroidism, hypoadrenalism, hypothyroidism or diabetes mellitus. A third group are those in which the cellular immune process is non-specifically depressed in the presence of an underlying malignant process such as leukaemia or Hodgkin's disease. Children with chronic candidiasis associated with neonatal thymic dysplasia show complete failure of cell-mediated immunity in that they cannot reject skin allografts or be sensitized with dinitrochlorobenzene (DNCB). They also show a primary lymphocyte deficiency and their lymphocytes cannot be transformed into lymphoblasts *in vitro* by phytohaemagglutinin (PHA). Patients with primary endocrine deficiency may have lymphocytes which respond to PHA, although they do not respond to candidin *in vitro*. Such patients also may not respond to other antigens, such as tuberculin, mumps, histoplasmin, coccidioidin and streptococcal antigens, as well as being unable to be sensitized *in vivo* to DNCB. Some of them show a different defect in that there is a failure of production of the chemical mediators of cellular immunity by lymphocytes *in vitro*. In these patients lymphocytes respond normally by transforming into blast cells in the presence of candida antigens, tuberculin or allogeneic lymphocytes. The association of chronic mucocutaneous candidiasis with a number of different endocrine defects brings to mind the failure of certain aspects of cellular immune processes in mice born with a congenital defect in growth hormone and thyroxine production.

Cutaneous lesions associated with neoplastic disorders. Two cutaneous conditions have been found frequently to occur associated with diffuse neoplastic disease. These are dermatomyositis and the so-called chronic annular erythema. In the case of dermatomyositis antibodies have been found in the serum which react with extracts of the tumour. At the same time immunoglobulins can be demonstrated on the surface of striated muscle and on the surface of collagen bundles in the skin. It is possible that tumour antigen is released into the circulation and fixes on to muscle and collagen, where antibody reacts with it and sets up a chain of events leading to the full clinical picture. It is now felt that if dermatomyositis begins in a patient over the age of 40, it may indicate the presence of carcinoma within the body. Dermatomyositis may remit once the tumour is removed. Chronic annular erythemas are also considered to be hypersensitivity reactions in many cases to circulating antigens derived from an internal carcinoma, although similar cases may be associated with hypersensitivity to fungal antigens such as trichophytin. Where the annular erythema is related to the presence of an internal carcinoma, it often clears up once the tumour is removed by surgical means.

Sézary syndrome is the name given to a generalized erythroderma associated with a lymphoproliferative disorder that has many of the characteristics of a T-cell leukaemia. The large cells in the circulation have some of the features that allow their identification as T-cells. They form E-rosettes with sheep erythrocytes and do not bear immunoglobulin on their surfaces. Similar cells are found infiltrating the skin lesions.

Immunological reactions in the skin due to physical agents. Physical agents such as cold, pressure and different wave lengths of light can modify the tertiary structure of skin proteins in such a way that the body may not be able to recognize its own tissue proteins as "self" and they become antigenic, in much the same way as if a foreign chemical grouping are attached to the molecule. The body can react with either an urticarial reaction or with delayed hypersensitivity to the application of ice to the skin, if a patient has become sensitized in this way. In the case of cold urticaria, skin sensitizing antibodies (reagins) can be demonstrated in the serum of the patients. If these are transferred to the skin of a normal individual and cold is applied they will react with the skin proteins whose tertiary structure has been modified by cold. Occasionally cryoglobulins may precipitate in the cold and complex in the periphery, inducing a reaction which has been described as urticarial. If these proteins are transferred to the skin of another individual and cold applied, a similar reaction will develop. This would appear to indicate that the complexing of the abnormal IgG molecules under the influence of cold are sufficient to institute the chain of events leading up to the release of histamine and the urticarial reaction.

In some patients the application of pressure directly to the skin will produce a reaction similar to the Arthus phenomenon with erythema and swelling taking 4–6 hours to develop (Pressure Urticaria). This condition must not be confused with dermatographism in which histamine is released into the skin within 15 minutes of drawing a hard object across the surface of the skin and is probably due to the direct release of pharmacological agents as a result of the pressure. Although it has many features in common with the Arthus reaction, there is no direct evidence that pressure urticaria is immunologically induced.

Ultra-violet light can induce either delayed hypersensitivity or urticarial reactions in sensitive subjects. Urticarial sensitivity can be transferred locally by skin sensitizing antibodies. Certain chemical substances attached to the body's proteins are only recognized as antigens when activated by light of particular wavelengths. These are generally drugs which are absorbed systemically. Examples of such photosensitizing drugs are chlorpromazine, tetracycline, sulphonamides and chlorpropamide. The drugs bind to skin protein and are activated when light of the correct wavelength is shone on the skin. The response is usually a cell-mediated type of immune reaction taking 24–48 hours to develop with erythema induration and vesiculation. After a heavy exposure to light the reaction in the skin may persist for a week or more before resolving.

Atopic eczema (atopic dermatitis). This condition which has a very marked hereditary element usually starts in early childhood. The eczematous condition appears characteristically more marked on the face and in the distal flexures. Histologically there is a vascular dilatation and marked infiltration of the dermis with lymphocytes, with occasional macrophages and plasma cells. The condition is invariably vesicular and usually secondarily infected. Children with this disease tend to be predisposed to develop asthma in adolescence or early adult life. Patients with this disease readily develop skin sensitizing (reaginic) antibodies in their serum to a wide range of different allergens. There is also a high incidence of raised levels of IgE and IgG in patients with this condition. On the other hand they have a lowered resistance to the viruses of herpes simplex and vaccinia, and are readily susseptible to secondary infections. Although there is a high incidence of skin sensitizing antibodies in the serum of patients with atopic eczema, these do not appear to play a role in the pathogenesis of the disease. This is indicated by the observation that atopic eczema can occur in children, with agammaglobulinaemia, who were found not to be able to produce skin sensitizing antibodies.

Little is known about the aetiology of atopic eczema, however the evidence to hand seems to indicate that this syndrome is associated with a number of functional abnormalities of the antibody-producing mechanism, probably of hereditary origin. The high incidence of skin sensitizing antibodies, raised levels of IgE and IgG, associated with the marked susceptibility to infection would indicate that there could be a functional over-production of certain antibodies, associated with a reduced production of other types of antibodies. The hypothesis that atopic eczema is the result of a malfunctioning antibody-producing mechanism or dysgammaglobulinaemia is confirmed by the regular occurrence of this skin condition in the Wiskott-Aldrich syndrome. The Wiskott-Aldrich syndrome which consists of eczema, thrombocytopenia and frequent severe infections is a sex-linked recessive disease in which there is a high mortality from infection. Although normal levels of immunoglobulins are found in the serum, the patients behave clinically as agammaglobulinaemics in that they are unable to produce antibodies readily and frequently have low levels of isohaemagglutinins in the serum. If the cause of this disease was associated with a failure to make normally reacting antibodies, a similar failure might well be related to the cause of atopic eczema in other children. A high incidence of atopic eczema may be associated with other immunodeficiency states. These include selective IgA deficiency and ataxia telangiectasia.

Histologically, the skin lesion in atopic eczema shows a strong mononuclear infiltration. This suggests that there might be a non-specific increase in delayed hypersensitivity. However so far there is no consistent evidence of an increase in contact sensitivity, and cellular immunity to certain viruses appears reduced. So, in conclusion, the findings are consistent with an overactivity of some aspects of the immune response with decreased activity of other functions.

Discoid lupus erythematosus. The aetiology of discoid lupus erythematosus is as obscure as that of most skin diseases. Transition from discoid L.E. to systemic L.E. occurs in less than 5% of cases. This together with the fact that the sex ratio of female to male patients differs in the two conditions, suggests that the genetic predisposition to the two diseases is different. In the less than 5% of patients with discoid L.E. who develop systemic L.E., it has been suggested that the individuals are genetic carriers for both diseases. The incidence of autoimmune phenomena in patients with discoid lupus erythematosus are high, despite a complete absence of systemic disease. As many as 35% may have anti-nuclear antibodies in their serum and both rheumatoid factor and anti-thyroid antibodies may be found.

Histological examination of the skin reveals degenerative changes in the basal layer of the epidermis and marked oedema of the dermis at the dermo-epidermal junction. This can also be shown to be the site of deposition of immunoglobulin and complement in the skin indicating that an immunological reaction is occurring at this site. The systemic absorption of both drugs and bacterial antigens have been suggested as being predisposing factors in this disease. In one patient a definite relationship has been found between bacterial infection and the absorption of bacterial antigens, and exacerbations of this disease. Moreover a histologically proven plaque of discoid lupus erythematosus has been found to develop at the site of a delayed hypersensitivity reaction caused by the intradermal injection of a dead suspension of bacteria to which the patient was allergic.

In other patients with discoid lupus erythematosus the intradermal injection of a suspension of their own mononuclear cells has been found to produce delayed hypersensitivity reactions in the skin. It is not known however, whether this was a reaction to bacterial or drug antigens carried in the macrophages or a direct autoimmune reaction of the lymphocytes against the skin. The cause of the actual lesions of discoid lupus erythematosus is thus not known; however, there is evidence of marked immunological activity at the site of the lesions. It would also appear that both humoral and cellular immune mechanisms might be involved. It is most unlikely that the reaction is a pure autoimmune condition, although secondary systemic autoimmune phenomena are common in these patients. It could well be that the disease is primarily an immunological reaction to foreign antigens of bacterial or drug origin, absorbed systemically almost continuously and reacting with both humoral and cellular immune mechanisms at the dermo-epidermal junction. The presence of the associated autoimmune phenomena may be no more than might be expected in such a long lasting and diffuse disease caused by an immunological reaction with antigens of external origin.

Autoantibodies in bullous diseases of the skin and Behçet's syndrome. The association of autoantibodies directed against different parts of the epidermis in the serum of patients, with various bullous diseases, is well documented. However, the significance of these antibodies is far from clear.

Autoantibodies are present in the serum of patients with pemphigus vulgaris, pemphigus foliaceous and pemphigus vegetans. These antibodies are directed against the intercellular substance of the stratum spinosum (prickle cell layer) of the epidermis. This is the site in the epidermis where these diseases develop, as pathologically they are associated with degenerative processes involving the intercellular bridges between the cells of the prickle cell layer of the epidermis. This causes loss of contact between the cells and results in the formation of the bullae. The difference between the different types of pemphigus is related to the level in the epidermis at which this process occurs. In pemphigus vulgaris the process occurs deeper in the epidermis and the prognosis in this variant of the disease is worse than in the other forms. Pemphigus vulgaris can be controlled by treatment with corticosteroids and under these conditions the level of circulating antibody can be found to diminish.

Bullous pemphigoid is a far less serious disease which is associated with separation of the basement membrane from the epidermis. This disease is also associated with autoantibodies in the serum directed against a constituent of the epidermis. However, whereas in pemphigus vulgaris the antibodies are directed against the intercellular substance of the prickle cell layer, in bullous pemphigoid antibodies are directed against the basement membrane of the epidermis, again the site of the primary lesion in this disease. The presence of autoantibodies appears to be related to the severity of the disease. One hint as to the relation of these antibodies to the pathology of the disease is that in some cases they are not demonstrable in the serum until the disease has been present for some time, although γ-globulin can be demonstrated bound to the epidermis. Antibodies are generally not present at a stage in the disease when no skin lesions can be demonstrated. Dermatitis herpetiformis, which is often indistinguishable from bullous pemphigoid histologically, can be distinguished from it immunologically as it has not so far been found associated with the development of autoantibodies against the epidermal basement membrane. Complement as well as Ig can, however, be detected bound to the basement membrane. The relation of this to the lesion that develops is not clear, although complement levels in blister fluid is depressed, implying that it is used up in the development of the lesion.

The pathological significance of these autoantibodies is a matter for discussion. The intradermal injection of serum from a patient with pemphigus vulgaris back into his own skin does not cause the development of a bulla, the only lesion which is found is the typical weal and flare of a local anaphylactic reaction in the skin. High titres of these antibodies are found in the serum of patients with endemic Brazilian pemphigus foliaceous in which an arthropod-borne infectious agent is thought to be an aetiological factor in the disease. Sera from patients who have recovered from severe burns have also been described as having antibodies in their serum, similar to those found in patients with pemphigus. Both these phenomena would indicate that these antibodies are not primary aetiological agents in these diseases. It is well known that one can induce autoantibodies in the serum of experimental animals without causing any disease in the target tissue to which they are directed. It is likely that these bullous diseases are of infective origin, possibly due to a virus. In this case the autoantibodies could develop as a result of exposure of antigens by the disease process. It is of particular significance that they can increase or decrease with the intensity of the disease. Whatever the causes of the various forms of bullous diseases of the skin, it is more than likely that the development of autoantibodies results from the disease rather than causes it.

Dermatitis herpetiformis is a blistering disease that occurs in patients with gluten sensitive enteropathy (coeliac disease) and the skin lesions are directly related to gluten ingestion. The disease is characterised by subepidermal bullae that are infiltrated with polymorphs and eosinophils. Immunologically the disease is associated with anti-reticulin antibodies that can be detected by immunofluorescence. In addition over one-third of the patients have antinuclear antibody in their serum. Although there are no antibodies against basement membrane, immunoglobulin deposits may be detected below the basement membrane in both involved and uninvolved skin. In the majority of cases the deposits are of IgA and in a few IgG. In addition the deposits may contain C3. The reticulin antibodies disappear when the patients are placed on a strict gluten free diet and there is a suggestion that they cross react with gluten. Patients with dermatitis herpetiformis have a high incidence of HLA antigens B1, B8 and DW3.

Another disease of the skin and mucous membranes associated with the development of autoantibodies in the serum is Behçet's syndrome. This condition consists of ulcer formation in the mouth and on the genitals as well as urethritis and in some cases encephalitis. Histologically the lesions show mainly non-specific inflammation in the dermis. Autoantibodies against cells derived from oral mucous membranes are found in the serum of patients with focal oral ulceration as well as those with the complete disease complex of Behçet's syndrome. The antibodies do not appear to be organ specific but cross react with foetal skin and colon. In at least one form of Behçet's syndrome, that with herpetiform lesions, an infective agent has been suggested, as inclusion bodies consistent with being of viral origin have been found in the nuclei of cells within the lesion. Moreover the disease responds to treatment with tetracycline. Mycoplasma has also been suggested as the causative factor in other forms of the disease. It may be therefore that in Behçet's syndrome as in bullous diseases of the skin, the production of autoantibodies is secondary to the exposure of antigen as a result of infection possibly of viral origin.

Autosensitization and the skin

The concept that autoimmune processes are the cause for a widespread number of conditions of the skin has been current among dermatologists for many years. The term "autosensitization" was coined by a dermatologist thirty-five years before the present interest in auto-immunity was stimulated by work on systemic lupus erythematosus and Hashimoto's thyroiditis. It was believed that the secondary spread of eczema whether due to contact sensitivity or due to varicose ulcer was due to the patient becoming sensitive to breakdown products of his own skin. In a recent investigation of 81 patients with stasis eczema associated with secondary rashes, no evidence of circulating antibody was found against the skin in all but four patients. A much more likely explanation for the phenomena considered by many dermatologists as due to autosensitization, is the systemic absorption and dissemination of antigens whether of bacterial origin or due to attachment of a chemical sensitizer such as a drug to tissue proteins. In other cases it is probable that autoantibodies develop secondary to tissue damage due often to an infective agent and play little part in the pathogenesis of the disease. It is probably only in lupus erythematosus that tissue damage can occur as a result of an immune reaction with an autoantigen and this is probably exposed either by the action of an infective agent or as a result of a drug hypersensitivity reaction.

Bibliography

Books

Fry, L. & Seah, P. P. (eds) (1974), *Immunological aspects of skin diseases*. Lancaster: MTP.
Immune mechanisms in cutaneous disorders. Special Issue. *J. invest. Derm.*, **67**, 301–482 (1976).

Articles

Beck, J. S. & Rowell, N. R. (1966), "Discoid lupus erythematosus."*Quart. J. Med.*, **35**, 119.
Cream, J. J. & Turk, J. L. (1971), "A review of the evidence for immune-complex deposition as a cause of skin disease in man." *Clin. Allergy*, **1**, 235.
Lehner, T. (1967), "Behçet's syndrome and autoimmunity." *Brit. med. J.*, **i**, 465.
Turk, J. L. (1970), "Contribution of modern immunological concepts to an understanding of diseases of the skin". *Br. med. J.*, **3**, 363.
Turk, J. L. (1971), "Autoimmunity in skin diseases," in *Modern trends in Dermatology* (Ed., P. Borrie), p. 176. Butterworths.

Chapter XII

Related Organ-specific Immunological Diseases—
Thyroid, Adrenals, Parathyroids and Stomach

In this chapter immunological diseases of the thyroid and adrenal glands, parathyroid glands and gastric mucosa will be discussed together. This is because there is a high degree of correlation between immunological diseases of one of these organs with diseases of one of the others to be discussed. However, no strong case exists for thinking that there is any underlying general defect of the central immune mechanism causing these diseases. More likely there is a genetic predisposition to the development of one or more of these diseases and the primary lesion is as likely to be in the organ or organs affected which could have been the site of virus or chemical damage.

Organ-specific immunological diseases are associated with the presence of humoral antibodies in the serum. However, no evidence exists that these autoantibodies are the cause of the disease process, although similar diseases can be produced in experimental animals by the injection of homologous or heterologous organ-specific antigens. These diseases are therefore autoimmune in that the body is reacting abnormally against its own tissues with what might be called an immunological rejection process as though it were not part of "self". The mechanism by which such phenomena could be stimulated have been discussed in an earlier chapter and they may occur secondary to a primary disease process in the target organ or another organ. It must therefore be emphasized that the presence of humoral autoantibodies in the serum does not necessarily indicate disease of the organ to which these antibodies are directed.

It is logical to start a discussion of these diseases with the thyroid gland as the recognition of autoantibodies against thyroglobulin in the serum of patients with Hashimoto's disease in 1956 started much of the present interest in the role of immunological processes in disease.

Diseases of the Thyroid Gland

I. *Hashimoto's disease—chronic lymphadenoid goitre*

(a) *Clinical picture.* This disease which occurs more frequently in the female is associated with an enlargement of the thyroid gland which may be such that it obstructs the airway. The gland feels rubbery and histologically the typical glandular structure is replaced by lymphoid tissue. Depending on the amount of normal thyroid tissue which is replaced the patient may show symptoms of myxoedema. The disease may go on to fibrosis resulting in a disease which used to be known as primary hypothyroidism without goitre.

The lymphoid tissue consists mainly of small lymphocytes and histiocytes but typical germinal centres are found frequently in the lymph follicles and plasma cells can be found among the lymphocytes in close proximity to the germinal centres. Lymph follicles and germinal centres are also found in the thymus indicating that the mechanism behind the disease is not limited to the thyroid itself.

Humoral antibodies in the serum of patients with Hashimoto's disease are directed against the cellular elements of the thyroid gland as well as against thyroglobulin. Cytoplasmic thyroid antibodies are detected by the complement fixation technique (Chapter II) and give a better correlation with disease of the gland than antibodies against thyroglobulin. It is considered that a complement fixation titre of $>1:32$ is indicative of Hashimoto's disease. Thyroglobulin antibodies are however found much more ubiquitously and a titre of $1:2,500$ or greater is usually necessary before a diagnosis can be made, under such conditions these antibodies can be detected by the relatively crude technique of precipitation of thyroglobulin in an agar plate. Despite these limits it is considered by many that a complete diagnosis of Hashimoto's disease cannot be made without a needle biopsy of the thyroid gland and histological confirmation.

Hashimoto's disease is treated by a ten-day course of 60 mg/day prednisolone followed by thyroxine. This treatment produces a dramatic reduction in size of the thyroid gland. Treatment with thyroxine alone is used but is slower.

(b) *Experimental thyroiditis—possible mechanism of the disease.* The mechanism of chronic "auto-allergic" thyroiditis has been studied extensively in experimental animals. A disease similar to that found in the human can be produced in experimental animals by the injection of homologous or heterologous thyroid tissue in an adjuvant mixture. The disease thus produced consists of a marked lymphocytic infiltration of the gland with small lymphocytes and histiocytes. However, it differs from the human disease histologically in that there is a relative scarcity of plasma cells and true germinal centres are not found in the gland.

The disease in experimental animals has been thought by many to be completely cell-mediated, as it is associated with the development of a state of delayed hypersensitivity to the intradermal injection of an extract of thyroid tissue and the disease cannot be transferred passively with serum containing autoantibodies to the glandular tissue. Similar skin reactivity can be found in patients with Hashimoto's disease. However, there have not been consistently positive reports of the ability to transfer the disease passively with lymphocytes, although no difficulty exists in transferring skin reactivity from a sensitized to a normal animal. Currently it is considered that the disease is caused by an interaction of humoral and cell-mediated immune mechanisms. The role of humoral mechanism in the causation of the disease in the human is highlighted by the frequency of plasma cells in the gland and germinal centres in both the target organ and in the closely adjacent thymus.

How the immune mechanisms are stimulated to react against thyroid tissue is not known, but a possibility exists that antigens may become more readily immunogenic as the result of the action of viruses or chemical agents.

There is no doubt that genetic factors can cause a predisposition to chronic thyroiditis. There is a markedly high incidence of thyroid disease, both Hashimoto's disease and thyrotoxicosis in the families of patients with Hashimoto's disease. Moreover, Hashimoto's disease has been described in both members of two pairs of uniovular twins. Thyroid disease has also been described in a number of patients with congenital diseases associated with abnormalities of the X chromosome. Two patients who had Turner's syndrome with an enlarged or drumstick X chromosome, were also found to have Hashimoto's disease, and two patients with Klinefelter's syndrome, a disease also associated with an abnormal X chromosome were discovered to have thyroid dysfunction.

Hashimoto's disease has been found associated with a number of other diseases. These include chronic hepatitis, rheumatoid arthritis, Sjögren's disease, systemic lupus erythematosus and Addison's disease. One of the more striking associations is between immunological disease of the stomach and the thyroid. Pernicious anaemia is found in about 6% of patients with thyroid disease. About a third of patients with immunological disease of the thyroid have antibodies to gastric parietal cells and about a half have antibodies to gastric intrinsic factor in their serum.

(c) *Significance of thyroid autoantibodies.* Low levels of thyroid autoantibodies, usually directed against thyroglobulin rather than the cytoplasmic components of the thyroid have been found in 4% of normal subjects. A higher incidence has been found, in the absence of overt thyroid disease, in other unrelated immunological diseases such as systemic lupus erythematosus, and chronic hepatitis. Raised levels of thyroid autoantibodies have also been found in leprosy and other long standing chronic infections. This would indicate that patients with chronic diseases, where there is continuous stimulation of the central immunological mechanisms, develop the property to react with higher levels of antibodies than normal people to available antigens. This is probably a non-specific event similar to that produced in experimental animals with Freund's adjuvant.

The significance of antibodies to cytoplasmic components of the thyroid in apparently normal people is different as these have been shown in post-mortem studies to be related to the presence of focal thyroiditis that was not detected in life.

II. *Thyrotoxicosis*

The immunological basis of this disease has only recently been clarified. It has been known for some time that about 40% of patients with thyrotoxicosis have antibodies to thyroglobulin in their serum, thus it was reasonable to suspect that some immunological process was in progress during this disease. However, it had been known for even longer that these patients contained a substance in their serum which stimulated thyroid function in experimental animals. Stimulation of thyroid function was assayed by the release of radioactive iodine from the thyroid glands of animals which had been labelled previously with radioactive iodine, and in whom pituitary thyroid stimulating hormone (TSH) had been suppressed by pretreatment with thyroxine. This stimulator is an IgG antibody and has been called "long acting thyroid stimulator" (LATS), as it takes longer to act than TSH. Recently it has been shown that this LATS is an immunoglobulin of type G (IgG). LATS is found in the serum of about 40% of patients with thyrotoxicosis and there is a strong correlation between the presence of LATS and anti-thyroglobulin antibodies. The incidence of LATS was even higher in the serum of patients with exophthalmos.

The role of TSH in the pathogenesis of thyrotoxicosis has been re-examined in the light of these more recent findings. It has been found that, far from being increased in thyrotoxicosis, the level of TSH in the blood is usually less than that found in normal individuals, and only increases in thyrotoxic patients following treatment. The secretion of TSH by the pituitary is inhibited by a normal "feed back" mechanism due to the excessive amounts of thyroxine in the blood. Thus it is accepted now that thyrotoxicosis is not due to an excessive stimulation of the thyroid by pituitary TSH. Moreover there is an inverse ratio between LATS and TSH in the blood.

The role of LATS in causing thyrotoxicosis has been emphasized by the finding of thyrotoxicosis in babies born from mothers with a high level of circulating LATS. LATS antibody has been found to be thyroid specific and probably combines with an antigen on the thyroid cell surface. Antigen–antibody interaction on the surface of the cell could then stimulate cell metabolism. Evidence of acceleration of cell metabolism can be found from electron microscopical examination of these cells, which show evidence of increased protein synthesis and an increase in the size of the Golgi apparatus which would be associated with the increased secretion of thyroglobulin. Increased metabolic activity of cells as a result of antigen–antibody interaction at the cell surface has been found in a wide range of different experimental systems. Another possible explanation for the action of LATS, which has been suggested, is that it could remove an inhibitor of enzyme activity in the thyroid and in this way increase thyroid activity.

As mentioned above LATS antibody is not found in the serum of all patients with thyrotoxicosis. This would suggest that there could be other causes for this disease. This appears to be confirmed by a study of the response of patients with thyrotoxicosis to the drug carbimazole. Carbimazole was only found to be effective in a proportion of patients treated, and this was found to be the group which did not have LATS antibody in their serum. Patients which did not respond to carbimazole, had LATS antibody and antithyroglobulin in their serum and had a strong family history of thyroid disease.

The presence of antithyroid antibodies in the serum of patients with thyrotoxicosis has been assessed in relation to the form of therapy that patients with thyrotoxicosis have been receiving. It has been found that a certain proportion of patients with thyrotoxicosis become hypothyroid following treatment with radioactive iodine or partial thyroidectomy. Examination of thyroids post-operatively showed that those patients which developed hypothyroidism after surgery had marked lymphocytic infiltration of the thyroid, some with germinal centres. Moreover, there was also a higher incidence of cytoplasmic complement fixing antibody in the serum of these patients indicating a co-existing Hashimoto's disease. As a result of this surgeons have learnt to remove less of the thyroid gland at operation if they find co-existing macroscopic evidence of lymphadenoid disease of the thyroid gland. However, no correlation between the level of antithyroglobulin antibodies and anti-thyroid cytoplasmic antibodies has been found with the development of the hypothyroid state after treatment with radioactive iodine. It has been suggested that the development of hypothyroidism following treatment with radioactive iodine is the result of an immunological reaction. However, there does not appear at the present to be any support for this concept. The level of antithyroid antibody is also of no value in predicting the response of patients to antithyroid drugs.

As mentioned above there is a higher incidence of LATS antibody in the serum of patients with thyrotoxicosis with exophthalmos than in the serum of those without. Although exophthalmos can occur in the absence of circulating LATS, it has been suggested that this antibody may facilitate the development of this condition. However, the association of LATS with pretibial myxoedema in thyrotoxicosis is even stronger. Since there has been an association between exophthalmos and LATS, prednisolone (10–45 mg/day) has been used as an immunosuppressive agent to combat this condition. Exophthalmos improved and LATS disappeared from the serum in all cases.

Adrenal glands—Addison's disease

Although it is recognized that a certain proportion of cases of Addison's disease are due to destruction of the adrenal gland by tuberculosis, there has always been a considerable group where there was atrophy of the gland due to an unknown cause (idiopathic Addison's disease). The immunological nature of this disease has been suggested by the finding of lymphocytic infiltration of the gland and antibody in the circulation directed mainly against the cells of zona glomerulosa in the cortex of the gland. Some cases of adrenal atrophy have been associated with insufficiency of the anterior pituitary gland, in which case there has also been infiltration of the anterior pituitary with lymphoid tissue containing germinal centres. Antibodies against the steroid producing cells of the adrenals cross-react with other steroid producing tissues such as placental trophoblast cells, ovarian corpus luteum cells, and the interstitial cells of the testis. It is interesting that the antigen has the same cytoplasmic localization as the antigen in the thyroid cells to which there are antibodies in the circulation in Hashimoto's disease.

Similar lesions of the adrenal glands can be produced in experimental animals by the injection of homologous or autologous adrenal tissue in an adjuvant mixture. The disease thus produced is associated with the presence of antibodies against adrenal tissue in the serum of affected animals. As in the human disease antibodies are directed against the cortex and not against the medulla. Immunoglobulins are found fixed in the diseased cortex. However, failure to transfer the disease passively with either cells or serum alone would suggest that as most experimental organ specific immunological diseases, the lesions are the result of the interaction of both humoral and cell-mediated immunological mechanisms.

It has been suggested that immunological adrenal disease in the human is not limited to the adrenal gland, but is part of a more widespread "polyendocrinopathy". This is because of the high incidence of thyroid disease, hypoparathyroidism, diabetes mellitus and atrophic gastritis with this disease. These other conditions are not associated with Addison's disease due to tuberculous adrenal insufficiency. It is of interest that patients with immunological Addison's disease have a high incidence of antibodies to gastric intrinsic factor and gastric parietal cells in their serum but a low incidence of pernicious anaemia. This disease complex may also include steatorrhoea.

Although immunological Addison's disease has a high degree of association with immunological disease of the thyroid gland, the thyroid gland disease itself has a low incidence of association with Addison's disease. Thus although a patient with thyroiditis has a good chance of having atrophic gastritis, the chance of his having adrenal disease is low. However, if he has adrenal disease the chance of his having thyroid disease is high. The association of thyroid disease and gastric disease appears to be one immunological disease entity, and the "polyendocrinopathy" associated with adrenal disease, which may contain thyroid disease, would appear to be a different independent and rarer disease entity.

Hypoparathyroidism

Idiopathic hypoparathyroidism with circulating antibodies against the parathyroid gland can occur in the absence of Addison's disease or pernicious anaemia. However, it cannot yet be determined whether this is an independent disease entity or a variation of the "polyendocrinopathy" discussed above, in which the balance of the disease is directed more to the parathyroid glands rather than directed against a number of different organs at the same time. The high incidence of parathyroid disease with other disease suggests the second possibility, although, as with thyroid disease, hypoparathyroidism could occur as a separate disease entity.

Atrophy of the parathyroid gland can be produced as an independent entity in experimental animals by the injection of parathyroid tissue in an adjuvant mixture, in the same way as experimental allergic thyroiditis and adrenalitis.

Immunological disease of the stomach—pernicious anaemia

Castle and his colleagues postulated in 1930 that pernicious anaemia was due to a failure of absorption of an "extrinsic factor" in the diet coupled to an "intrinsic factor" present in normal gastric secretions. Since then the dietary extrinsic factor has been identified, chemically characterized and synthesized and is now known as Vitamin B12 (cyanocobalamin). The failure of absorption of Vitamin B12 giving rise to the typical megaloblastic anaemia has also been known to be associated with a marked disturbance of gastric function. This has been classically demonstrated by a lack of hydrochloric acid in the gastric secretions. Atrophy of the gastric mucosa is associated with both a loss of the chief cells and a reduction in the number of gastric parietal cells. The association of atrophy of the mucosal cells of the stomach with marked infiltration with lymphoid tissue containing germinal centres has suggested that the deficiency in gastric intrinsic factor might be caused by an immunological mechanism.

Two phases occur in the absorption of Vitamin B12. The first is the coupling of Vitamin B12 to intrinsic factor and the second phase is the uptake of the Vitamin B12-intrinsic factor complex by the intestinal mucosa. Antibodies have been detected in the serum of patients with pernicious anaemia, that can inhibit both these phases. In fact two types of antibody have been detected in the serum. The first combines with the gastric intrinsic factor and can block the attachment of

Vitamin B12 to intrinsic factor (type 1: blocking antibody). The second type of antibody, which is less common binds the Vitamin B12—intrinsic factor complex (type 2: binding-site antibody) and can prevent the uptake of the complex by the intestinal mucosa.

Although these antibodies are present in the serum of a high proportion of patients with pernicious anaemia and are found in the IgG fraction of the serum, it is recognized that their mere presence in the serum does not explain the mechanism of the disease. The finding of antibodies in the gastric juice against intrinsic factor would be more important in explaining the mechanism of the failure of absorption of Vitamin B12, than the mere presence of these antibodies in the serum.

Antibodies against the gastric parietal cells can be detected in a higher proportion of patients with pernicious anaemia than antibodies against intrinsic factor. This may be because the techniques used to detect these antibodies are more sensitive. However, the role of both antibodies against intrinsic factor and antibodies against the parietal cells in the pathogenesis of the disease is obscure. This is especially so as these antibodies are detected predominantly in the serum, although they may also be detected in gastric secretions. It may be that the primary lesion is atrophy of the gastric mucosa as a result of both cell-mediated and humoral antibody mechanisms. This would then cause a reduction in the amount of intrinsic factor secreted into the gastric juices. The presence of antibodies in the serum may be a parallel phenomenon and not the direct cause of the malabsorption of Vitamin B12 and the resultant megaloblastic anaemia. Antibodies against gastric parietal cells can occur in hypothyroid states without any evidence of pernicious anaemia although this antibody is rarely found in patients with a histologically normal gastric mucosa. Intrinsic factor antibodies are never found in the absence of pernicious anaemia.

Some idea of the mechanism of pernicious anaemia can be obtained from the response of these patients to treatment with prednisolone (40 mg/day). This enhanced Vitamin B12 absorption, and the histological appearance of the gastric mucosa began to return to normal, during treatment, with the result that parietal cells began to be seen in gastric biopsies. Both intrinsic factor and acid reappeared in the gastric juice. Serum antibody levels against intrinsic factor and gastric parietal cells was reduced in only a proportion of the patients treated. In these studies it was suggested that antibody against gastric parietal cells were stimulated by the release of antigen from damaged gastric mucosa and that their presence was secondary to the actual disease process. It was apparent that antibodies against intrinsic factor were also a secondary event and not the cause of the changes in gastric secretion and Vitamin B12 absorption, as might have been suggested by earlier studies.

As mentioned above there is a striking association between disease of the thyroid, especially primary myxoedema, which is now accepted as due to the results of an immunological disease of the thyroid, and pernicious anaemia, and a high incidence of atrophic gastritis in hypothyroid patients. There is an even higher incidence of antibodies against gastric parietal cells in patients with Hashimoto's disease and other forms of chronic thyroiditis, without actual clinical evidence of pernicious anaemia. Similarly a high proportion of patients with pernicious anaemia have antibodies against thyroid cytoplasmic antigens or thyroglobulin or both in their serum, without clinical evidence of thyroiditis. It has been suggested that gastric mucosa and thyroid tissue have certain features in common. They both concentrate iodide, and are embryologically related. It is therefore possible that there may be a common factor in diseases of these two tissues. It is not known what this factor is and if such a common factor is discovered, much will have been done to elucidate the mechanism of these two diseases.

Bibliography

Books

Buchanon, W. W. & Irvine, W. J. (eds.) (1967), *Symposium on Autoimmunity and Genetics. Clin. exp. Immunol.*, **2**, suppl.
Irvine, W. J. (ed.) (1967), *Thyrotoxicosis—Proceedings of an International Symposium, Edinburgh, May 1967*. Edinburgh: Livingstone.
Royal College of Physicians, Edinburgh (1967), *Symposium, Thyroid Disease and Calcium Metabolism*.
Wright, R. (1977), *Immunology of gastrointestinal disorders and liver diseases*. London: Edward Arnold.

Articles

Blizzard, R. M., Chee, D. & Davies, W. (1966), "The incidence of parathyroid and other antibodies in the sera of patients with idiopathic hypoparathyroidism." *Clin. exp. Immunol.*, **1**, 119.
Blizzard, R. M., Chee, D. & Davies, W. (1967), "The incidence of adrenal and other antibodies in the sera of patients with idiopathic adrenal insufficiency (Addison's disease)." *Clin. exp. Immunol.*, **2**, 19.
Irvine, W. J., Stewart, A. G. & Scarth, L. (1967), "A clinical and immunological study of adrenocortical insufficiency (Addison's disease)." *Clin. exp. Immunol.*, **2**, 31.
Jeffries, G. H., Todd, J. E. & Sleisinger, M. H. (1966), "The effect of prednisolone on gastric mucosal histology, gastric secretion and vitamin B12 absorption in patients with pernicious anaemia." *J. clin. Invest.*, **45**, 803.

Chapter XIII

Diseases of the Intestinal Tract, Respiratory Tract, Liver, and Amyloidosis

Coeliac disease

Coeliac disease or idiopathic steatorrhoea is a gluten sensitive enteropathy. Sensitivity is to a polypeptide in the α gliadin fraction of gluten. Permanent remission may be obtained if the patient is kept on a gluten free diet. Clinically the disease may be associated with dermatitis herpetiformis, fibrosing alveolitis, diabetes mellitus, selective immunoglobulin (IgA) deficiency and lymphoreticular atrophy affecting the spleen and lymph nodes. Patients are found to have antibodies in their serum against gluten. Fifty per cent of adults and all children with the disease have antibodies against reticulin. These disappear when the patients are placed on a strict gluten free diet. Following gluten challenge there may be low levels of circulating complement and C3 indicating the possibility of an immune complex aetiology. However increased numbers of lymphocytes may also be found in the lamina propria in a jejunal biopsy, suggesting a role for cell-mediated immunity. Patients with these conditions have a high incidence of HLA—B1 and B8, and HLA DW3.

Crohn's disease and ulcerative colitis

These conditions may be considered to form two ends of a spectrum of chronic inflammatory bowel disease. In Crohn's disease the lesion is a localised sarcoid like granuloma with epithelioid cells, giant cells and lymphocytic infiltration. In ulcerative colitis there is ragged ulceration over a wide area with a diffuse infiltration with polymorphs, eosinophils, lymphocytes and plasma cells. Crohn's disease has therefore the appearance of a condition in which cell-mediated immunity underlies the pathological features of the disease, whereas in ulcerative colitis the lesions are more consistent with the involvement of humoral antibody processes. Both diseases may be associated with a number of clinical features that suggest additional circulating immune complex aetiology. These include arthritis, anterior uveitis and erythema nodosum. Ulcerative colitis is associated with autoantibodies against human colon, smooth muscle, mitochondrial and thyroid cytoplasmic antigens as well as gastric parietal antibodies, antinuclear factor and antireticulin antibodies. It has been suggested that both conditions are abnormal immune responses to a common infective agent.

Autoantibodies in ulcerative colitis react with a polysaccharide antigen which can be extracted from *sterile foetal* human colon. This antigen was also found to be present in sterile foetal rat colon and could also be extracted from the bacterium *E. coli* 014. The incidence of this autoantibody, however, is low only occurring in the region of 15% of patients with ulcerative colitis and no obvious relationship exists between the presence of the antibody and the duration or severity of the disease. A similar antibody to that described in human ulcerative colitis has been produced in experimental animals. Rabbits immunized with *E. coli* 014 will produce antibodies which react with an antigen present in rat colon, with the same distribution in the colon as the antigens, against which the autoantibodies from patients with ulcerative colitis react.

The autoantibodies found against human colonic mucosa in patients with ulcerative colitis are not cytotoxic for the colon cells *in vitro*. However, evidence exists that autoimmune cell-mediated immunological mechanisms could be involved in the disease. Peripheral blood leucocytes from patients with ulcerative colitis can be shown to be cytotoxic to human foetal colon cells in tissue culture. It might therefore be that a colon-specific hypersensitivity reaction could be important in the formation of tissue lesions in ulcerative colitis. However, these immune reactions involving the cytotoxic action of lymphocytes are not likely to be exclusively, or even primarily, responsible for the tissue damage observed in the diseased colon.

Another suggestion is that both allergy to some factor in the diet and an autoimmune cell-mediated immune reaction could interplay to produce the disease entity, ulcerative colitis. A further immunological process could also be involved and that is an immune reaction of the body against the bacteria which form the normal flora of the colon. The presence of these bacteria would protect the colonic mucosa from other organisms which are capable of damaging it. It is known that the flora of the colon in ulcerative colitis is different from that of the normal colon. In ulcerative colitis there is a predominance of *Streptococcus faecalis* and *E. coli* is often absent. Results in experimental animals have shown that if a strain of *E. coli* specific for the particular animal is eliminated from the colon either by immunization with this organism or by treatment with antisera against the specific organisms, lesions develop in the colon similar to those in ulcerative colitis. The disease, however, can be stopped if the specific strain of organism is given by mouth and recurs if the treatment is stopped.

Thus the interplay of possible allergy to food, change in the normal colonic flora, whether the result of a dietary change or immunological processes, and autoimmune processes in the pathogenesis of ulcerative colitis has yet to be sorted out. The final disease appears to be associated with such a complex of different and varied immunological processes that it is difficult to dissociate one from the other and decide which events are associated with the primary disease process and which events develop secondarily.

It has been suggested that certain cases of excessive gastro-intestinal protein loss in children could be the result of an allergic disease of the gastro-intestinal tract. Some of these cases improve dramatically on an elimination diet, specifically on a milk-free diet. When milk is reintroduced into the diet diarrhoea, vomiting, peripheral eosinophilia and the intestinal protein loss become worse again. Such patients may have precipitating antibodies in the serum to milk and have other allergic manifestations such as asthma, eczema and persistent rhinitis which were aggravated by the intake of milk. It is of interest that treatment with corticosteroids has the same effect as withdrawing milk from the diet, in reducing the excessive protein loss from the gastro-intestinal tract.

Diseases of the Respiratory Tract
"Cot death"—sudden death in infancy

Allergy to cows' milk protein is not only considered to be a significant cause of gastro-intestinal upsets associated with diarrhoea in infancy, but can also be the cause of acute respiratory distress and under certain circumstances has been postulated to be the cause of sudden death in infancy between the age of one and six months. Under experimental conditions it has been possible to produce sudden death from anaphylaxis in experimental animals by introducing a small quantity of cows' milk into lightly anaesthetized animals which had been previously sensitized to cows' milk. Histologically there is desquamation of the columnar or cuboidal epithelial cells of the bronchioles so that they are deposited in large numbers in the lumen as single intact cells, many of which show no degenerative change. This picture is identical to that observed in the bronchioles of human infants dying suddenly of unknown cause, where the lumen of the bronchioles is also filled by large numbers of single epithelial cells. It is of interest that death from anaphylaxis in the lightly anaesthetized animal, equivalent to deep sleep in the human infant, was silent, sudden and without violence, as might be expected if it was analogous to cot death and this was due to inhalation of gastric contents in a sleeping infant which was highly sensitive to cows' milk. Although the degree of anaphylactic sensitivity to cows' milk in infancy is not known, conventional antibodies against cows' milk can be found in the serum of infants as early as six weeks of life and significantly higher levels were found in serum of bottle-fed than in breast-fed babies at six weeks of age.

The demonstration of precipitating antibodies in the serum against cows' milk antigen could be taken to indicate that immunological processes other than anaphylaxis might play a role in pulmonary disease due to the inhalation of food antigens. The hypothesis has been current for some time that "cot death" in infants might be due to an anaphylactic reaction following the inhalation of cows' milk protein. However, the role of an Arthus reaction contributing to this condition should be considered. Inhalation of cows' milk and a resulting immune complex disease in the lungs may also underly other forms of chronic pulmonary disease.

The role of the Arthus reaction in causing chronic pulmonary disease

The role of IgE antibodies or reagins in the causation of pulmonary disease, such as bronchial asthma, due to inhaled antigens has been accepted for a long time. However, it has only recently been suggested that certain chronic diseases of the lungs leading to diffuse fibrosis can be attributed to persistent Arthus-type reactions occurring in the alveoli. The term "diffuse fibrosing alveolitis" has been given to a condition of the lung associated with cellular thickening of the alveolar walls with a strong tendency to fibrosis and the presence of mononuclear cells within the alveoli, leading to fibrotic destruction of the lung architecture with occasionally lymphoid follicles or epitheloid granulomas. This condition has been known as diffuse interstitial fibrosis of the lungs, interstitial pneumonia or pneumonitis, or Hamman-Rich disease.

Fibrosing alveolitis is occasionally found accompanying more generalized diseases associated with autoimmune phenomena, such as rheumatoid arthritis, Sjögren's syndrome, or diffuse systemic sclerosis. However, a key to the pathogenesis of this condition can be found in the observation that it develops as a late stage in certain allergic diseases due to the inhalation of organic dusts containing fungal or other antigens. These diseases have been found to be associated with a high level of antibodies of the IgG type in the serum, skin sensitivity of the Arthus type to the inhaled antigen and an allergic reaction in the lung which was also shown to be due to an Arthus-type of reaction.

The first of these diseases of the lung (extrinsic allergic alveolitis) associated with an Arthus reaction to inhaled antigens, to be investigated was "Farmer's lung". In Farmer's lung the antigens were found to be thermophilic actinomycetes in mouldy hay. Similar antigens in mouldy overheated sugar cane bagasse and mushroom dust were found to be the cause of similar conditions called "Bagassosis" and "mushroom picker's lung". Weevils in wheat-flour provide antigens which cause the same disease in workers with wheat-flour. In pigeon and budgerigar keepers, serum proteins in the birds' faeces cause the same disease (bird fancier's lung), and inhalation of bovine and porcine pituitary and serum protein antigens can produce the disease in those taking pituitary snuff for diabetes insipidus.

When patients who present with pulmonary symptoms, allergic

alveolitis with or without asthma, are skin tested, the reaction that develops is usually an Arthus-type of reaction—oedema and erythema, maximal three to four hours after the test. However, if there is an asthmatic component in the disease there may also be an immediate weal and flare reaction. Histological examination of the skin test site and the lung at the height of the disease will show that both IgG and complement are deposited in the region of small blood vessels as might be expected for an Arthus-type reaction due to the formation of immune complexes. Inhalation of the antigen causes dyspnoea, cough, malaise, and pyrexia after about seven hours. Histologically, as well as the deposition of immune complexes and complement, there is an exudate of mononuclear cells in the interstices between the alveoli and mixed mononuclear cells and polymorphonuclear leucocytes into the alveoli. Recently it has been suggested that cell-mediated immune processes may also play a role in the pathogenesis of these conditions.

The association of lung disease with rheumatoid arthritis and anti-nuclear factor. 30% of patients with fibrosing alveolitis in which no extrinsic cause can be found have rheumatoid factor in their serum. Of these about a third have obvious rheumatoid arthritis. Complexes of IgG and rheumatoid factor (IgM anti-IgG antibodies) have been found along the alveolar walls of one of these cases which has been investigated very fully, suggesting that these immune complexes could be related to the pulmonary disease process. Antinuclear factor has been found in the serum of patients with fibrosing alveolitis but without joint symptoms. Whether these develop secondary to the disease process as in other chronic diseases, or are part of the primary disease complex is not known.

A high incidence of rheumatoid arthritis has been described associated with other chronic diseases of the lungs such as pneumoconiosis (Caplan's syndrome) and progressive massive fibrosis in coal miners. However, there is no evidence, as yet, in these patients that the two diseases have a common aetiology. It may be that rheumatoid arthritis develops more readily in patients with widespread long-standing chronic inflammatory diseases. Similar observations are the reports of an increased incidence of arthritis in patients with psoriasis and ulcerative colitis. However, the arthritis associated with chronic pulmonary disease differs from that occurring in psoriasis and ulcerative colitis. In arthritis with chronic pulmonary disease there is a high incidence of rheumatoid factor in the serum; whereas in patients with arthritis associated with psoriasis and ulcerative colitis rheumatoid factor is not present in the serum.

Goodpasture's syndrome. The association of diffuse pulmonary haemorrhage with glomerulonephritis was first described by Goodpasture in

1919. Since then there have been a number of reports of this disease. In the later stages of the disease there may be diffuse mottling of the lungs due to deposition of haemosiderin. As mentioned in the chapter on the kidney, there is evidence that the renal lesions are caused by an immune process which some have thought to be autoimmune. On immuno-histological examination of the kidney, immunoglobulin and complement can be demonstrated deposited in a smooth pattern along the basement membrane of the glomerulus. The deposition is of a different character to that found in other forms of glomerulonephritis, serum sickness and systemic lupus erythematosus, where it has a discontinuous "lumpy-bumpy" distribution, associated with the deposition of immune complexes in the form of aggregates on the glomerular basement membrane. Similar deposits of immunoglobulin or complement can be detected in the lung along the alveolar basement membrane.

Virus-like particles have been seen by electron microscopy in the kidney. This has suggested that the disease is of infective origin. The virus could also be present in the blood stream and be deposited on the glomerular and alveolar membrane, where it would react with antibody and complement. An immune reaction on the glomerular membrane would then cause renal damage as in other forms of glomerulonephritis. The smooth deposition of immunoglobulin and complement could be due to an initial smooth deposition of virus antigen. However it is more likely that the virus could modify the antigenicity of the basement membrane in some way so that an auto-antibody is produced against it.

Thus it has been proposed that the syndrome of pulmonary haemorrhage and glomerulonephritis may represent a primary virus disease with involvement of the lung and, perhaps secondarily, the kidney. The host antibody response and the deposition of antibody and complement which is fixed on the basement membrane in the kidney and lung could be a direct response to the virus or to host antigen modified by the virus. The immune reaction which then develops will cause a secondary glomerular inflammation.

Sarcoidosis

Sarcoidosis is a granulomatous disease, in which the granuloma consists mainly of mononuclear cells associated with the presence of occasional giant cells. Typically the giant cell granulomas of sarcoidosis do not caseate and break down as do those in chronic tuberculosis. Sarcoid granulomas are found typically in the lungs, skin, lymph nodes and spleen. However in many cases it may present in the eye as a uveitis. As many as 50% of cases start as erythema nodosum in the skin.

In the past it has been suggested that sarcoidosis was an abnormal form of tuberculosis. This view is not at the present held by many investigators. However the cause of this granulomatous disease is not known and hardly anything is known about the pathogenesis of the condition. The onset of the disease is explosive at the same time as the patient shows signs of erythema nodosum in the skin, granulomas may also be found in the lymph nodes, spleen, bone marrow and lungs.

About two-thirds of patients with sarcoidosis have a marked deficiency of cell-mediated immunity, although there is no abnormality in humoral antibody formation. There is marked reduction in delayed hypersensitivity to tuberculin, histoplasmin, candidin, trichophytin or mumps antigen injected intradermally, and patients fail to convert to tuberculin positivity when immunized with BCG. Similarly, they cannot be sensitized to develop contact sensitivity to chemical sensitizing agents such as 2,4-dinitrochlorobenzene. Surprisingly they appear to be able to reject homografts normally. These patients also show a defect in the reactivity of their lymphocytes to be transformed by antigens *in vitro* into "blast" cells.

On top of this selective deficiency in cell mediated immunity the patients respond with a particular skin reaction to the intradermal injection of extracts of spleen or lymph node of other patients with sarcoidosis (Kveim Test). The reaction, which occurs takes up to four to six weeks to develop, morphologically takes the form of a hard red nodule in the skin. When fully developed biopsy will show a follicular epithelioid granuloma, the appearance of which closely resembles the granuloma of sarcoidosis itself. The nodule once developed will take a long time to resolve. It has been thought that the Kveim reaction, as the actual lesions of sarcoidosis, are immunological in nature. The Kveim reaction is not a typical manifestation of delayed hypersensitivity. However it might be that the disease is due to a particular form of the cell-mediated immune response in which abnormal reactions are produced against an antigen present in sarcoid tissue. If this is so sarcoidosis could be considered to have two aspects. The first is the presence of a specific antigen, possibly infective, in the sarcoid granulomatous tissues. The second is the state of the cell-mediated immune reaction to this antigen. Patients with sarcoidosis do not appear to be able to show a normal cell-mediated immune reaction to certain antigens. However, they are still able to react to the agent which will produce the Kveim reaction with the typical granulomatous, possibly immunological, reaction. The histological appearance of the Kveim reaction is very similar to that of granulomas which develop to beryllium or zirconium, which are thought to be a special type of cell-mediated response against the metals in people who have become sensitive. A similar specific allergic granuloma is the appearance of a papular late reaction, showing histologically a sarcoid pattern, to small doses of tuberculin which occurs in a small proportion of tuberculin positive individuals.

A histological appearance similar to that seen in the tissues in sarcoidosis can be found in peripheral tissues and lymph nodes when there is a particular balance between the cell-mediated immune response and the level of antigen in the tissues. An example of this is the sarcoid appearance in lymph nodes draining certain carcinomas. Sarcoid appearances may also be found in the skin and lymph nodes of patients at a particular point of the immunological spectrum of leprosy. Such an appearance is found in "borderline tuberculoid" leprosy. It may not be found in "polar tuberculoid" leprosy where the cell-mediated immune response is so great that most of the antigen is eliminated from the tissues nor in other forms of leprosy on the low-resistance side of this point on the spectrum where specific cell-mediated immunity to *Myco. leprae* may be minimal or absent.

It could well be, therefore, that "sarcoid" appearances, far from being those of an individual disease, do no more than reflect the tissue damages which occur following a chronic hypersensitivity reaction at a particular point on a disease spectrum when the potential is there to eliminate most, but not all, of the antigen or infecting organism. Under these conditions it may be difficult as in tuberculoid leprosy to demonstrate the infectious agent. In some experiments claims have been made to demonstrate a transmissible agent in sarcoidosis. The question remains what form of disease, if any, does this agent produce where the balance between cell-mediated immunity and the infectious agent is outside the particular limits within which a "sarcoid" tissue reaction occurs?

At the present time little is known about the nature of the disease entity called sarcoidosis or these other granulomas, although it is suspected that these reactions are variations of or deviations from the normal cell-mediated immunological response. Fractionation of extracts from the spleen of sarcoidosis patients has shown that the active principle producing the Kveim reactions is probably present in the subcellular organelles associated with phagocytosis (lysosomes). This suggests that the agent causing the reaction could be an infective organism. However, it is highly resistant to powerful chemical and physical agents, unlike most infective agents. Much will be learnt about the nature of this disease, if this agent can be identified.

So far it has been shown that sarcoidosis responds to treatment with steroids (20 mg Prednisone daily) which will inhibit the development of the Kveim reaction, although it will not block a reaction if started 4-6 weeks after injection. Other immuno-suppressive agents have not yet been described as being useful in this disease.

Diseases of the Liver

(a) *Acute viral hepatitis.* Two viral diseases of the liver are generally considered under this heading, Hepatitis A and Hepatitis B. The more severe illness is that produced by the Hepatitis B virus. Hepatitis B is associated with the presence of the surface antigen of the virus in the circulation. This antigen used to be referred to as the Australia (Au antigen) and is now referred to as HBsAg; the core antigen of the virus is referred to as HBcAg. HBsAg may be detected in the serum of patients during the incubation period and early clinical course of Hepatitis B infection by precipitation with specific antisera, haemagglutination or the more sensitive radiommunoassay. It is now known that it consists of 7 to 9 polypeptides of molecular weight ranging from 19,000 to 120,000.

HBsAg is generally detected in the serum within one month of exposure to the virus. Its presence precedes elevation of the transaminases which are first noted at two months. Subsequently antibodies —both antiHBs and antiHBc are found. Cell-mediated immunity (leucocyte migration inhibition and lymphocyte transformation) as well as antiHBs generally develop after symptoms have resolved. AntiHBs is not found in persistent carriers who continue to have HBsAg in the circulation. The persistence of antiHBc usually indicates active disease. Hepatitis B disease may be associated with a number of extrahepatic manifestations resembling serum sickness. These are suggestive of an immune complex aetiology. Aggregates of pleomorphic particles and tubules have been detected in the serum by electron microscopy. These have been interpreted as being immune complexes in antigen excess. Other particles have been interpreted as being in antibody excess or have been seen unaggregated. The extrahepatic manifestations include erythematous macular papular rashes, urticaria, polyarthralgia and arthritis. These may be associated with transient fall in CH50, C3 and C4. There may also be cryoprecipitins in the serum containing HBsAg and antiHBs. Immune complexes may also be found in the joint fluid. Polyarteritis nodosa may develop in Hepatitis B infection in the absence of liver disease and this may be so severe as to lead to renal failure. In this condition HBsAg, IgM, IgG and C3 may be detected in the vessel wall. Chronic glomerulonephritis may also develop. In this case HBsAg-antibody complexes may be found deposited on the glomerular basement membrane with a nodular pattern. Persistence of Hepatitis B virus and HBsAg in the circulation in chronic infections has been considered to be due to a defect in cell-mediated immunity. The mechanism of hepatocellular damage is still controversial. It is not known whether this is due to direct viral damage, immune complex injury or to a cell-mediated immune reaction. Knowledge of immune reactions in Hepatitis A infection is not so well developed as that in Hepatitis B. However an HA Ag has been isolated and immunological assays worked out for its detection.

(b) *Chronic active hepatitis.* This is a disease where there is persistent destruction of liver parenchymal cells leading to the development of coarse nodular cirrhosis. Histologically, masses of plasma cells and lymphocytes can be seen surrounding and infiltrating nodules of liver tissue. The plasma cells can be shown to be making IgG, and two-thirds of cases have a high level of IgG in the serum. This disease used to be known as "plasma cell hepatitis". Forty per cent of patients have antibodies to DNA and other nuclear constituents in their serum and 16% actually have L.E. cells in the blood. Thyroid autoantibodies are also found commonly in the serum of patients with this disease. As a result of the high incidence of antinuclear antibodies and L.E. cells, this disease has been thought by many to be a variant of systemic lupus erythematosus and called "lupoid hepatitis". A peculiar auto-antibody that can be found by immunofluorescence in the serum of a large proportion of patients with chronic active hepatitis is one which reacts with smooth muscle. This antibody can be differentiated from other anti-tissue antibodies and is not present in the serum of patients with systemic lupus erythematosus. The presence of this antibody as well as the much lower incidence of other autoantibodies formally distinguishes this disease from SLE. In addition there are autoanti-bodies against bile canaliculi and antimicrosomal antibodies. The commonest systemic complication is arthritis, although occasional cases of renal involvement and arteritis in the skin have been described. Ulcerative colitis has also been described in association with this condition. This disease has a high incidence in people with HLA group B8.

This is thus a disease in which there is a progressive relentless destruction of liver tissue with eventual complete failure of function, probably as a result of an immunological interaction. The destruction of the liver cells is thought to be an autoimmune process, probably triggered off by a virus infection as in 25% of cases there is a suggestion of a history of virus hepatitis.

Confirmation of the role of immunological processes in the patho-genesis of this disease is obtained by the response of patients to treat-ment with immunosuppressive drugs. Prednisolone causes pronounced improvement but large doses have to be used, which in themselves cause toxic symptoms. Better results have been obtained with pro-longed courses of 6-mercaptopurine (50–100 mg daily) or azathioprine (100–200 mg daily) for over a year. During this time liver function was found to return to nearer a normal level. Whether these drugs act in their anti-inflammatory capacity or as true immunosuppressive agents is not known.

(b) *Primary biliary cirrhosis.* Primary biliary cirrhosis is another disease of the liver where it is thought that immunological processes might play a part in tissue destruction. There is chronic intrahepatic cholestasis as a result of chronic non-suppurative inflammation and destruction of the intrahepatic bile ducts. This is thought to occur as a result of some immunological reaction as there is mononuclear cell infiltration round the bile ducts and some of the mononuclear cells can be shown to contain IgM, there is also an increased level of IgM in the serum of 80% of patients with this disease.

This condition is associated with a high incidence of different auto-antibodies in the serum. Over 90% of patients have IgG antibodies which react with mitochondria, whether of the liver, gastric parietal cells or renal tubules. These antibodies are not however pathognomonic of primary biliary cirrhosis as they also occur in the serum of 30% of patients with active chronic hepatitis. The antigen against which these antibodies are directed has been found to be part of the mitochondrial inner membrane. Since this has a similar structure to the coat of some viruses and bacteria, it has been suggested that these antibodies indicate a cross reaction with a microorganism. Patients with primary biliary cirrhosis also have a high incidence of antinuclear antibodies and thyroid autoantibodies in their serum. The relation of these different autoantibodies to the disease process is not known, but it is thought that they could be a reflection of the release of antigens as a result of liver damage which could itself be the result of an unrelated immuno-logical process or an, as yet, unidentified toxic agent.

Granulomas similar to those seen in sarcoidosis have been found in lymph nodes throughout the body in 40% of patients with primary biliary cirrhosis. Over half of the patients show a depression in their response to contact sensitization with 2·4 dinitrochlorobenzene and this is associated with a diminution in the ability of lymphocytes from these patients to respond to stimulation with phytohaemagglutinin. So far, the defect in cell-mediated immunity in this condition cannot be tied in with any particular pathological process. It would appear that the defect in cell-mediated immunity, as the presence of autoantibodies, are secondary to an as yet unidentified primary pathological process.

Amyloidosis

The deposition of amyloid material in the spleen, liver, kidneys and other organs of patients with chronic infections such as tuberculosis, osteomyelitis, and bronchiectasis as well as in rheumatoid arthritis and myelomatosis has been studied for a considerable time. These diseases have in common that they are associated with continuous immuno-logical activity. This association was confirmed by the finding that γ-globulin (IgG) could be found consistently in these deposits. However, IgG is not the only, and not even the major component of amyloid. Immunochemical analysis of this material has revealed the presence of complement components, α-globulin, lipoprotein and fibrinogen. The presence of both IgG and complement components suggests that the site of the deposition of this material could have been at some time the site of a reaction due to the deposition of immune complexes. Ninety-five per cent of amyloid consists of fibrils which contain a specific protein that is not related to any of the well known serum proteins. This protein is known as AA (amyloid A) protein and has a molecular weight of 8,500. Using antiserum directed against this protein it has been possible to detect an antigenically related protein of large molecular weight in the serum. This protein is known as SAA (Serum A-related protein). The concentration of SAA in the serum is generally low (less than 200 ng/ml) and it is mainly present as a complex in combination with albumin. The level of this component rises in patients with amyloidosis, cancer, infections, rheumatoid arthritis, multiple myeloma, macro-globulinaemia and lymphomas. In leprosy the level of SAA is higher in the lepromatous form of the disease and rises during the development of erythema nodosum leprosum in parallel with the rise in polymorpho-nuclear leucocytes.

The immunoglobulin found in amyloid tissue has been shown to react with cell membranes of human cells. This suggests that the deposition of amyloid could be an autoimmune phenomenon. The reaction between the cell wall antigen, antibody and complement could bind the serum lipoprotein and these complexes could then trap fibrinogen. In the case of myelomatosis the whole process could have been initiated by the deposition of aggregated immunoglobulins produced by plasma cells in the myeloma which would fix complement and then cause the deposition of the other components of amyloid tissue.

The deposition of amyloid in human disease can be reproduced in experimental animals by the daily injections of an antigen. The more antigenic the substance, i.e. the greater the immune response produced, the more rapidly deposits of amyloid can be found in the tissues. The rapid development of amyloidosis in experimental animals after the repeated injections of a strongly antigenic substance is associated with marked depletion of lymphocytes from the spleen and lymph nodes and some degree of thymic atrophy. Lymphocyte depletion in the spleen has a perifollicular distribution and it is in this area that the amyloid material is deposited. The deposition of amyloid is followed by infiltration of the areas immediately adjacent with plasma cells and histiocytes and giant cells. Plasma cell proliferation in the area appears to be secondary to the deposition of amyloid rather than preceding it. The cellular infiltration is no different from that found in other chronic inflammatory states. During the induction of amyloidosis by daily injection of antigen into experimental animals, the antigen is initially deposited in areas in the spleen where amyloid formation would be expected to occur, i.e. in the marginal zone of the red pulp. This is the same area in which antigen is normally taken up in immune animals secreting specific antibody. This distribution of antigen suggests that amyloid results from the local secretion of the fibrous protein, which is a specific finding in all amyloid deposits, possibly by reticulum cells, as a result of long continued exposure of these cells to the presence of immune complexes. The relation to deposition of immune complexes over a long period of time is consistent with the occurrence of amyloid in diseases where there is continuous immunological activity such as rheumatoid arthritis or in chronic infections. It could also be, as has been suggested, an autoimmune phenomenon in which the antigen lies in the cell membrane. The association of amyloidosis with prolonged states of rheumatoid arthritis would also be consistent with this being a secondary autoimmune phenomenon. This could be another example of the occasional occurrence of autoimmune phenomena as non-specific events secondary to long-term chronic inflammatory processes in the body. Little is known about the cause of primary amyloidosis. However, a number of cases of primary amyloidosis have been described in which there is a monoclonal rise of the immunoglobulins associated with Bence-Jones proteinuria. Conversely 15% of cases of multiple myelomatosis are complicated by amyloidosis. This would suggest that primary amyloidosis could be basically due to an abnormality of immunoglobulin production, a plasma cell dyscrasia.

There are however a number of instances which suggest that amyloidosis is not primarily an immunological phenomenon. Amyloidosis has been reported to occur in patients with agammaglobulinaemia. Moreover amyloid disease can still be induced in mice by the injection of casein, after they have been made immunologically tolerant to that antigen. Amyloidosis has also been shown to occur in mice thymectomized within the first 24 hours of life. These mice develop a progressive nephritis at four to eight months of age which is associated with a parallel development of massive deposits of amyloid in the spleen. It has thus been suggested that the primary lesion in amyloidosis is impaired or deficient glomerular filtration and that the functional incapacity of the kidneys to eliminate endogenous or exogenous material could result in the deposition of amyloid.

It appears that there are two phases of amyloid formation. Mice given casein injections together with nitrogen mustard, cortisone or anti-lymphocyte serum during the early phase of treatment will not develop amyloid disease. Whereas if cortisone, nitrogen mustard or X-irradiation is given late in the course of amyloidogenic treatment, the disease is actually enhanced. The first phase of the disease appears to be diminished by immunosuppressants, suggesting that it has an immunological origin, despite the enhancement by thymectomy and the fact that it occurs in agammaglobulinaemic patients. The second phase may well depend on renal function.

Bibliography

Books

Pepys, J. (1969), *Hypersensitivity diseases of the lungs due to fungi and organic dusts.* Monographs in Allergy, **4**. Basel: Karger.
Scadding, J. G. (1967), *Sarcoidosis.* Eyre and Spottiswoode.
Wright, R. (1977), *Immunology of gastro-intestinal disorders and liver diseases.* London: Edward Arnold.

Articles

Franklin, E. C. (1976), "Amyloid and amyloidosis of the skin." *J. invest. Derm.*, **67**, 451.
Gunther, M., Aschaffenburg, R., Matthews, R. H., Parish, W. E. & Coombs, R. R. A. (1960), "The level of antibodies to the proteins of cow's milk in the serum of normal human infants." *Immunology*, **3**, 296.
Markowitz, A. S., Battifora, H. A., Schwartz, F. & Aseron, C. (1968), "Immunological aspects of Goodpasture's syndrome." *Clin. exp. Immunol.*, **3**, 585.
Miescher, P. A. & Grabar, P. (eds.) (1968), "WHO Conference on use of antimetabolitis in disease associated with abnormal immune responses." *Immunopathology Vth International Symposium.* Basel: Schwabe and Co.
Parish, W. E., Barrett, A. M. & Coombs, R. R. A. (1960), "Inhalation of cow's milk by sensitized guinea pigs in the conscious and anaesthetized state." *Immunology*, **3**, 307.
Sherlock, S. (1970). "The Immunology of Liver Disease." *Amer. J. Med.* **49**, 693.
Turner-Warwick, M. (1967), "Auto-allergy and lung diseases." *J. roy. Coll. Phycns. Lond.*, **2**, 57.

Chapter XIV
Haemolytic Diseases and Thrombocytopenic Purpura

Rhesus Haemolytic Disease of the Newborn

It is well known that haemolytic disease of the newborn is due to isoimmunization of an Rh-negative mother by erythrocytes from a Rh-positive foetus containing one of the Rh antigens. However, only 10% of Rhesus-negative women become sensitized, and the first evidence of sensitization is not found until six to eight weeks after the birth of the first Rhesus-positive baby. Foetal red cells are known to pass across the placenta in small numbers in all normal pregnancies, but appear only to cause antibody production after parturition. In 80% of pregnancies that cause the production of Rhesus antibodies, both mother and child show ABO compatibility. It is thought that in an ABO incompatible pregnancy the small number of foetal cells that cross the placenta are rapidly haemolysed intravascularly by an excess of maternal antibody. Thus if there is ABO incompatibility in the first or subsequent pregnancies the mother will be protected from Rhesus immunization until she carries an ABO compatible foetus.

As antibody does not begin to be found until 6–8 weeks after delivery, it has been suggested that immunization occurs as a result of a massive transplacental haemorrhage at the time of delivery, which could be due to a particularly traumatic delivery. However, no correlation can be found between trauma at delivery and Rhesus sensitization. In fact a large proportion of mothers who have been sensitized do not have a large bleed at delivery. There is no doubt that there is a proportion of mothers who have a higher risk of becoming sensitized and this can be correlated with the presence of foetal cells in the maternal circulation after delivery. It is very likely that in the majority of cases these are derived from a number of small undetectable haemorrhages at delivery or earlier.

In many cases antibody is not detected in the serum after the first sensitizing pregnancy but develops during the second pregnancy. This is not that the mother was not sensitized as a result of the first pregnancy but developed only a small primary response in which the level of antibody produced was below the level that could be detected in the serum. During the second pregnancy the mother would get a second antigenic stimulus and then develops a secondary antibody response, in which the level of antibody is higher and can be detected in the serum.

It has been suggested that mothers do not develop antibodies in the serum during the course of the first sensitizing pregnancy. However, if

sensitive enough techniques are used, an increased incidence of early
sensitization can be detected. There is no doubt that foetal cells pass
across the placenta in small numbers throughout pregnancy. This level
could be insufficient to immunize and to produce a primary response
during the first pregnancy, but sufficient to maintain a temporary state
of immunological tolerance. Around the time of parturition the level of
cells might rise to that which could produce a primary immunological
response. As a result of this, antibody will be detected in the sera of
some of the mothers 6–8 weeks after delivery. In other mothers, subliminal sensitization will occur so that in the second pregnancy the dose
which was sufficient to maintain a temporary state of tolerance in an
unsensitized person will produce a secondary immune response with a
detectable level of circulating antibody.

It is now accepted that if anti-Rh serum is given passively to an Rh-
negative mother immediately after delivery of an Rh-positive infant, it
will suppress Rhesus immunization of the mother. A few cases have been
described where the passive administration of anti-Rh serum has prevented antibody production after the patient had received large volumes
of Rh-positive blood ($\sim$ 200 ml). However, an equal number have been
described where there was a failure to prevent immunization after such
a massive stimulus. It is suggested that in the latter cases the dose of
anti-Rh given was insufficient to prevent primary immunization and
that if the dose of anti-Rhesus serum given is too low, it might actually
augment the primary antibody response, rather than depress it. Anti-Rh
serum is prepared by Rh immunization of healthy Rh negative men or
healthy post-menopausal or sterilized women. Only two-thirds of subjects will actually respond with the production of anti-Rh antibodies
when immunized. A donor is bled when he has 20–30 μg antibody per
ml plasma and 100 ml of plasma is removed at a time, reinjecting the
red cells back into the donor (plasmaphoresis). Pure IgG is then prepared
and the final solution contains 10 g IgG/100 ml. The antibody is administered to the mother by the intramuscular route in doses of 120–
300 μg antibody. Under experimental conditions, it has been shown that
a dose of 75 μg will suppress primary immunization by 1 ml Rh-positive
red cells and a dose of 267 μg will suppress the response to 13 ml Rh-
positive red cells. It has been estimated that a single intramuscular injection of 3200–4000 μg anti-Rh is probably effective in suppressing the
response to transfusion with 500 ml of citrated Rh-positive whole blood.

It is now recommended by the WHO that all Rh-negative women
whose pregnancy terminates after more than 12 weeks' gestation should
be given 200–300 μg of anti-Rh by intramuscular injection. Following
abortion within the first 12 weeks of pregnancy the dose may be reduced
to 50 μg. In Rh-negative subjects inadvertently transfused with Rh-
positive blood, Rh immunization can probably be suppressed by giving
a total dose, intramuscularly, of about 25 μg of anti-Rh per ml of red

cells. It is possible that the passively injected antibody acts as a negative feed-back in turning off antibody production, rather than just destroying the foetal cells present in the circulation. It could be, however, that the passively administered antibody combines with the antigen and prevents it from combining with similar receptors on cells potentially capable of becoming antibody producers against this specific antigen. The dose of antibody necessary to suppress antibody formation is known to be greater than that necessary to clear the number of foetal cells present in the maternal circulation just after delivery. Thus, passive antibody must be in excess and of high activity in order to prevent the antigen from stimulating the antibody-producing system to start a primary response.

"Autoimmune" Haemolytic Anaemias

In many cases of haemolytic anaemia antibody is found either in the serum directed against the patient's own red cells, or antibody and complement either together or alone can be detected on the surface of the circulating red cells themselves. In one-third of the patients auto-immune haemolytic anaemia is described as being "secondary", that is, it is associated with another disease process. In the other two-thirds of patients there is no other disease specifically associated with the anaemia and these are described as being "idiopathic", although in time it is likely that a number of different causes will be found for these anaemias as well.

(i) *Mechanism of the disease process.* The haemolytic anaemias and the thrombocytopenias so often associated with them are so far the only group of diseases where it can be definitely stated that tissue damage develops from a direct reaction between autoantibodies and the body's own cells. The anaemia is caused by the reaction of autoantibody with or without complement with antigens on the surface of the red cells. As a result of this in severe cases agglutination or phagocytosis by blood monocytes can occur to the cells when actually in the circulation. However, the anaemia is almost completely due to the cells being sequestrated by macrophages in the spleen or the liver. The degree to which actual haemolysis occurs in the circulation is not known, but it is not thought to contribute significantly to the disease process. The severity of the disease can be assessed by labelling the patient's red cells with radioactive ^{51}Cr. Whereas transfused red cells normally survive in the circulation with a half life of the order of 25 days, in autoimmune haemolytic anaemias it has been estimated that normal red cells survive in the circulation with a half life of as little as five days.

(ii) *Type of antibody.* In one-quarter of cases the red cells can be found to agglutinate spontaneously *in vitro* when the temperature of the blood is dropped to room temperature or lower. The antibodies in these cases are known as "cold agglutinins" and agglutinate red cells of the same specificity as the patient's in saline when left in the cold. These antibodies are IgM macroglobulins. They have a poor avidity and can be readily dissociated from the surface of the cells, so that frequently only complement can be detected on the cell surface with an anti-globulin reagent.

In the majority of cases of haemolytic anaemia, the patient's red cells do not agglutinate normally *in vitro*. However, globulin can be detected on the surface of washed cells by the use of anti-globulin serum, which agglutinates the cells (Direct Coombs' test). The anti-globulin serum is prepared against normal human globulins generally in rabbits. Anti-globulin serum will agglutinate red cells with immunoglobulins or complement on their surface. The serum from patients with auto-immune haemolytic anaemia can be shown to react *in vitro* with red cells of the same specificity and following the reaction they can also be agglutinated by the anti-globulin serum (Indirect Coombs' test). These antibodies, which are IgG, only react with the red cells at 37°C and are known as "warm auto-antibodies". They are immunoglobulins of the type IgG. In half the cases both antibody and complement can be detected on the red cell surface by the direct Coombs' test. However, in the other half only IgG alone or complement alone can be detected. As these antibodies do not cause agglutination directly and can only be detected by the agglutination of cells, with which they have reacted, by antiglobulin serum, they are sometimes referred to as "incomplete antibodies". If the antibodies are only weakly avid and easily dissociable their reaction with the cells can still be detected by the presence of complement on the cell surface.

(iii) *Antigenic specificity of haemolytic autoantibodies.* In 30% of patients with haemolytic anaemia due to "warm autoantibodies", the specificity of some of the antibodies is directed against one or two of the Rhesus antigens on the surface of the red cells, commonly anti-e or anti-c. The sera of these patients will thus be able to react with red cells from normal subjects which have the same antigen on their surfaces. In the other 70% of patients, the antigen on the red cell surface with which the autoantibodies react has not been identified and is thus referred to as "non-specific" because it does not have Rhesus specificity. In the majority of patients, which have antibodies that are directed against antigens with a Rhesus specificity, there are also antibodies present in the serum with a further unidentified specificity, similarly referred to as "non-specific" antibodies. The term "non-specific" used for these antibodies is not immunologically correct, as all antibodies must have a specificity of reaction. It would thus be better to refer to them as "antibodies of as yet undetermined specificity". As the antigens against which these antibodies are directed are present on the surface of all human red cells, some authors still prefer to retain the term "non-specific". Further investigation of so-called "non-specific" "warm" haemolytic autoantibodies showed that these had some degree of specificity in that they would react with a series of different primate red cells but not with non-primate red cells. A strong correlation was found between the ability of these red cells to be agglutinated by anti-Rh serum and their ability to be agglutinated by warm autoantibodies. It has been suggested, therefore, that all warm autoantibodies have a specificity related to the Rhesus antigen system. Autoantibodies with Rhesus specificity differ qualitatively from the isoantibodies which develop in normal people as a result of direct Rhesus sensitization. The reaction between autoantibodies and the Rhesus antigen is said to be "imperfect", referring to the fact that there they do not fit the Rhesus antigen as well as the isoantibodies and are thus less avid and more easily dissociable.

A large number of "cold" IgM agglutinins in the sera of patients with haemolytic anaemia react with an antigen known as the I antigen present on the surface of the red cells of most normal people. This antigen is not present on the red cells at birth. These antibodies are found more commonly in "secondary haemolytic anaemia" associated with the primary atypical pneumonia due to *Mycoplasma pneumoniae*. A few patients with haemolytic anaemia associated with reticulum cell sarcoma or reticulosis have been found to have cold agglutinins which react only with foetal red cells or those from the rare normal adults that do not carry the I antigen on their red cells. These are often referred to as anti-i antibodies.

Another type of "cold autoantibody" causing haemolytic anaemia but with a different specificity is that associated with the disease "Paroxysmal cold haemoglobinuria". This antibody reacts in the cold with the patient's own red cells or red cells from other normal subjects containing the blood group P antigens. Reaction between the antibody and the red cells only occurs in the cold, but lysis of the sensitized red cells can only take place at 37°C since complement can only lyse sensitized red cells at this temperature. This complicated mechanism accounts for the odd nature of the disease. Haemoglobinuria as a result of massive intravascular lysis of erythrocytes always follows a set pattern. The patient is exposed to cold and then after a pause of a few minutes up to several hours symptoms begin to occur. There is a rigor followed by high fever and the passage of urine containing a high concentration of haemoglobin. The whole episode may last for only a few hours, but occasionally it may persist for a day or more. Following an attack the patient may become jaundiced and the spleen enlarges as a result of the massive haemolysis and sequestration of red cells. The clinical picture may be associated in some cases with Raynaud's phenomenon. In many cases this autoantibody is developed as a result of a syphilitic infection, although a number of cases have been described where there was no history of syphilis. It has been suggested that the autoantibody against the P antigen could develop as a result of tissue changes incidental to infection with *Treponema pallidum*, viruses or perhaps crush injuries. This might result in the release of altered antigen from damaged tissues, as the P antigen has been found not only on red cells but platelets and other human tissue cells. It therefore appears that all three types of erythrocyte autoantibodies have specificity against a blood group antigen. Two criteria are necessary before such antibodies can be classified as autoantibodies. Firstly, the antibody must have specificity for one of the erythrocyte isoantigens and secondly the erythrocytes of the patient must carry this specific antigenic determinant.

(iv) *The association of autoimmune haemolytic anaemia with other disease states.* The association of "cold autoantibodies" with a specificity against the I antigen, with infection due to *Mycoplasma pneumoniae*, and those with specificity against the P antigen, with infection with *Treponema pallidum* are now well established. A total of about one-third of autoimmune haemolytic anaemias are found associated with other disease. Of these a large proportion are associated with malignant disease of the reticuloendothelial system such as chronic lymphatic leukaemia, reticulosarcoma or other lymphomas. The majority of these are of the "warm antibody" (IgG) type, although a number do occur with "cold antibodies" (IgM). Autoimmune haemolytic anaemias can occur associated with other leukaemias or even epithelial neoplasms. Another large group occur associated with chronic infections such as tuberculosis or bronchiectasis, although an occasional case can occur associated with an acute virus infection such as measles or infectious mononucleosis. Systemic lupus erythematosus is not infrequently associated with haemolytic anaemia of the "warm antibody" (IgG) type, and occasionally autoimmune haemolytic anaemia may occur with rheumatoid arthritis, but this can be of either the "warm antibody" type or the "cold antibody" type.

Drug Induced Haemolytic Anaemia

Haemolytic anaemia has been described as a result of treatment with a number of drugs. These include para-amino salicylic acid, phenacetin, quinidine, quinine, chlorpromazine, stibophen and penicillin. The drugs are capable of binding onto the surface of the red cell and the patient's serum is capable of agglutinating normal compatible red cells in the presence of the drug. In some cases the cells can be lysed when complement is added. In some cases it appears that the immune complexes formed between the drug and the antibody are bound onto the surface of the red cell after the formation of the complexes. Haemolytic anaemia can also occur after penicillin therapy. Haemolytic anaemia due to penicillin only occurs after treatment with massive doses in the region of 10 mega-units or more daily. The antibody that causes haemolysis is generally an IgG type. In this case benzylpenicilloyl groups bind to the red cells *in vivo*. The cells are then lysed by antibody in the circulation directed against the benzylpenicilloyl hapten. Immunoglobulin (IgG) can also be detected on the surface of the cells by the direct antiglobulin test. In some cases a proportion of the antibodies bound to the red cells are not directed against the benzyl penicilloyl group but have a specificity as yet undetermined. Whether these antibodies are autoantibodies or have a specificity directed against a minor determinant derived from penicillin is not known.

Certain drugs appear to be able to induce an autoimmune haemolytic anaemia possibly in the same way as viruses. The earliest cases of this phenomenon described was due to certain insecticides (chlorinated hydrocarbons: heptachlor and dieldrin) which produced not only antibodies which would react with the drug bound to the red cell but also antibodies which would react with normal compatible cells in the absence of the insecticides.

Drug induced autoimmune haemolytic anaemia has however been studied most fully in patients on treatment with α methyl DOPA (Aldomet) for hypertension. The incidence of actual haemolytic anaemia following the use of this drug is low. However the direct antiglobulin test shows that as many as 20% of patients on this drug have antibody of the IgG type on the surface of their red cells. Positive direct antiglobulin tests begin to be found three months or more after the beginning of treatment. Thus sensitization does not develop before three months. The incidence of sensitization appears to be dose-dependent. It occurs in less than 11% of patients treated with 1 g. or less of the drug a day. Whereas if they are treated with over 2 g. a day the incidence of sensitization rises to 36%. If patients do not develop antibody after 6 months treatment, it appears that they are in the group that will never be sensitized. If the patient is taken off Aldomet the direct antiglobulin test becomes negative showing that antibody ceases to bind to the red cell surface. L-DOPA used in the treatment of Parkinsonism has also been found to induce similar autoantibodies that react with erythrocytes and show some degree of Rh specificity.

The next fascinating aspect of sensitization of the red cells by Aldomet is that, when the antibody is eluted from the red cells, up to 95% show Rhesus specificity similar to that shown by the autoantibodies in autoimmune haemolytic anaemia of the warm type. So far only IgG has been found on the surface of the red cells. Complement does not appear to be bound by this antibody.

The mechanism of action of this drug is obscure, but when worked out, it might well provide the clue for the mechanism of a number of autoimmune phenomena, especially those associated with drugs or virus infection. It is conceivable that the drug or the virus could modify a normal antigen in such a way that the body were to make antibodies against its own tissues. Aldomet (α methyl dopa) has the formula shown in Figure 1. *In vivo* it could be converted by the enzyme tyrosinase to a DOPA quinone and then by the same enzyme into a melanin pigment. The amount of the quinone present in the body at any particular time will be only a small fraction of the material ingested. However quinones bind onto proteins are powerful sensitizing agents and DOPA quinone could well bind onto the surface of red cells. If the DOPA quinone was to bind onto the peptide chain carrying the Rhesus antigen, antibody could be induced to an antigen in which the quinone was the hapten and the Rhesus antigen the carrier. The antibody would have specificity for both the quinone and the Rhesus antigen, although the antibody would not fit as well with the Rhesus

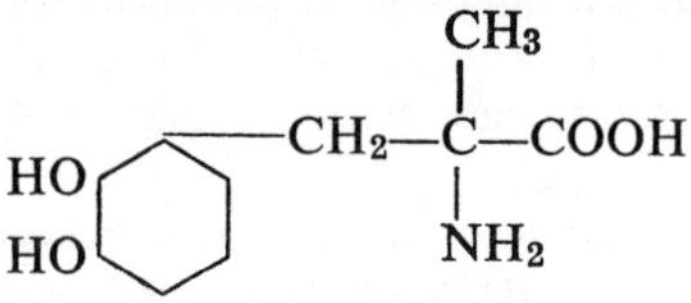

Fig. 1.

antigen as an isoantibody induced by direct immunization of a Rhesus negative individual with Rhesus positive blood. It is well known that Rhesus autoantibodies are less avid than isoantibodies and are more readily dissociable. This would be due to the poorness of fit of the antibody to the antigen.

The reason α methyl dopa takes as long as three months to sensitize, could also be related to the fact that it binds to the Rhesus antigen. The Rhesus antigen is only found on the surface of red cells. If the hapten did not decrease the life-span of the circulating red cells it could take three months before these cells are removed by the reticulo-endothelial system and for sensitization to occur. Another alternative hypothesis is that the α methyl dopa being an amino acid is incorporated into the Rhesus antigen when the red cells are being made. The red cells will then have an abnormal amino acid in their Rhesus antigens which would cause a failure of the Rhesus antigen to be recognized as "self".

It also appears that α methyl dopa will enhance the antigenicity of cell nuclear components, as some patients on this drug for three months or more, will develop antinuclear factor in their serum. The development of antinuclear antibodies does not correlate with the presence of anti-red cell antibodies, nor is it dependent on the dose of drug given, as is the development of antinuclear antibodies. The significance of the antinuclear antibodies is not known as patients on Aldomet do not develop systemic lupus erythematosus as do those on hydralazine. The presence of antinuclear factor in the serum of patients treated with Aldomet has been used as evidence suggesting that the drug acts on the central immune mechanisms directly and increases responsiveness to self-antigens. The respective roles of altered antigenicity and stimulation of the central immune mechanisms in producing autoimmune phenomena will have to be worked out for this as for other agents.

Thrombocytopenic Purpura

Although the cause of thrombocytopenic purpura is not known in many cases and is classed clinically as "idiopathic" in a proportion of patients, the disease can be shown to be associated with other immunological phenomena as in systemic lupus erythematosus. About 50 % of patients with "acquired" haemolytic anaemia have a low circulating platelet count, although in many cases this is not low enough to produce clinical purpura. If purpura supervenes in a patient with autoimmune haemolytic anaemia the prognosis is considered to be grave. In some cases where idiopathic thrombocytopenic purpura has been treated by splenectomy, this is followed by the development of an autoimmune haemolytic anaemia. The term immuno-pancytopenia has been coined to describe autoimmune haemolytic anaemia associated with leucopenia and thrombocytopenia. The presence of antibodies against the platelets in autoimmune thrombocytopenia is very difficult to demonstrate because few platelets can be demonstrated in the blood of these patients to allow for an equivalent of the antiglobulin test to be performed. However, thrombocytopenia has been produced in normal subjects by the transfusion of plasma from patients with idiopathic thrombocytopenia, indicating that there are circulating anti-platelet antibodies present in the blood stream.

The humoral factor in the plasma causing idiopathic thrombocytopenia has been shown to react with platelets. It is a conventional immunoglobulin of molecular weight 150,000. Immune complexes formed by the interaction of platelets with this autoantibody will react with complement. If platelets labelled with radioactive ^{51}Cr are transfused into patients with thrombocytopenic purpura, they can be shown to be eliminated more rapidly from the circulation. Similarly if labelled platelets are transfused into a normal individual followed by plasma from a patient with idiopathic thrombocytopenic purpura, they can also be shown to be eliminated more rapidly. Labelled platelets infused into patients with thrombocytopenic purpura can be shown to be sequestered in the liver and in the spleen. However, it appears that more are sequestered in the liver than in the spleen. This is of interest in view of the fact that some of these patients are cured by splenectomy. Thus the removal of the spleen in thrombocytopenic purpura must be effective because of the removal of a major site of antibody production, rather than because one is removing a major site of sequestration of platelets coated with autoantibody.

Thrombocytopenic purpura is a well known complication of drug therapy. It occurs with a wide range of different drugs including sedormid, quinidine, quinine, digitoxin, sulphadimidine, sulphafurazole, insulin, aspirin, codeine, phenobarbitone, butobarbitone, novobiocin, chlorthiazide and hydrochlorthiazide, antipyrin (phenazone), amidopyrine and sodium aurothiosulphate. Of these quinine and quinidine are also known to cause haemolytic anaemia.

A considerable amount of research has been done on thrombocytopenic purpura especially due to sedormid. Antibodies can be detected in the serum of patients, who have had purpura, which react with the drug bound onto the surface of platelets as a hapten. Immune reaction on the surface of the platelets can be shown to cause agglutination or lysis of the platelets and fixation of complement. If the antibody is present in high concentration in the serum, the addition of the drug will cause immune precipitation *in vitro*, although this is rare. If a patient is allergic to a drug such as sedormid, which causes thrombocytopenic purpura, the application of the drug to the skin will cause a local area of purpura due to the local absorption of the drug through the skin.

The dose of drug which may cause purpura in a sensitive subject may be very large or very small. As little as 0·1 mg of a drug daily for 6 days is enough to drop the platelet count to one-third of the normal in a highly sensitive subject.

The Treatment of Autoimmune Haemolytic Anaemia and Thrombocytopenic Purpura

(i) *Corticosteroids*. Corticosteroids are the first line of defence in the treatment of autoimmune haemolytic anaemia and thrombocytopenic purpura. Prednisone in a dose of 40–80 mg daily appears to be able to control the disease in about 40% of patients with haemolytic anaemia and will be effective in producing a rise in the circulating platelets in 60% of patients with thrombocytopenic purpura.

In a small proportion of patients clinical improvement is associated with a decrease in the amount of circulating antibody and in some the level of antibody may become undetectable in the serum. Thus the drug appears in these patients to be having a true immunosuppressive effect in reducing or abolishing the amount of antibody produced. Suppression of antibody production takes about one week to develop. This is the same time as it takes for the circulating platelet level to return to normal in patients with thrombocytopenic purpura treated with steroids. The reduction in circulating antibody can be shown to be associated with a reduction in the general level of circulating immunoglobulins, so the effect of steroids does not appear to be on the production of the specific autoantibody alone. The effect of steroids on the antibody level in haemolytic anaemia would appear to be the result of a general effect on the suppression of the immune response of the individual by an effect on the central immunological mechanisms. Steroids can also be shown to reduce the level of circulating antibodies to a number of antigens in certain experimental animals.

In a proportion of patients clinical improvement occurs in the haemolytic anaemia on treatment with steroids without any drop in the circulating antibody or with a drop in antibody level insufficient to account for the clinical improvement seen. Steroids can be shown to inhibit the phagocytosis of sensitized red cells by leucocytes *in vitro*. Thus it is possible that in the majority of patients, where there has not been a marked reduction in the level of circulating antibody, the clinical effect of steroids could be in preventing the phagocytosis of antibody coated red cells by the cells of the reticulo-endothelial system in the liver, spleen and bone marrow.

Prolonged use of corticosteroids produces intolerable side-effects in a large proportion of patients. These include osteoporosis resulting in pathological fractures, gastrointestinal bleeding and psychotic disorders. Also a proportion of the patients never respond to steroids at all. Thus corticosteroids may not be able to be used in treatment alone. In these cases, the possibility of splenectomy or the use of other immuno-suppressive drugs must be considered.

(ii) *Splenectomy.* The value of splenectomy in autoimmune haemolytic anaemia is very much a subject for debate. It is thought that splenectomy has little influence on the course of the disease, although it may produce a temporary remission. As the spleen is one of the major sites in the reticuloendothelial system where antibody coated red cells are sequestered, removal of this organ may reduce the number of cells being sequestered. As mentioned above, the transfusion of radioactive chromium (^{51}Cr) labelled red cells into a patient with haemolytic anaemia will show that the red cells are sequestered mainly in the liver and spleen. In a proportion of patients sequestration is greater in the spleen than in the liver. It is in these patients that it has been recommended that splenectomy be used. If sequestration is greater in the liver than in the spleen, it is thought that splenectomy will be less effective.

In some cases autoimmune haemolytic anaemia is the first sign of a more general disease of the immunological mechanisms and may later be associated with thrombocytopenic purpura, or even the whole symptom complex of systemic lupus erythematosus. The development of thrombocytopenic purpura or systemic lupus erythematosus has been described as a complication of splenectomy for autoimmune haemolytic anaemia. It is not known however, whether these conditions would have supervened normally at about the time the splenectomy was performed or whether the splenectomy accelerated the naturally occurring disease process.

Splenectomy appears to be much more successful in the treatment of autoimmune thrombocytopenic purpura than haemolytic anaemia. In this condition it has been shown that sequestration of platelets is almost completely in the liver with little removal by the spleen. This would suggest that, in both haemolytic anaemia and thrombocytopenic purpura, splenectomy does not act by removing a major area of phagocytosis of antibody coated red cells or platelets, but has some other action. Although the removal of the spleen in experimental animals has little effect on the production of circulating antibody, splenectomy has been shown in certain cases to cause a marked reduction in the level of circulating antibody in autoimmune haemolytic anaemia. This suggests that it is in fact an important source of antibody production in some of these cases. Moreover under experimental conditions it has been shown that splenectomized individuals fail to produce circulating antibody to transfused foreign red cells. Thus it appears that in the human the spleen is an important organ for producing antibodies to red cells and also platelets. The success of splenectomy in causing remissions of autoimmune haemolytic anaemia and thrombocytopenic purpura would thus be due to its removal as an antibody producing organ rather than as a major site of phagocytosis. Relapses after splenectomy would be due to the production of antibody being taken over by other areas of lymphoid tissue throughout the body.

(iii) *Immunosuppressive drugs.* 6-mercaptopurine and 6-thioguanine both potent immunosuppressive drugs have been used in the treatment of autoimmune haemolytic anaemia and thrombocytopenic purpura and have produced marked remissions of the disease. Azothioprine (1·5–2·5 mg/kg daily) and cyclophosphamide (200 mg daily) have also been used with some success. Cyclophosphamide has been shown to suppress the haemolytic anaemia which occurs in the autoimmune disease resembling systemic lupus erythematosus in mice which develops possibly as a result of infection with a virus-like organism. These drugs have been used alone in human disease. Current practice is to use them in patients who show marked side-effects from corticosteroids. It is usual to continue the steroids but at a dose which does not produce toxic side-effects (as little as 5 mg prednisone per day). Combined therapy with imuran (azathioprine), 6-mercaptopurine or cyclophosphamide, together with the lower dose of prednisone seems to be the treatment of choice in patients with autoimmune haemolytic anaemia in whom the level of prednisone necessary to control the disease produces toxic symptoms or in patients with idiopathic thrombocytopenic purpura who have had a relapse following splenectomy.

The mode of action of immunosuppressive drugs in these diseases is not completely understood. An impairment in the ability of patients, under treatment, to form certain types of antibody can be readily demonstrated. However, it appears that there is no correlation between the presence, absence or extent of the suppression of the antibody response and the clinical response of the patient. Thus patients may improve clinically with little demonstrable effect on antibody production while others in whom antibody production is suppressed may show little clinical improvement.

As with the corticosteroids the effect of these drugs may to some extent be on the ability of the reticulo-endothelial system to phagocytose antibody coated red cells or platelets. It has also been suggested that there could be an effect on one of the nine components of complement which actually produce the damage to the cells following reaction with antibody and are involved in "preparing" the cells for phagocytosis. Immunosuppressive drugs appear to act on a number of different processes in the body and could block the immune reaction at any level between antibody production and the final phagocytosis of the damaged cell.

Bibliography

Books

Dacie, J. V. (1963), *The Haemolytic Anaemias—Congenital and Acquired. Part 2. The Autoimmune Anaemias*. Second edition. London: Churchill.
Dodd, B. E. & Lincoln, P. J. (1975), *Blood Group Topics*. London: Edward Arnold.
Pirofsky, B. (1969), *Autoimmunization and the Autoimmune Hemolytic Anaemias*. Baltimore: Williams & Wilkins.
Prevention of Rh. Sensitization (1971), *Wld. Hlth. Org. techn. Rep. Ser.*, No. 468. Geneva: WHO.

Articles

Ackroyd, J. F. (ed.) (1964), "The diagnosis of disorders of the blood due to drug hypersensitivity caused by an immune mechanism." *Immunological Methods*. Oxford: Blackwell.
Breckenridge, A., Dollery, C. T., Worlledge, S. M., Holborow, E. J. & Johnson, G. D. (1967), "Positive direct Coombs tests and antinuclear factor in patients treated with methyl dopa." *Lancet*, ii, 1265.
Mollison, P. L. (1968), "Suppression of Rh immunization by passively administered anti-Rh." *Brit. J. Haematol.*, **14**, 1.
Swanson, M. & Schwartz, R. S. (1967), "Immunosuppressive therapy. Relation between immunological competence and clinical responsiveness." *New Engl. J. Med.*, **277**, 163.

Chapter XV

Immunological Processes Affecting the Eye and Nervous System

The Eye

Any discussion of immunological processes as they affect the eye must be prefaced by a discussion of those anatomical and physiological factors which make the reactions in the eye differ somewhat from that which would be expected in any other area of the body. The main points of difference between the eye and other tissues are—

1. The presence of components which lack a conventional blood supply. These are the lens, the cornea and the vitreous. The lens, moreover, is surrounded by a capsule which prevents antigen entering it and leaving it, under normal physiological conditions.
2. Under normal conditions there is a limitation in the passage of cells and proteins from the blood stream into the aqueous or the vitreous. Similarly if an antigen enters the aqueous or the vitreous it forms a depot from which the material will diffuse out only very slowly.
3. There is no lymphatic drainage of the tissues lying within the eye. Whereas in other tissues antigens drain through the lymphatics down into the local lymph nodes, antigens drain away from the eye into the blood stream. Thus there is no local draining lymph node for the eye.
4. The lens contains very strong organ specific antigens but scarcely any species specific antigens. However, none of the antigens in the vitreous are specific to this material but cross react with antigens in the liver, kidney and serum. The vitreous does not contain any antigens which cross react with antigens in the lens.

Experimental animals immunized with material from their own vitreous will form antibodies against this tissue—autoantibodies. These antibodies will also react with antigens in the vitreous of man and other experimental animals. The presence of these autoantibodies in the serum do not produce lesions in the eyes of animals in which they are in the circulation.

1. *Reactions of the eye to foreign antigens*

Because of the anatomical and physiological peculiarities of the eye, described above, the eye reacts differently to other tissues when injected with foreign antigens.

When antigen is injected into the vitreous, it leaks out only very slowly and forms a localized depot. Antigen cannot drain into the local lymphoid tissue. However, cells can migrate from the blood stream into the area of antigen deposition. Within one week there is an accumulation of lymphocytes and mononuclear cells, which is especially intense in the vascular tissues of the iris and ciliary body, forming what is known as a "spontaneous uveitis". Between the seventh and tenth days after antigen injection, some of the mononuclear cells begin to transform into cells of the plasma cell series and antibody is secreted locally into the tissues of the eye and spills over into the circulation. Often there are higher levels of antibody in the aqueous than in the peripheral blood. The inflammation will die down over a period of some months after which it is not possible to detect any evidence of the previous condition. The eye to all appearances is then normal. However, if the animal is injected with the same antigen, even six months to a year later, at a distant site in the body, an eye which has been the site of injection of that antigen and had a "spontaneous uveitis" will flare up and develop a condition resembling the clinical state of "recurrent non-granulomatous uveitis". This reaction is immunologically specific and only occurs when the animal has a second contact with the same antigen which was originally injected into the eye.

This flare-up is not due to the presence of residual antibody within the eye, but to a few sensitized "memory" cells which remain within the ocular tissues. These react with the antigen and cause a second micro-inflammation, as a result of which other cells enter the eye from extraocular centres such as the lymph nodes and spleen. These cells which infiltrate as a secondary event also transform into plasma cells as in the primary "spontaneous uveitis" and begin to secrete antibody locally into the eye which react with antigen coming in from the circulation.

It therefore appears that, although there is no lymphoid tissue to which antigen drains from the eye, lymphoid cells migrate into the eye following antigen instillation, undergo the same changes and produce antibody in the same way as they would in the central lymphoid tissues of the body. Under the correct conditions, the eye develops its own lymphoid tissue, whenever necessary. The "uveitis" which develops as a result of contact of the eye with antigen is directly analogous to the changes in lymph nodes which occur when antigen is injected into a tissue with a normal lymphatic drainage. A similar picture to the secondary uveitis found in the experimental animal, has been produced in man as a result of systemic absorption of tuberculin following a tuberculin test in the skin. In this case it is suspected that the primary "spontaneous uveitis" caused by tuberculoprotein had been subclinical.

Reactions similar to anaphylaxis, the Arthus reaction and delayed hypersensitivity can also be observed in the eye. If anaphylactic antibody is present in the circulation and antigen is injected into the vitreous, there is increased permeability of the blood vessels of the iris and contraction of plain muscle causing the pupil to contract. This occurs as a result of the local release of pharmacological agents such as histamine in the same way as in any other tissue. The reaction also occurs as rapidly as it would in other tissues.

Arthus reactions can also be produced in the eye in the presence of a high level of antibody. There is oedema of the iris and the ciliary body. The iris becomes hyperaemic and haemorrhages occur. The infiltration is with polymorphonuclear leucocytes which are also found in the aqueous. Proteinaceous material and fibrin strands are also evident in the anterior chamber. Unlike the Arthus reaction in the skin, where the reaction is maximal 4–8 hours after injection, the peak of the reaction in the eye is 24 hours after the antigen is injected into the vitreous. The polymorphonuclear leucocytes become superseded by mononuclear cells, as in the reaction in other tissues, and eventually plasma cells are found in the infiltrate. Immune complex uveitis can be induced in rabbits by the systemic injection of foreign serum proteins. The uveitis develops in conjunction with immune complex damage to the renal glomeruli. Similar uveitis can be induced by repeated injections of streptococcal antigens. Damage to the uvea by an intravitreous injection of endotoxin can cause a recurrence of immune complex uveitis. In man uveitis is regularly associated with other evidence of immune complex disease such as arthritis, and cutaneous vasculitis.

In delayed hypersensitivity reactions to the intravitreous injection of antigen there is a violent inflammation maximal at 24 hours, in which the iris is hyperaemic and there is proteinaceous material, fibrin strands and inflammatory cells in the anterior chamber. The iris and ciliary body are infiltrated with mononuclear cells and there is a perivascular infiltration round the blood vessels of the choroid (focal choroiditis). The injection of tuberculin into the vitreous of a tuberculin sensitive animal produces a mixed Arthus and delayed reaction. The instillation of antigen such as tuberculin or vaccinia virus or a simple chemical sensitizer into the conjunctival sac of a sensitized animal or individual will evoke a severe delayed hypersensitivity reaction, not only in the cornea resulting in opacification, but also resulting in a severe uveitis. This must be considered a significant hazard for anyone working with these materials. The eye itself can be sensitized directly by putting antigen into the conjunctival sac of an animal, which has not been previously sensitized with the antigen. This process is similar to the primary spontaneous uveitis which develops when antigen is injected into the vitreous. Sensitization takes 3–4 weeks to develop and results in the development of a severe iritis. This may be the mechanism behind the development of endogenous uveitis in man and could be due to pollens, drugs or other allergens present in the air contaminating the conjunctival sac.

2. *Infectious uveitis*

Infectious agents probably produce severe and serious disease in the eye more as a result of antigenic stimulation than as a result of a direct cytopathogenic effect. This may occur especially with viruses such as vaccinia and herpes simplex, fungi such as in histoplasmosis and protozoa such as *Toxoplasma gondii*. The direct cytopathogenic effect of herpes simplex virus is to produce a simple dendritic ulcer of the cornea. However, this is often superseded by a disciform keratitis and iritis in which there is no detectable virus. Hypersensitive animals show a higher incidence of disciform keratitis than non-immune animals.

The pattern of the lesions in the eye is often typical for the organism causing the disease. This is probably the result of the particular localization of the antigen in the eye. Thus in one series, in 94% of patients where the disease took the form of disciform detachment of the macula without haemorrhages, and discrete choroidal lesions with a clear vitreous, the disease was shown to be due to histoplasmosis, histoplasmosis being associated with only 25% of other lesions of the uveal tract. In 94% of patients with focal exudative retino-choroiditis, the disease was associated with toxoplasmosis, which was present in only 23% of other uveal lesions. In most cases of uveitis no organism can be isolated, suggesting that the pathogenic process is one of hypersensitivity rather than direct damage caused by the organism.

The only endogenous uveitis of domestic animals is that found in horses associated with leptospirosis. In this condition antibody is found against the organism in the aqueous, and the level of antibody in the aqueous is often 10–2,000 times as high as that in peripheral blood. Leptospiral uveitis has also been found in man with higher levels of antibody in the aqueous than in the peripheral blood. Similarly cases of uveitis associated with tuberculosis and toxoplasmosis have been described occasionally with levels of antibody in the aqueous higher than that in the serum. This suggests that the uveitis is due to direct antigenic stimulation of the eye with local antibody production and is similar to that which can be produced with simple protein antigens in the experimental animal. This "spontaneous" induced hypersensitivity reaction is due to direct contact with antigens derived from the organism in the eye itself or is a secondary uveitis to antigen, derived from the organism present in the circulation, in an eye where there has been a subclinical primary uveitis.

Uveitis occurs frequently with joint diseases such as ankylosing spondylitis, infectious arthritis, Still's disease and Reiter's syndrome. This type of uveitis shows a strong association with HLA-B27. One hypothesis which would cover this relationship is that both uveitis and arthritis are manifestations of diseases where there are circulating immune complexes. The antigen causing the disease might be of bacterial, viral or mycoplasmal origin. Immune complexes would tend to stick in the uvea and joints because of common peculiarities of the blood vessels which would cause them to localize at these sites and cause inflammatory reactions in both places at the same time.

3. *Autoimmune uveitis—sympathetic ophthalmia*

Experimental animals can be made to develop uveitis when immunized with an homogenized suspension of homologous uvea in an adjuvant mixture (Freund's adjuvant, a water-in-oil emulsion containing tubercle bacilli). The disease is a transient one starting with vitreous opacities followed by cells in the aqueous. Deposits are seen on the anterior lens capsule and the posterior surface of the cornea. There is mononuclear cell infiltration of the ciliary body with extension into the adjacent vitreous, iris and choroid. The external layers of the retina are also involved secondarily. Plasma cells are prominent in the infiltrate and in severe reactions there are many polymorphonuclear leucocytes and macrophages. Precipitating antibody can be demonstrated in the serum against uveal tissue antigens. The animals also show delayed hypersensitivity reactions in the skin when injected intradermally with soluble extracts of the uvea. As the uvea contains antigens in common with other tissues delayed hypersensitivity reactions can also be evoked when the animals are skin tested with extracts of homologous spleen.

The disease seen in the experimental animals appears analogous to human clinical uveitis starting as a cyclitis but eventually spreading to the whole uvea. However, the most important condition which it resembles is that form of uveitis known as sympathetic ophthalmia. This condition follows injury to the eye, generally penetrating wounds which involve the uveal tract, especially the ciliary body and the root of the iris. Uveitis develops in the non-injured eye between two weeks and three months after injury. There is a massive cellular infiltration of the iris and ciliary body; the choroid only being involved later. Cellular deposits are found on the back of the cornea and granulation tissue develops in both the injured and non-injured eyes at the same time. In 20% of cases both eyes recover, but in the other 80% the disease is progressive and both eyes become permanently blind. However, if the original damaged eye is removed in time the condition will resolve. The condition can be controlled by prompt and intensive corticosteroid therapy in 64% of cases, though in a number there is a recurrence on stopping steroids. There is one case reported where corticosteroids were given prophylactically following injury to the eye and sympathetic ophthalmia developed soon after steroid treatment was stopped. The incidence of sympathetic ophthalmia is low and occurs only in the region of 0·5% of injuries to the eye.

Under normal conditions antibodies against uveal antigens can be detected in the serum by the complement fixation reaction during the time when a uveal wound is healing. If the patient develops such antibodies sympathetic ophthalmia does not develop. However, in a small proportion of patients delayed hypersensitivity reactions can be demonstrated when they are skin tested with uveal antigens, these patients do not develop circulating antibodies and then proceed to develop sympathetic ophthalmia. Patients with antibodies in their circulation against uvea do not develop delayed hypersensitivity skin test reactivity and do not develop sympathetic ophthalmia. There is thus a direct correlation between delayed hypersensitivity to uveal antigens and sympathetic ophthalmia. The presence of circulating antibodies to uvea appears to preclude the development of delayed hypersensitivity to these antigens and the development of the autoimmune disease state. This is one example where there appears to be a direct relationship between delayed hypersensitivity to the tissue involved and the development of autoimmune tissue damage.

4. *Lens-induced inflammations of the uveal tract*

Lens-induced hypersensitive reactions of the uveal tract follow operative or traumatic injury which liberates lens protein into the rest of the eye. If there has been previous subclinical release of lens protein, the reaction takes 24–48 hours to develop. If, however, there has been no previous release of lens protein the inflammatory reaction takes 10–14 days to develop. If the reaction is a mild one it has been referred to by ophthalmologists as "phacotoxic uveitis" and, if severe, as "endophthalmitis phacoanaphylactica".

Lens-induced uveitis is an autoimmune hypersensitivity reaction to organ-specific antigens present in the lens, which normally do not come into contact with cells of the lymphoid system, as the lens is surrounded by a capsule which prevents antigens leaving it under normal physiological conditions. Lens-induced hypersensitivity can induce a secondary sympathetic ophthalmia in the undamaged eye and this can be cured by simple extraction of the damaged lens. Patients with lens-induced uveitis will show positive skin reactions when injected intradermally with lens protein, indicating the presence of a generalized hypersensitivity to this antigen. Such reactions are not shown by patients with glaucoma developing as a result of simple degeneration of the lens and direct block of the outlet of the aqueous (phacolytic glaucoma). This condition appears to be a result of simple mechanical changes rather than due to immunological reactions as does the uveitis.

Skin sensitivity to lens protein may be found in patients with cataract. If lens material is left behind during operation in these patients there is a risk of uveitis developing. However, if all the lens material is removed at operation, the post-operative course will be uneventful.

Hypersensitivity to lens protein does not occur in patients with normal eyes. A small percentage of patients with cataracts develop hypersensitivity to lens protein. Such a state of hypersensitivity will cause a predisposition to the development of uveitis if any lens material is left in the anterior chamber of the eye at operation.

Lens-induced uveitis is observed mainly as a complication of accidental injury or extracapsular extraction of the lens. It appears to occur only rarely following spontaneous rupture of a swollen cataract under pressure. This could be because, under these conditions, the lens proteins have lost their specific antigenicity. The inflammatory reaction of lens-induced uveitis is mainly round the lens in the anterior chamber or in the vitreous, as might be expected. Disintegrating lens tissue is surrounded by polymorphonuclear leucocytes and round these may be found mononuclear cells, granulation tissue and plasma cells. The iris becomes firmly adherent to the inflammatory tissue and is itself infiltrated with mononuclear cells and plasma cells. Antibody is formed locally in the iris and may be found in the aqueous.

5. Uveitis developing as a result of allergic disease of the central nervous system

In most cases where eye disease is produced experimentally, this has been done by direct manipulation of the eye or by sensitization of the animal with uveal tissue. One observation of potential importance as a cause of endogenous uveitis in man, is the finding that uveitis has been observed in animals with experimental autoimmune allergic encephalomyelitis produced by the sensitization of the animal with antigens derived from the central nervous system. The reaction may be due to antigens in myelin present in the nerves which supply the iris and ciliary body, or else due to a possibility that uveal tissue contains antigens which cross react with those in the central nervous system. Another possibility is that inflammation of the iris and ciliary body is secondary to inflammation of the retina, itself a nervous tissue.

The acute encephalomyelitis associated with measles and other exanthemata is considered to be an allergic reaction to central nervous tissue. It is therefore of interest that bilateral uveitis has been described as a complication of measles, mumps and chickenpox. There are also other conditions in which eye disease has been found together with involvement of the central nervous system. Thus it may be that some cases of endogenous uveitis of unknown aetiology may be the outward manifestations of a subclinical allergic encephalomyelitis.

Central Nervous System

Immunological diseases of the central nervous system can be divided basically into two groups. In the first, the brain could be damaged by an auto-allergic process in which immunologically active cells or antibody react with the brain or peripheral nervous tissue. In the second group brain or peripheral nervous tissue could be damaged as a result of an immunological reaction between cells or antibody and a foreign antigen. In this case tissue damage is secondary to the immune reaction rather than a direct result of it.

1. *Autoimmune allergic encephalomyelitis*

This condition can be produced with ease in experimental animals by injecting them with homologous or heterologous brain tissue in the standard water-in-oil emulsion containing tubercle bacilli (Freund's adjuvant). The disease begins to develop 10–14 days after the intramuscular injection of this mixture and is fatal in a high proportion of the animals. It generally takes the form initially of a paralysis of the hind limbs and recto-vesical incontinence. Histological changes may be seen in the brain as early as six days after the injection of the brain mixture. The inflammatory lesion originates as a focal collection of lymphocytes, histiocytes, plasma cells and occasional polymorphonuclear leucocytes in the adventitial sheath of small veins. Although these cells go on to invade the surrounding brain tissue their distribution remains predominantly perivascular. Quite frequently during the acute phase of the disease there is marked inflammation of the meninges of the brain, brain stem and spinal cord. In some cases the choroid plexus is also involved in the inflammatory reaction. The brain tissue shows marked demyelination which is quite circumscribed and perivascular in distribution. Rarely fusion of several areas result in a diffuse type of demyelination, but this is never as extensive as that seen in multiple sclerosis.

The relative role of humoral antibodies and cell-mediated immune reactions in producing these lesions has been discussed frequently. Originally it was thought that autoimmune allergic encephalomyelitis was a pure manifestation of the cell-mediated immune reaction. In the experimental animal the disease is often associated with a state of delayed hypersensitivity to brain tissue which can be demonstrated by intradermal injection of a purified extract of the tissue. The reaction in the brain is one of perivascular mononuclear cell infiltration rather like the tuberculin reaction in the skin. Moreover the disease process cannot be transferred to a normal animal by the injection of serum from an affected animal. This impression was confirmed by the finding that disease could be transferred by lymph node cells from affected animals. However, such a transfer could only take place if the transfer was performed in histocompatible inbred animals or under other conditions where the cells transferring the disease survived in the recipient for a long period of time. Thus the transferred disease could not be due to the direct action of the transferred cells on the brain tissue. It would therefore seem that the cells need to persist in the host for a period of time to elaborate a factor which was necessary to produce the disease.

These donor cell suspensions would contain cells both capable of initiating a cell-mediated immune reaction but also cells capable of synthesizing humoral antibodies. Thus it would seem likely that the actual disease is caused by the combined action of both cell-mediated immune processes and humoral antibody. There is no doubt that cell-mediated immune processes probably form the major component of the immunological reaction, but it is extremely probable that they need the supplementary action of humoral antibodies to produce the full clinical effect. This combined action of both cell-mediated and humoral immune processes in the production of disease is probably a more general phenomenon in the initiation of auto-immune processes than has been previously realized. Recently this combined action has been demonstrated conclusively to cause the lesions in experimental auto-immune allergic orchitis, and in the future other similar immunological disease states will be shown to be the results of the interaction of cell-mediated immune processes with the effect of humoral antibodies.

Autoimmune allergic encephalomyelitis may occur in man following a course of injections with rabies vaccine. This vaccine can be prepared against the virus in rabbit spinal cord and the patient is then injected with heterologous spinal cord antigens. The incidence of this disease following rabies vaccination is between 1:1000 and 1:4000. However, the antigen is injected without adjuvant. Clinical neurological signs appear 7 to 20 days after the first injection of the vaccine and consist of meningeal signs associated with involvement either of peripheral nerves or the spinal cord. There is numbness, paraesthesiae and flaccid or spastic paralysis mainly of the lower limbs with rectal and bladder incontinence. Sometimes the symptoms and signs ascend rapidly to the trunk and upper limbs. In these cases death usually supervenes due to respiratory paralysis. In Japan the disease has been described as taking what is called the "cerebral" form. These cases occur 5 to 8 weeks after vaccination, and are associated with psychiatric disturbances and epileptic fits. Motor disturbances occur in one-third of cases and visual disturbances in four-fifths of cases. This condition is, however, rare. Histologically the disease is associated with perivascular collections of mononuclear cells often together with some plasma cells. The brain and spinal cord show localized areas of demyelination with a perivascular distribution similar to that seen in experimental animals with autoimmune allergic encephalomyelitis. The distribution of lesions does not appear to be related to the clinical form which the disease takes whether the more common spinal form or the rare cerebral form. The optic chiasma and optic nerves are often affected.

2. *Diseases of the central nervous system associated with virus infections*

Encephalitis is a well known, although infrequent, complication of many infective exanthemata of virus origin. These include measles, rubella and varicella. A similar process has been described following mumps and vaccination. Neurological symptoms appear 7–10 days after the febrile stage of the infection. Owing to the presence of perivascular infiltration with mononuclear cells and a similar distribution of areas of demyelination throughout the central nervous system, it has been suggested that these conditions are analogous to the state of allergic autoimmune encephalomyelitis that can be produced in experimental animals. However, disease of the central nervous system is not restricted to the viruses enumerated above, and it is probable that the underlying causative mechanism of the actual disease process is similar in a much wider group of neurological conditions associated with virus infection. In many other virus diseases such as poliomyelitis and the encephalitis due to arthropod-born viruses such as dengue, and Western equine encephalomyelitis, neurological symptoms are preceded one to two weeks earlier by evidence of a generalized viraemia, in the form of a mild febrile illness.

It has been estimated that in poliomyelitis and arthropod-born virus infection neurological symptoms appear in only between 0.1% and 10% of patients infected. Neurological symptoms begin to appear in patients at about the same time as they develop significant levels of antibody in the circulation. It has therefore been suggested that in these conditions neurological disease could well be due to a hypersensitivity reaction to the virus proliferating in the central nervous system rather than to the direct toxic effect of virus multiplication.

The effect of immunological reactions in causing disease of the central nervous system, during virus infection, has been studied extensively in one particular experimental model—lymphocytic choriomeningitis of mice (LCM) (Fig. 1). LCM is a naturally occurring virus disease of mice. However, disease caused by this virus has occurred in humans, in whom it takes the form of a mild febrile respiratory disease followed a week or so later by a severe meningitis. The time scale of the infection is similar to that which occurs in other virus infective diseases with neurological complications. The biological course of infection of the mouse with this virus will be described at some length, as it illustrates the way in which pathological changes in the central nervous system can be produced by immune reactions against the virus rather than by the direct toxic action of the intracellular growth of the virus in cells of the central nervous system. In its most severe form the disease is fatal with maximum mortality about eight days after intracerebral inoculation of the virus. There is meningitis, encephalitis and myelitis. However, other organs especially the liver and kidneys are often affected. Histologically there is marked lymphocytic infiltration of the central nervous system as well as the other organs affected.

It was observed quite early that some colonies of mice might carry

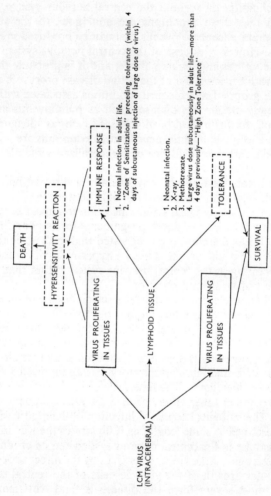

Fig. 1. Lymphocytic choriomeningitis infection in the mouse (after Hotchin, 1962). An example of the interaction of virus and immunological mechanisms in the brain.

this virus without developing any signs of disease, and mice infected with LCM virus *in utero* would not develop the disease, although virus could be isolated from them in adult life. A similar state of tolerance to the virus could be induced by injecting the virus intracerebrally into the newborn mouse within the first 24 hours of birth. Under these conditions the virus would propagate in the mouse without causing any harmful effects. If such a mouse was challenged by the intracerebral injection of virus it would not develop disease, in the same way as a mouse which had not received the virus *in utero* or in early neonatal life. Tolerance could be induced in adult life by giving the virus intracerebrally associated with treatment with immunosuppressive agents such as X-irradiation or methotrexate. Treatment with corticosteroids will modify the disease caused by the virus. Tolerance can also be induced in the adult mouse by giving virus subcutaneously, rather than intracerebrally and allowing it to proliferate for more than four days. If the mouse is challenged intracerebrally with the virus after four days it will be found to be tolerant. However, before four days while the virus is proliferating to a level at which the immune mechanisms become tolerant, the mouse goes through a phase of enhanced sensitization and if challenged intracerebrally during this period will develop the fatal disease more rapidly. This phenomenon in which the adult animal passes through a phase of sensitization before becoming tolerant to high doses of antigen has been described with a number of other antigens and is now a well recognized immunological phenomenon. Originally it was thought that the hypersensitivity response against LCM virus was of the cell-mediated type. However, the virus in the blood has been shown to be in the form of immune complexes combined with IgG and complement. Moreover, study of the glomeruli of these mice shows a progressive accumulation of IgG, complement and viral antigen in irregular deposits along the capillary wall and mesangia after the first three weeks of life. It has therefore been suggested that the meningitis in LCM infection is also of immune-complex origin rather than cell-mediated.

Prior sensitization with inactivated virus vaccines has been found in certain cases to increase the intensity of the disease produced by subsequent infection with live arthropod-born viruses and also to decrease the incubation time of the development of the neurological disease, indicating the probable immunological nature of the process. Although humoral antibody neutralizes viruses *in vitro* and under most conditions *in vivo*, evidence is accumulating, especially in arthropod-born virus infections, to show that the passive injection of humoral antibody at the right time after infection actually enhances the lesions in the central nervous system. It would therefore appear that humoral antibodies play a far greater role in producing hypersensitivity reactions in virus infections than has been previously appreciated.

The actual distribution of lesions in the central nervous system would appear to depend on which cells are particularly susceptible to the infecting virus. Thus a different distribution of lesions in the central nervous system will be found in poliomyelitis, vaccinia and disease due to the arthropod-born viruses. The nature of the lesion will also vary depending on whether cell-mediated or humoral antibody mechanism predominates, although the site of the inflammatory reaction is generally perivascular, indicating the involvement of blood-born immunological factors in these diseases. Neurological complications occur infrequently following infections with other viruses such as influenza, adenovirus or herpes zoster. The interval between the onset of the febrile illness and the development of neurological complications may vary between one and 100 days. The form which the disease might take is that of an encephalitis, transverse myelitis or polyradiculopathy. In the latter cases, the disease may show a clinical picture characteristic of the Guillain-Barré syndrome and may be severe enough to cause respiratory paralysis. Such patients may respond rapidly to treatment with corticotrophin. It may well be that these conditions are manifestations of an allergic reaction to the virus which caused the initial illness. An allergic reaction to virus antigen should always be considered as a mechanism in similar disease states.

3. *The possible role of immunological processes in other demyelinating diseases*

The demonstration that an acute demyelinating disease could be produced in experimental animals by an autoimmune process, suggested that a similar mechanism might underly multiple sclerosis (MS) and other demyelinating diseases in man. Much work has been undertaken to try and find an immunological aetiology for multiple sclerosis. In the acute phase of multiple sclerosis the foci of demyelination have the same perivenous distribution as the experimental allergic disease and there is also the same perivascular infiltration with mononuclear cells. However, in chronic multiple sclerosis lesions are larger and often bear no relation to blood vessels, with very few mononuclear cells in the perivascular space. Moreover the progress of the disease is very different from that found in experimental demyelinating disease. In the experimental disease there is either acute death or recovery, whereas in multiple sclerosis the disease has remissions and relapses lasting as much as 20–25 years. This is associated with the appearance of fresh concentric rings of demyelinization on the margin of old lesions, and marked proliferation of astrocytes.

It has been suggested that multiple sclerosis is due to a virus which grows very slowly in the brain. This suggestion has occurred as a result of research into the disease "scrapie", a condition of the central nervous system which occurs in sheep. This disease can be transferred to other sheep or to mice by direct intracerebral inoculation. The transmitted disease has an incubation period of up to three years in sheep and of four to five months in mice. The agent of scrapie is much smaller than that of a normal virus. Following up this suggestion that a slow proliferating virus similar to scrapie could cause multiple sclerosis, brain from patients with multiple sclerosis have been injected intracerebrally into normal sheep and mice. Initial reports of a scrapie like disease in these animals remains unconfirmed. However the possibility that MS could be produced by a "slow" virus still remains.

A less chronic sclerosing disease of the brain where both a virus and allergic aetiology have been considered is subacute sclerosing panencephalitis (SSPE). This condition is due to a chronic infection with measles virus which has been isolated from the brain cells of patients with this disease, in tissue culture. Some patients with this disease have abnormally high levels of both IgM and IgG antibodies against measles virus in the cerebrospinal fluid as well as in the serum. An increased reactivity of the lymphocytes to respond *in vitro* by "blast" transformation has also been described in the presence of measles virus. In many of the patients the disease was preceded by measles up to 14 years previously, suggesting that the virus might have been latent in the brain. Another possibility that has been suggested is that the disease occurs following a second infection with measles virus in a patient who already is highly sensitive to the virus. It has been suggested that this condition is due to an impairment of the cell-mediated immune processes against the virus allowing it to remain latent in the body for so long after infection. Evidence for such an impairment is at present lacking, especially as specific lymphocyte reactivity may not be impaired. The possible immunological background for this disease is supported by the finding that the disease is associated with enlargement of the thymus and that marked improvement of the disease has occurred in one case treated by thymectomy and in another case the progressive disease process has been arrested by treatment with corticosteroids.

Following the association of measles virus with SSPE there have been a number of reports of increased levels of anti-measles antibodies in MS. The significance of these findings is not clear and it is thought that increased titres against this antigen could be the result of immunological hyperreactivity rather than persistent infection with this virus. Currently it is considered that MS could be due to infection with a slow virus similar to that causing scrapie, and that persistence of infection might be the result of an immune defect. Tissue damage would be the direct result of toxic viral damage or due to an allergic reaction.

Multiple sclerosis research is very much one of rash claims and unconfirmed reports. Unfortunately this occurs as frequently in the immunological as in other fields. As a result a certain amount of scepticism must be employed in assessing results, especially in the field of therapy. Claims of success using immunosuppressive agents such as azathioprine and anti-lymphocytic globulin or transfer factor must therefore be treated with extreme reservation.

Despite these observations important new information has begun to accumulate in the association of histocompatibility antigens with the incidence of multiple sclerosis. The serologically defined HLA antigens A3, B7 and B18 occur with increased frequency in patients with MS. More recently an association has also been found with the lymphocyte activating determinant DW2 at the D locus that can be demonstrated by mixed lymphocyte reactions. The pathogenetic significance of these associations is as yet unknown. However the association of the major histocompatibility complex (MHC) with the immune response (Ir) genes suggests a basis for a primary immunodeficiency against a specific infectious agent.

It would appear possible that a wide range of diseases of the central nervous system are due to immunological processes. These are not necessarily against the brain tissue itself. It appears more likely that brain damage occurs as a result of hypersensitivity reactions probably against viral antigens occurring in close relation to brain tissue and causing the acute or chronic damage. The tissue which more often is affected by these processes is myelin. However other tissues are affected, presumably dependent on to which tissue the viral antigen has a particular affinity.

Myasthenia gravis. Myasthenia gravis has been associated for many years with hyperplasia and germinal centre formation in the thymus. A number of cases have also been described associated with neoplastic growths of the thymus—thymomas. The immunological association between myasthenia gravis and thymic pathology was confirmed by the finding of antibodies in the serum of a proportion of patients with this disease which reacted *in vitro* with the alternate striations of skeletal muscle and the myo-epithelial cells of the thymus. Similar antibodies have also been found in the serum of patients with thymomas but without any clinical evidence of myasthenia gravis. Although these antibodies occur most frequently in myasthenia gravis, there is no complete correlation between their presence and the disease.

An experimental model of myasthenia gravis has been produced in the guinea pig, following the injection of bovine thymus or muscle in Freund's adjuvant (containing mycobacteria). These guinea pigs developed an abnormal accumulation of lymphocytes round the Hassall's corpuscles in the thymus associated in about half the cases with a neuromuscular block similar to that found in myasthenia gravis in man. The response of the guinea pig muscle to nerve stimulation reverted to normal after treatment with neostigmine. Antibodies were found in the serum of animals, immunized with muscle, which reacted with the striations of skeletal muscle and the myoepithelial cells of the thymus. However these antibodies did not develop in guinea pigs immunized with thymus, despite their development of a myasthenic type of neuro-muscular block. Thymectomy after immunization with muscle or thymus prevented the development of the myasthenic neuromuscular block. It has been suggested that in myasthenia gravis there is an excessive release of an inhibitor of neuromuscular transmission from the epithelial cells of the thymus. The excessive release of this hormone may be stimulated by an immunological reaction directed against the cells or as a result of their neoplastic proliferation. The production of autoantibodies against muscle might occur secondary to the primary disease process and not be related to the development of the neuromuscular block.

Further experiments have shown that calf thymus contains a soluble substance which when injected daily for 10 days into guinea pigs would produce a myositis and a neuromuscular block that could be improved with neostigmine and aggravated with d-tubocurarine. It has been suggested that this substance, which has been called "thymin", is the hormone released in increased amounts from the diseased thymus which induces the chronic changes at the neuromyal junction as well as the direct myopathic changes which have also been described in severe cases of myasthenia gravis.

Bibliography

Books

Kies, M. W. & Alvord, E. C. (eds.) (1959), *Allergic Encephalomyelitis*. Springfield Ill.: Thomas.
Maumenee, A. E. & Silverstein, A. M. (eds.) (1964), *The Immunopathology of Uveitis*. Baltimore: Williams and Wilkins.
Multiple Sclerosis Research. Eds. A. N. Davison, J. H. Humphrey, A. L. Liversedge, W. I, McDonald & J. S. Porterfield. Her Majesty's Stationery Office, London (1975).
Rahi, A. H. S. & Garner, A. (1976), *Immunopathology of the Eye*. Oxford: Blackwells.

Articles

Burnet, F. M. (1968), "Measles as an index of immunological function." *Lancet*, **ii**, 610.
Goldstein, G. (1968), "The thymus and neuromuscular function." *Lancet*, **ii**, 119.
Goldstein, G. & Whittingham, S. (1966), "Experimental autoimmune thymitis." *Lancet*, **ii**, 315.
Goldstein, G. & Whittingham, S. (1967), " Histological and serological features of experimental autoimmune thymitis in guinea pigs." *Clin. exp. Immunol.*, **2**, 257.
Hotchin, J. (1962), "The biology of lymphocytic choriomeningitis infection: virus induced immune disease." *Cold Spring Harbor Sympos.*, **27**, 479.
Legg, N. J. (1967), "Virus antibodies in subacute sclerosing panencephalitis: a study of 22 patients." *Brit. med. J.*, **iii**, 350.

Oldstone, M. B. A. & Dixon, F. J. (1968), "Immunohistochemical study of allergic encephalomyelitis." *Am. J. Path*, **52**, 251.

Strauss, A. J. L. & Van der Geld, H. W. R. (1966), "The thymus and human diseases with autoimmune concomitants, with special reference to myasthenia gravis." *The Thymus: Exper mental and Clinical Studies*. Eds. G. E. W. Wolstenholme & R. Porter. London: Churchill.

Webb, H. E. & Gordon Smith, C. E. (1966), "Relation of immune response to development of central nervous system lesions in virus infections in man." *Brit. med. J.*, **ii**, 1179.

Chapter XVI

The Immunology of Cancer

The role of immunological processes in the control and development of cancer has been recognized since the work of Paul Ehrlich at the turn of the century. However, the mechanisms by which immunological processes act have only been appreciated in the last few years. Much of the stimulus for advances in the field of tumour immunology have come from the revival in interest which has occurred in the general field of experimental immunology, stimulated by the large amount of information and conceptual advances resulting from modern interest in transplantation immunology. The advances in the past ten years in tumour immunology in the laboratory have far outstripped our ability to apply the knowledge gained, to the patient. However, if one can draw a lesson from the advances in clinical transplantation, one can expect that there will be a similar application in the next ten years of concepts derived from the laboratory to the treatment of cancer. Already work in the laboratory has increased our knowledge considerably about what makes a cancer cell different from other cells in the body and the methods by which the body controls the growth and even eliminates colonies of cancer cells without the help of the physician or surgeon. In fact advances in the treatment of cancer in the future will result from our ability to enhance or supplement the body's own reaction. This however, cannot be done scientifically until we understand completely the changes in both the cancer cells and the body's defences which allow them to interact. This chapter will be divided into three parts. The first will be a discussion of those changes which occur in the cancer cell which makes it different from other cells. Then it will be possible to discuss the inborn defence mechanisms of the body against the uncontrolled proliferation of such cells. Finally an attempt will be made to indicate in which way these inborn defence mechanisms can be enhanced or supplemented in the human. This will lead us to a final assessment and a possible rational approach to what may be called the "immunotherapy of cancer".

1. Immunological Changes in the Cancer Cells

Cancer cells do not appear to be recognized immunologically by the body completely as part of "self". Two processes appear to be involved. One is the loss of some of the normal tissue specific antigens. The other is that the tumour cells appear to gain new tumour specific antigens which were not previously present in the cells from which they were derived. The loss of normal tissue specific antigens appears to be associated with the functional differentiation which is associated with the neoplastic changes which occur within the cell. The cancer cell becomes biochemically different from the tissue from which it is derived, in that it can lose tissue specific enzymes associated with specific functions and will at the same time lose certain antigenic characteristics, which identifies it with that tissue. An example of this may be found in thyroid carcinomata in man, where a loss of tissue specific thyroid auto-antigens has been demonstrated in a proportion of the tumours examined.

As well as a loss of certain tissue specific antigens neoplastic cells have been found to develop new antigens. Two types of antigen are found, those which are recognised by the host as being foreign and are referred to as tumour specific transplantation antigens (TSTAs), and those which are not antigenic in the host but can be recognised by their antigenicity in other species. These latter antigens are mainly the so-called onco-foetal antigens.

(i) *Tumour specific transplantation antigens*

Although there has been little success in the precise definition of tumour specific antigens in human tumour systems, this has been a field for extensive research in animal models. It is useful to discuss these, as the failure to demonstrate similar antigens in man is due to a lack of suitable assay models that are so readily available in experimental systems using inbred strains of animals. Viruses which induce tumours such as Rous sarcoma in chickens, polyoma virus in mice, the SV40 virus in monkeys and hamsters and certain adenoviruses in a wide selection of animals, will induce TSTAs in the transformed neoplastic cells. These antigens are specific to the virus inducing the neoplastic transformation irrespective of the species or strain of animal in which the tumour develops. These TSTAs remain within the proliferating cells, after the virus which induced the neoplastic transformation can no longer be detected. However this does not exclude the possibility that genetic material from the original infecting virus has not been incorporated in the DNA of the transformed neoplastic cells. TSTAs cause the rejection of the tumour if it is transplanted into a syngeneic host.

Whereas all tumours induced by a particular virus share antigenic specificity and do not cross-react with other virus-induced tumours, the antigenicity of non-viral tumours is much more complicated. In the case of chemically-induced cancers there is no relation between the antigenic nature of the tumour and the chemical-inducing agent even in two tumours induced by the same agent in the same animal. This lack of relationship between the chemical carcinogen and the antigenicity of the tumour is emphasized by work on tumours induced by films of cellophane. This material, which does not bind to the tissue cells and thus cannot induce neoplastic changes in the recipient cells simply by changing surface antigenicity by chemical reaction, is still capable of inducing the presence of new tumour specific antigens. The antigenicity of these tumours is in fact so great that they are rejected by syngeneic animals unless their ability to reject the tumours by immunological means is blocked in some way.

Altered antigenicity appears to be a general characteristic of all tumours. Some of these antigens can be shown to cross react with embryonic tissues. Others are unique to the particular tumour and are independent of species or carcinogen inducing the tumour. New antigens can be shown to appear very early in the process of carcinogenesis. This may occur even in the "precancerous" stage, even before a hyperplastic cell line has taken on the full characteristics of a true metastasing neoplasm. One of the hypotheses for the appearance of these "new" antigens is that all cells have the genetic ability to produce all these antigens. All but a few of these potential tissue antigens are lost or do not have the chance to appear during the normal process of tissue differentiation. However, during the process of tissue dedifferentiation associated with neoplastic change, any one of a large number of these antigens may develop apparently spontaneously. Another possibility that has been put forward is that these antigens could be due to mutation during the process of carcinogenesis, but this process is considered to be less likely than the mechanism described above.

In man the best evidence for tumour associated antigens is in Burkitt's lymphoma of African children where all the evidence to date points to this tumour being caused by a virus referred to as the Epstein-Barr (EB) virus. This virus is ubiquitous in the general population. However, higher titres of anti-EBV antibodies are found in patients with Burkitt's lymphoma and infectious mononucleosis. The main target of the EB virus is the B-lymphocyte. Burkitt's lymphoma occurs most commonly in Africa but has been found in other areas of the world. It is considered that EB virus is also the aetiological agent in infectious mononucleosis, and in certain nasopharyngeal carcinomas. The reason why this virus produces different disease forms in different patients is as yet poorly understood. However, epidemiological observations have shown a striking parallelism between the distribution of Burkitt's lymphoma and malaria in Africa. This has suggested that malarial infection could act as an aetiological co-factor in the development of these tumours by temporary depression of the immune response. Another tumour in which a specific antigen can be demonstrated is melanoma. Studies of this tumour have revealed a common cytoplasmic antigen that is not present in normal skin. Evidence for tumour specific antigens in man is extremely scanty. This has led to doubts as to whether human tumours are antigenic in the same way as animal tumours and whether a spécific immune reaction can aid in their elimination.

(ii) *Onco-foetal antigens and other antigenic markers of tumour activity*
Onco-foetal antigens are antigens found in association with neoplasms but are not antigenic in the host. They can only be detected by the use of antisera prepared in other species.

(a) *Carcinoembryonic antigen (CEA)*. This antigen is present in color-ectal carcinomas and is absent from normal adult colonic epithelium. It is present in foetal intestinal epithelium up to six months of gestation. CEA is not found in other tumours of the gastro-intestinal tract. CEA may be detected by radioimmunoassay in the plasma of all individuals but is significantly raised in patients with tumours or inflammatory conditions of the bowel. The highest levels are found in those with tumours, especially with metastases. The level of CEA in the plasma generally falls after surgical removal of the tumour. Increased levels of CEA have also been found in patients with breast cancer and neuro-blastoma.

(b) *α fetoprotein (AFP)*. Raised levels of α fetoprotein, which is normally found in foetal plasma is found in 90% of patients with primary hepatomas. Positive results may also be found with hepatitis and liver cirrhosis especially in children. AFP is also raised in patients with teratomas and yolk sac carcinomas and the test is useful in distin-guishing these tumours from seminomas. Raised levels of AFP are found in amniotic fluid and maternal blood if the foetus has abnorm-alities such as spina bifida.

(c) *Human chorionic gonadotrophin (HCG)*. Although strictly not an onco-foetal antigen, estimation of HCG in the plasma by radio-immunoassay is useful in the diagnostic and follow up of patients with choriocarcinoma or hydatidiform mole. It is also of value in deter-mining the presence of syncytiotrophoblast in ovarian and testicular tumours.

2. The Immunological Reaction Against Tumours
As has been discussed in the previous section some tumours carry anti-gens which are not normally carried by healthy cells within the body. The tumour cells will then be treated by the central immunological mechanisms of the body as not being part of "self". The reaction will be to the foreign antigenic determinant in the same way as the body would react against any of its own cells or macromolecules to which a foreign chemical grouping has been bound artificially.

The reaction of the body against its own tumour is very similar to the reaction of the body against an allogeneic tissue graft, since the tumour, although being isogeneic tissue, is considered by the body to be allogeneic. The ability to reject tumour tissue as though it was a graft from another animal can be demonstrated by experiments involving active immunization. Animals can be immunized against tumours from syngeneic animals (inbred animals which are genetically identical, in the same way as identical twins, and which can accept normal tissue grafts one from the other). Active immunization with tumour tissue has to be undertaken under the right conditions. The injection of live tumour cells will immunize the host, but the immune response will not be great enough to eliminate the rapidly proliferating tumour cells. In this case the presence of the immune state can be demonstrated by passive transfer studies, described below. Dead or disrupted cells do not appear to be able to immunize the host against a transplant of a tumour of the same antigenic specificity, even if injected together with adjuvants. This may be due to a weakness of antigens on these cells, in producing an immune response. Another possibility is that there might be a lability of the tumour specific antigens in the dead cells, so that they are more susceptible to destruction by tissue enzymes. Active immunization with tumour cells can only be undertaken following X-irradiation of these cells prior to injection, so that the tumour specific antigens are not destroyed but the cells become incapable of proliferation and spread. In the case of virus-induced tumours it is possible to immunize the animal actively with the virus, in which case they become resistant to subsequent challenge with tumours induced by the same virus. In some cases tumours may show spontaneous regression and this can be shown to be due to an immune response on the part of the host, as the host now becomes resistant to further transplants of the tumour.

Studies on the mechanism of immunity, which develops to tumours, have been undertaken using the passive transfer of serum and cells. Actively immunized animals contain antibodies in their serum which are cytotoxic to tumour cells *in vitro*. However, transfer of such serum *in vivo* has not been found to eliminate established tumours. In some cases transfer of serum, from actively immunized animals, alone actually enhances the growth of the tumour. Serum antibodies bound to the tumour specific antigens are capable of protecting the tumour cells from cell-mediated immune processes. The role of cell-mediated immune processes in the protection of animals from tumour growth is however far from clear. The intravenous injection of lymphocytes from the thoracic duct of rats specifically immunized against a tumour has been found to protect other rats from the growth of the specific tumour transplanted into them. This was at first thought to be evidence that cell-mediated processes similar to those involved in normal tissue graft rejection was involved in the rejection of tumours. It was later found that a similar state of immunity could be transferred with cells from other species immunized with the same tumour and even with extracts of disrupted cells. These studies are analogous in many ways to those which have been made on the passive transfer of "cellular immunity" to bacteria. It can thus be stated that at the present time, although there is evidence that serum antibodies are not the only factors involved in the defence of the body against tumours, no evidence exists that these tumours are controlled by cell-mediated immune processes alone. Moreover, nothing is known about the nature of the cell-mediated immune processes involved, as no studies of the transfer of immunity have been made in which it can be categorically stated that the injected cells or even their progeny are the cells which recognize the tumour specific antigens and interact with them in such a way as to result in the elimination of the tumour cells. Perhaps the most important evidence, that cell-mediated immune processes are involved in the defence mechanisms of the body which cause the elimination of mutant neoplastic cells, is that there is a significant increase in the incidence of neoplastic tumours in mice, in which the cell-mediated immune response has been specifically abolished or reduced by treatment of the animals with antilymphocyte serum or by neonatal thymectomy. Although some humoral antibodies will enhance the growth of tumour cells by protecting the tumour specific antigens, it is probable that the immune reaction of the body against tumour cells is due to the specific synergistic action of other types of humoral antibodies with cell-mediated immune processes. It is also probable that these specific immunological processes interact non-specifically with macrophages to control the spread of the tumour. Histological examination of tumours in the human which are spreading slowly reveals that these tissues are surrounded by a broad infiltrate of lymphocytes and macrophages. In those tumours which are spreading rapidly there is a striking absence of such an infiltrate with "inflammatory cells".

In a discussion of the defence of the body against tumours, one should not ask why tumours proliferate but why they are capable of growing at all in the face of what appears to be a very strong inbuilt immune process. The natural thing for the body's immune process would be to reject all neoplastic cells as soon as they appear before they spread throughout the body. Such cells should be recognized as being "not self" because they contain these tumour specific antigens. It is now considered that neoplastic dedifferentiated cells develop continuously throughout life probably by mutation. As soon as they develop they are eliminated by the body's immunological processes. The adaptive immune response as we know it in the human has been shown to have developed phylogenetically at the same time as tumours, capable of metastasing, first appeared. Both metastasing tumours and an adaptive immune response are first found together in primitive vertebrates. It is thought that the adaptive immune response has been retained by natural selection to cope with neoplastic cells which develop throughout life. Thus if most neoplastic cells are eliminated by immune processes, what are the factors which cause neoplastic growth to break away from the body's immunological control?

Once a tumour has already developed in the body, it develops a state of equilibrium with the immunological defence mechanisms directed against it. This state of equilibrium can be considered in most cases to be favourable to the tumour, or otherwise it would be eliminated completely. However, the balance is such that a certain amount of control exists over the uncontrolled proliferation of the tumour. One might consider that a balance exists between the tumour on the one side and the body's immunological mechanisms on the other side, in which the scales are always tipped to some extent in favour of the tumour (Fig. 1). However, if the balance is tipped only slightly in favour of the tumour, the body's immunological mechanisms will be able to keep some control over the tumour and prevent rapid dissemination all over the body. The time that a patient survives, once he develops a neoplastic tumour, will depend very much on the strength and quality of his immunological response as well as upon the virulence of the tumour. Both of these factors will determine the rapidity of growth and dissemination of the tumour. If the balance is tipped further in favour of the tumour and immunological defences are weak, growth and dissemination will be rapid, resulting in an earlier fatal result. Factors which decrease the immunological reaction will encourage the development of tumours in the first place by stopping the normal elimination of neoplastic cells before they proliferate into colonies of cells, and secondly will allow tumours that have managed to establish themselves to proliferate in an uncontrolled manner. In other cases, highly neoplastic tumours in the human have been known to resolve spontaneously under conditions where the only possible explanation could have been a rapid increase in immunological resistance, such that the balance has swung away from being even slightly in favour of the tumour.

There is an increasing awareness that an immunological spectrum of host response occurs with some tumours that is analogous to that which occurs in chronic infectious diseases such as leprosy. This is particularly exemplified by the investigation of two tumours in Africa—Burkitt's lymphoma and Kaposi's sarcoma. Positive delayed hypersensitivity reactions have been found to extracts of autologous Burkitt lymphoma cells in patients with Burkitt's lymphoma in clinical remission. These positive responders had longer remissions than those patients with negative skin tests. Patients with Kaposi sarcoma can also be divided into two groups; those with a relatively stationary form of the disease and those in which the disease runs a fulminating course to early death. Patients with the fulminating form of the disease show a striking impairment of response to sensitization with dinitrochlorobenzene and respond poorly to chemotherapy. Those with the relatively stationary form of the disease are more amenable to chemotherapy. This would suggest that chemo-

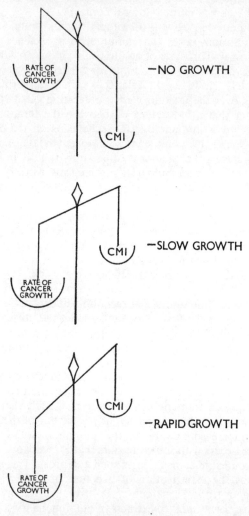

Fig. 1. Interaction between cell-mediated immunity (CMI) and the rate of neoplastic growth.

therapy or radiation can only act in conjunction with the body's immune response by helping to tip the immunological balance, possible by reducing the load of antigen which is producing either a state of immunological tolerance or causing the production of enhancing antibody.

Specific breakaway from immunological surveillance

(a) *Immunological tolerance.* Immunological tolerance has been demonstrated very clearly in certain virus induced tumours. The ability to develop these tumours is transmitted from mother to offspring either across the placenta in the case of certain leukaemias, or in mother's milk as in the case of an agent causing the development of mammary cancers. The virus then remains in the animal as it grows up and is not eliminated because it is not recognized as being "self". An increased incidence of certain lymphomas can be produced by injecting the virus in neonatal life under similar cirumstances. Such tolerance can be broken by the injection of normal lymphoid cells from a syngeneic donor which had not become tolerant in neonatal life.

(b) *Immunological enhancement.* Under certain circumstances immunisation with soluble tumour specific antigens will cause an enhancement of tumour growth. This will be the result of the production of non-cytotoxic antibodies that can act by blocking the antigenic sites of the tumour, thus protecting it from cytotoxic cell-mediated immune destruction. These "blocking antibodies" can also reduce the strength of the cell-mediated immune response by a central action on the afferent limb of the immune arc, possibly interfering with antigenic recognition. It is thought that circulating immune complexes containing soluble tumour antigen can play a similar role.

(c) *Soluble tumour specific antigens.* Tumours may lose antigenicity with age and thus become less susceptible to immunological surveillance. In addition they may shed increasing amounts of soluble antigen into the circulation. As well as a decrease in tumour antigenicity there will be soluble tumour antigen in the circulation. Soluble TSTA can form a powerful specific inhibitor of the immune response, both alone or complexed with antibody. Free antigenic determinants can block the effector arm of cell-mediated immunity. In some tumours the quantity of antigen released will increase as the tumour grows. As a result there will be an increasing reduction in the immune response. This will lead to a progressive escape from immunological control. It is thought that local release of soluble antigen could also account for the initial escape event and the failure of immunological surveillance.

Non-specific defects in immunological control causing an increased incidence of cancer. The spontaneous development of tumours occurs more readily in experimental animals where there is a basic defect in the immunological defence mechanisms of the body. Chronic immunological injury can be produced in experimental animals in what is known as "graft versus host" disease. This condition is produced by injecting immunologically active cells into an unrelated recipient under conditions where the cells can react against the host but the host cannot reject the donor cells which are reacting against itself. This artificial condition produced in laboratory animals results in a general atrophy of the lymphoreticular system. Under these conditions there is a defect in the control of neoplastic cell proliferation. Mice with this immunological defect have been found to develop malignant lymphomas, if conditions are such that they are able to survive their immunological defect for over eight months. The tumours which develop all originate in the lymphoid tissue and have many of the features of Hodgkin's disease with Sternberg-Reed cells, being highly invasive and metastasing into the liver.

A similar immunological defect could occur in NZB mice which develop spontaneous autoimmune phenomena associated with virus infection. In these mice the autoimmune disease is associated with the vertical transmission of a virus from mother to offspring. The auto-immune phenomena—haemolytic anaemia, immune complex glomeru-lonephritis and lupus erythematosus cells in the peripheral blood are all due to overactivity of the humoral antibody-producing system. As a result of this there could be a defect in the cell-mediated immune component which protects the animal against the proliferation of colonies of malignant cells. It has been observed that these mice are more prone to develop spontaneous malignant neoplasms of the lymphoreticular system at about the age of 10–12 months. The incidence of these tumours can be increased five-fold following the administration of the carcinogen 2-aminofluorene.

There is increasing evidence of a general reduction of immune responses in certain acute infections. These include bacterial infections and especially protozoal infections such as malaria. It has been found that mice infected with malarial parasites develop an increased incidence of tumours when infected with a lymphoma-producing virus. It has therefore been suggested that Burkitt's lymphoma develops in patients infected with EB virus under conditions where the immune response has been suppressed by chronic infection with malarial parasites. A further example of an increased incidence of tumours occurring in association with a defect in the basic immunological control mechanisms, has been found in mice infected with Reovirus type 3. These mice develop what is known as a "runting disease" similar to that found in the "graft versus host" disease described above. This is associated with an atrophy of the central lymphoid tissue. When the spleen cells of these mice with chronic immunological injury are given to newborn mice of the same inbred strain (histocompatible), half of the recipients develop the "runting disease" found in the donors and some of those, which survive, develop a lymphoma. Thus the virus has transformed the donor cells into being able to react against the syngeneic lymphoreticular system and causes chronic immunological damage. One of the possible explanations for the spontaneous development of lymphomas in these recipients is that they have lost the immunological capacity of automatically rejecting neoplastically transformed cells, which develop from time to time in animals and which would normally be rejected as soon as they appear.

In man the incidence of cancer increases with age. It is also known that the ability to produce cell-mediated immune reactions such as the tuberculin reaction decreases with age. There is a remarkable parallel, which has been shown statistically, between the decrease in tuberculin reactivity with age and the increase in the incidence of cancer in the population with age. It has thus been suggested that in man the development of cancer is associated with a progressive inability to eliminate the colonies of malignant cells which normally appear in a random fashion throughout life. These malignant changes may occur as a result of spontaneous mutation, virus infection, or due to chemical or physical induction. The inability to eliminate these transformed cells can be considered to be due to a decrease in the efficiency of the immunological defence mechanisms of the body, which occurs with age. One observation, that is consistent with this hypothesis, is related to the skin reactivity of normal people to streptococcal antigens. Streptococcal antigens are ubiquitous and so four out of five people in the population can be shown to produce delayed hypersensitivity reactions to these antigens, injected intradermally. However, in patients with disseminated neoplasms, there is a marked defect in the ability to show cell-mediated immune reactions to these antigens. The incidence of reactivity has been found to drop down from four out of five people in the normal population to one out of five people with disseminated neoplasms. The non-specific defect in cell-mediated immunity in patients with malignant disease, not arising from the lympho-reticular system has certain interesting features. Thus, overall it has been found that these patients have a marked defect in response to tuberculin or to active sensitization with 2·4 dinitrochlorobenzene (DNCB). Little defect has been found in their ability to show delayed hypersensitivity to antigens derived from *Candida albicans*. A further difference is that patients with gastro-intestinal tumours have a poorer response to DNCB than those with other tumours, despite positive tuberculin reactivity. Patients with lung cancer may respond less well to mumps antigen than those with other tumours. It may be that the ability to manifest cell-mediated immune reactions is inhibited by the presence of diffuse neoplasia. However, there is an increasing opinion that the inability to control the development of neoplasms is a result of a fundamental defect on the part of the patient to produce cell-mediated immune reactions which could eliminate malignant cells as they appear rather than to control the local invasion and dissemination of malignant cells, once they have established themselves. It also appears that the cell-mediated defence mechanisms against the establishment of the malignant cells decreases in activity with age, consistent with the marked increase in the incidence of cancer between the age of 50 and 70.

Another example of the defect in what has been called the "host surveillance mechanism" can be found in mice and rats thymectomized in neonatal life. It is well known that neonatal thymectomy in these species abolishes the ability of the animals to respond in adult life with cell-mediated immunological responses. They are unable to reject tissue transplants in a normal way and are unable to show delayed hypersensitivity reactions. Neonatally thymectomized animals show a much higher incidence of tumours when these are induced by chemical or viral means, than normal animals which have been left with a functioning thymus in neonatal life.

Chemical or physical suppression of the immune response against cancer. Physical or chemical agents which are immunosuppressive would be expected to inhibit the immunological elimination of cells which have become neoplastic by mutation. X-rays and certain alkylating agents such as nitrogen mustard and busulphan are both carcinogens and immunosuppressive agents. Polycyclic hydrocarbons such as 3-methyl cholanthrene and 1,2-5,6-di-benzanthracene are also immunosuppressive as well as being potent carcinogens. These compounds have been shown to be destructive to lymphoid cells, producing inhibition of mitosis and chromosome abnormalities, which could account for their associated immunosuppressive activity. There is an interesting parallelism in that the strains of mice in which these carcinogens produce immunosuppression develop leukaemias, whereas leukaemias do not develop in those strains of mice in which these carcinogens are not immunosuppressive. It has been suggested that carcinogens may not only produce cancer by direct action on the target tissue to which they attach but also produce a chronic malfunctioning of the immunological tissues and thus cause a failure to eliminate the neoplastic cells, induced by that particular carcinogen, once they develop. Many chemical carcinogens actually induce an immune response against their own chemical groups attached to tissue proteins. However, as the tumour specific antigens are not related antigenically to the chemical nature of the carcinogen, this immune response will not play any role in the rejection of the tumour cells, once they are formed. It is of interest that the cell proliferation produced specifically in the central lymphoid tissue is proportional to the ability of the individual animal to produce a cancer in the target tissue to which the carcinogen attaches itself. The ability of lymphoid tissue to proliferate under an immunological stimulus would seem to be controlled by the same factors which control the ability of neoplastic tissues stimulated with a chemical carcinogen. Thus the effect of chemical carcinogens on immune processes is a very complex action which needs to be unravelled.

Other immunosuppressive agents which are not directly carcinogens in their own right can encourage the growth of neoplastic tissues by suppressing the immune response which would normally keep these neoplastic tumours under control. Most of these agents act by suppressing the proliferation of cells in the central immunological tissues. Many of these agents act non-specifically to suppress cell proliferation in all tissues, and as such had been used as cancer chemotherapeutic agents before being used as immunosuppressive agents. The ability of such agents as X-rays, alkylating agents, and antimetabolites to suppress cancer once it has already developed must depend on a balance between the effect in inhibiting the proliferation of cells in the cancerous tissue and the inhibition of proliferation of cells in the central immunological tissues. Many examples exist in clinical experience where treatment with these agents has encouraged the proliferation of the cancer and resulted in a more rapid deterioration of the patient's clinical condition. This turn of events would be explained by the agent having a more profoundly depressive effect on the central immunological tissues than on the cancerous tissue. Thus, in treatment of patients with cancer with X-rays, alkylating agents or antimetabolites, due notice must be taken of the ability of these agents to encourage rather than depress cancer growth, by their strong immunosuppressive action.

In two particular cancers Burkitt's lymphoma and choriocarcinoma, methotrexate has been found to have marked beneficial effects after a very short period of treatment. The dose used has been in the range of 20 mg orally for four to eight days only. This treatment has produced a remarkable high incidence of cures in these conditions. In the case of Burkitt's lymphoma cures have been obtained with one intravenous injection of methotrexate or cyclophosphamide. It has been suggested that the amount of drug given was insufficient to kill off, by any means, all the cancer cells. It is probable that in both these conditions there is a high degree of immunity against the cancer. The drug reduces the number of cancer cells and tips the balance in favour of the immune reaction which itself recovers quickly from the effects of the drug treatment. The body's own defence mechanisms are then in a position to eradicate the tumour and effect the cure.

In this connection it appears that a continuous antigen source is necessary to maintain the immune reaction until all the tumour is eradicated. It has been suggested that too radical a removal of a tumour and especially the removal of the draining lymph nodes producing an immune reaction to a tumour may in some cases reduce the defence mechanisms of the body against certain cancers. Radical surgery may thus potentiate the dissemination of neoplastic tissues by a direct effect in reducing the body's immunity against the cancer.

Effect of surgical resection of a primary growth on the immunological defence mechanisms against the neoplasm. It is a recognized clinical observation that surgical removal of the primary growth sometimes enhances the spread of secondary deposits and causes a rapid deterioration in the clinical state of the patient. However, in most cases removal of a primary carcinoma will improve the clinical state of the patient. It is thought that in these cases the presence of the primary tumour exerts an immunosuppressive effect. When the tumour is present the immune response may be weak or absent. In these cases it is often possible to demonstrate a heightened state of immunity on removal of the primary tumour.

However, under certain conditions, resection of a primary tumour causes a depression in the immune state, which encourages the rapid dissemination of metastases throughout the body. In such a case it is possible that a continuous antigenic stimulus from the primary tumour was necessary to maintain the immune state. Another possibility is that as well as reducing the cell-mediated immune reaction against the tumour, the removal of the primary growth has encouraged the production of humoral antibodies which react with the tumour-specific antigens and protect these antigens from the cell-mediated immune reaction which would prevent these cells from proliferating and even destroy them. These antibodies are those known as "enhancing" antibodies as they enhance the growth of the tumour rather than control it.

This suggests that the immune response against tumours is delicately balanced. A sudden change in the amount of antigen stimulating the response, as might be produced by removal of a primary tumour, could affect the quality of its expression and result in an encouragement of the spread of metastases. However, it is likely that in most cases the presence of the primary tumour is immunosuppressive and its removal improves rather than causes a deterioration in the clinical state of the patient. The results gained from experience of controlled experiments in animals are in keeping with the impression gained from clinical experience.

3. Immunotherapy of Cancer

As has been discussed above, cancers can develop and proliferate as a result of a failure in the equilibrium between the spontaneous proliferation of neoplastic cells and the ability of the body's immune mechanisms to control this process. In the case of tumours induced by virus and chemical agents, it is logical to attempt to restore the state of equilibrium by eliminating the cause of the development of mutant neoplastic cells. However, other cancers might appear to develop as spontaneous mutations and are allowed to proliferate owing to a defect in the body's immune mechanisms. Under these conditions it is logical to try to potentiate the body's immune mechanisms, in an attempt to restore the state of equilibrium. Potentiation of immune processes may be by non-specific or specific means. Specific means, by analogy with defence mechanisms against microorganisms, would entail a process of active or passive immunization. As the immunological reaction of a patient to a tumour may be a balance between a cell-mediated immune response and the production of "enhancing antibody", a possible approach in the future could be to find a means of turning-off the production of "enhancing antibody", and thus allow cell-mediated immune processes a fuller expression.

(a) *Non-specific increase in immunity*

Possible attempts at increasing the immune capacity of the body non-specifically can be attempted in a number of ways, again by drawing analogy with what is known about defence mechanisms against myco-bacteria. Treatment of experimental animals with BCG, *Coryne-bacterium parvum* or Zymosan (dried cell walls of yeast) is known to increase resistance to bacterial and viral infections. This was found to be due both to a non-specific increase in the immune response to a wide range of antigens, and also to an increased activity of the reticulo-endothelial system. In experimental animals treatment with these agents has been found to increase non-specific immunity to certain virus and chemically-induced tumours.

A trial of the effect of an increase in non-specific immunity induced by BCG has been made on human patients with acute lymphoblastic leukaemia. The technique being used is to scarify the skin every fourth day for one month, then every seventh day. Twenty scarifications each 5 cm long were made on each occasion and 2 ml of a BCG suspension (75 mg/ml dry weight) was rubbed into each site. Prolonged survival without relapse has been claimed, using this form of treatment.

(b) *Active specific immunization*

Active immunization of experimental animals against tumour cells has only been successful by the injection of live cancer cells whose ability to proliferate has been abolished by prior X-irradiation. The injection of dead cells even in standard immunological adjuvant mixtures (such as Freund's adjuvant) has been remarkably unsuccessful. In successful experiments with immunization using X-irradiated cells, the animals have been immunized before the transplantation of the tumour from a syngeneic animal. In man immunization would only be possible after the cancer has developed, as each individual cancer carries different tumour specific antigens. However, by this time the central immuno-logical processes would already have received a considerable antigenic stimulus. In some cases the concentration of antigen might be so large that a state of immunological tolerance could have been induced to that particular tumour antigen. Under these conditions further injection of tumour cells could not enhance any immune reaction that might have developed or been revoked.

Despite these objections active specific immunization has been attempted in patients with acute lymphoblastic leukaemias, using cells from a pool of other donors with acute lymphoblastic leukaemia. The cells were irradiated before injection. Prolonged remissions have been claimed using this technique. As it is possible that leukaemias are of virus origin, the injection of cells containing dead virus might have boosted the patient's immune response to tumour antigens of virus origin. There is evidence that active immunotherapy could be more effective if patients are first brought into remission with chemotherapy. This would effectively reduce the level of tumour antigen and prevent any block in the development of a cell-mediated immune response.

Another approach has been to assume that neoplastic cells have a low degree of immunogenicity and as a result of this the body has produced only a weak immune response. If the tumour cells were to be conjugated to a highly antigenic foreign molecule such as a foreign γ-globulin, the immunogenicity of the molecule would be increased and there would be an enhanced immunological response and increased immunity would develop against the tumour cell itself. Immunization of experimental animals, which had developed tumours, to excised portions of their own tumours, treated in this way, has produced evidence of retardation of tumour growth. This was indicated by increased mononuclear cell infiltration, necrosis of the tumour and fibrosis. This technique of immunization has been tried in man, but results from different centres have not confirmed earlier claims for this approach.

The number of patients in which successful active immunization has been reported has been too small to assess really whether these techniques will have a general effectiveness. However, these approaches demonstrate the general direction in which future attempts at active immunization to neoplastic cells could be made.

(c) *Passive immunization*

(i) *Serotherapy.* In experimental animals sera from syngeneic animals carrying lymphoid tumours or with leukaemia have been shown to be cytotoxic for the tumour cells *in vitro*. Such sera have been found to reduce the growth especially of leukaemia cells in mice *in vivo*, if the number of cells present was small.

In man reports have occurred of the effectiveness of "convalescent sera" from patients with Burkitt's lymphoma, which had regressed under treatment with nitrogen mustard or cyclophosphamide more than two years previously. When transfused into other patients with Burkitt's lymphoma, regression of the tumour was induced which lasted three weeks, which was consistent with the time a high concentration of antibody would have been maintained in the body.

Another possible approach to the passive immunotherapy of cancer using specific antibody is to link the antibodies to radioactive isotopes or cytostatic agents in the hope that these agents would be specifically localized at the sites of tumour cell proliferation.

There are three limitations to the serotherapy of tumours. The first is that high concentrations of cytotoxic or high affinity binding antibodies are rare in patients with cancer. The second is that humoral antibodies are retained in the body only for a limited period of time before they are eliminated from the circulation. Finally there is a likelihood of the presence of enhancing antibody in the serum used.

(ii) *Cellular transfer of adoptive immunity.* In experimental animals the development of neoplasms of virus origin can be prevented by the injection of sensitized syngeneic lymphoid cells from actively immunized donors.

In man it is difficult to obtain cells from a donor immunized with a tumour containing the same tumour specific antigens as the tumour, carried by the patient whom one wishes to treat. This could only be possible in the case of Burkitt's lymphoma and leukaemias which might have tumour specific antigens in common due to their virus origin. The other difficulty is that syngeneic cells cannot be obtained in man in the same way as in inbred strains of mice. Allogeneic cells would be rejected as a homograft.

Attempts have been made to give the patient total body irradiation to eliminate both the tumour (in this case leukaemias) and also the body's immune response. Replacement therapy has then been undertaken with normal bone marrow. These cells, however, react against the patient with a "graft versus host reaction", which in many cases is fatal. Another approach that has been tried is to transfuse the patient with leukaemia with normal allogeneic peripheral blood leucocytes. In many cases of leukaemia, the immune response is diminished, so that the transfused cells are not rejected immediately "Graft versus host" reactions occur, one sign of which is exfoliative dermatitis. This is associated with a remission in the neoplastic disease and when the body's normal immune mechanisms recover the transfused allogeneic cells are rejected and the "graft versus host" symptoms disappear. The difficulty in this general approach is that any treatment given to reduce the "graft versus host" disease would also reduce the immune response of the transfused cells against the neoplastic cells. Adoptive immunization with cells does not appear to give much hope for treatment in the future. It is more likely that any advances in the field of immunotherapy of cancer will come either raising the resistance of the body to cancer non-specifically or from active immunization of the patient with his own neoplastic cells, possibly rendered more immunogenic by conjugation with a foreign antigen or hapten.

Bibliography

Books

Currie, G. A. (1974), *Cancer and the Immune Response*. London: Edward Arnold.
Immunotherapy of Cancer. *Wld. Hlth. Org. techn. Rep. Ser.*, 344 (1966).
Trentin, J. J. (ed.) (1967), *Cross-Reacting Antigens and Neoantigens* (*With Implications for Autoimmunity and Cancer Immunity*). Baltimore: Williams and Wilkins.

Articles

Alexander, P. & Hamilton Fairley, G. (1967), "Cellular resistance to tumours." *Brit. med. Bull.*, **23**, 86.
Al-Sarraf, M., Wong, P., Sardesai, S. & Vaitkevicius, V. K. (1970), "Clinical immunologic responsiveness in malignant disease. I, Delayed hypersensitivity reaction and the effect of cytotoxic drugs." *Cancer*, **26**, 262.
Burnet, F. M. (1970). "The concept of immunological surveillance." *Progr. exp. Tumor Res.*, **13**, 1.
Epstein, M. A. (1971), "The possible role of viruses in human cancer." *Lancet*, **i**, 1344.
Gershon, R. K., Carter, R. L. & Kondo, K. (1968), "Immunologic defense against metastases: Impairment by excision of an allotransplanted lymphoma." *Science*, **159**, 646.
Haddow, A. (1965), "Immunology of the cancer cell: tumour specific antigens." *Brit. med. Bull.*, **21**, 133.
Klein, G. (1975), "The Epstein–Barr virus and neoplasia." *New Engl. J. Med.*, **293**, 1353.
Mathé, G. (1967), "The immunological approach to the treatment of cancer." *Ann. roy. Coll. Surg. Eng.*, **41**, 93.
Schwartz, R. S. & Beldotti, L. (1965), "Malignant lymphomas following allogeneic disease: transition from an immunological to a neoplastic disorder." *Science*, **149**, 1511.
Wedderburn, N. (1970), "Effect of concurrent malarial infection on development of virus-induced lymphoma in BALB/C mice." *Lancet* **ii**, 1114.

Chapter XVII
The Role of the Clinical Immunologist

As may be seen in the previous chapters, clinical immunology has an impact on virtually all branches of medicine. Clinicians in the various recognized specialities have now to possess a more than elementary grounding in immunological concepts as they impinge on their own interests. Thus, when a patient appears before the doctor with a vasculitis, nephritis or arthritis, the question to be answered is not only whether this is a disease involving immunological mechanisms, but whether these symptoms are caused by a cell-mediated immune process or by humoral antibodies. However, of far greater importance is the need to identify the antigen causing the immune reaction. In many cases the best therapy is directed towards eliminating an antigen from the body or avoiding future contact with the antigen. If this is not possible, consideration has to be given to techniques by which the immune response might be switched to one which does not cause such great local tissue damage. One of the greatest problems in clinical immunology at the present time is that although we may suspect an immunological process to be the cause of a disease and even have corroborative evidence as to the form of immunological process involved, in many cases we may not be able to identify the antigen and thus make the true diagnosis.

Many hospitals, especially those in a university environment are in the process at the present time of setting up a department of clinical immunology. There has therefore recently been much thought as to what role such a department should play and what qualities should be expected of a clinical immunologist. In the first place, there has been considerable controversy as to whether a clinical immunologist should be based primarily in the wards and take complete responsibility for patient care and therapy or whether he should be based primarily in the laboratory and only be called in for consultation to give advice in diagnosis, indicate what investigations should be performed and advise on therapy. Of course, the role taken by a clinical immunologist in a particular situation will depend partly on his own interests and partly on his environment. So far, very few clinical immunologists have been trained primarily as such. Those whose approach is patient oriented and start at the bedside may have been trained initially in other specialities allied to internal medicine or paediatrics. These include rheumatology, allergy, nephrology, dermatology and clinical haematology, or even in endocrinology or metabolic diseases. Others have been trained in surgery and developed an interest in clinical transplantation. A clinical immunologist whose interest stems from the laboratory rather than from the bedside may have had training in pathology, microbiology, clinical biochemistry or clinical physiology, or else he may have been trained in research methods in one of the departments of basic medical sciences.

Ideally a department of clinical immunology should contain at least two physicians, one whose interests are mainly patient oriented and one whose interests are mainly laboratory oriented. Under exceptional circumstances, it might be possible for one person to combine these two roles. However, the techniques used to investigate the immunological aspects of disease have become so complex that it might be difficult to find someone with sufficient training in both aspects of the field. As clinical immunology is such a new field in medicine, few of the techniques available can be considered to be routine and many are still in the developmental stage. For many patients it is still necessary to develop new techniques or apply techniques which are often difficult to reproduce from laboratory to laboratory, to the investigation of a particular clinical problem. Much of the investigation of most patients falls within the category of research rather than routine investigation. In this way, a laboratory of clinical immunology will differ considerably from a laboratory of clinical biochemistry or clinical haematology.

To some extent the laboratory of clinical immunology will take over the investigation of certain conditions which have previously been traditionally the province of other departments. Thus, the investigation of autoimmune haemolytic anaemias and certain aspects of disseminated lupus erythematosus is in many cases performed by a department of haematology. The disorders of serum proteins are usually studied in departments of clinical chemistry. Skin testing is generally performed by allergy or dermatology departments. Estimations of rheumatoid factor or antinuclear factor levels are often performed in a laboratory belonging to a department of rheumatology. However, so many new conceptual as well as technical approaches are available, that centralization of all these different interests in a department of clinical immunology is now necessary. Immunological disorders may be roughly divided into those which result from normal, abnormal or increased immunological activity, and those which result from decreased immunological activity. Into the first group may be put immune complex diseases, problems of infectious diseases associated with increased cell-mediated immunity, chemical contact sensitivity, so-called autoimmune diseases and problems of transplantation. Into the second category are immunodeficiency disorders whether non-specific in childhood or secondary to other conditions such as neoplasia and specific immunodeficiency states in infectious diseases. It is necessary therefore, not only to investigate for an increased immunological function but also to look for decreased immunological function, whether of lymphocytes or immunoglobulins, specific or non-specific. When one considers that lymphocyte function is as important as immunoglobulin function in the genesis of disease, the role of the clinical immunologist gains its right perspective. The techniques for the investigation of increased or decreased lymphocyte function are among the more difficult in biological sciences, often involving complicated radioactive counting techniques as well as skill in various aspects of cell and tissue culture. Many of these involve a considerable amount of expertise and are difficult to reproduce from laboratory to laboratory.

The Investigation of Cell-mediated Immune Function

The ability of a patient to show cell-mediated immunity may be investigated either *in vivo* or *in vitro*. *In vivo* techniques involve the use of skin tests to determine pre-existing sensitivity or by actively sensitizing the patient.

(a) *Determination of pre-existing sensitivity*

  (i) Tuberculin at a dilution of 1:10,000 (0·1 ml).
       If negative, repeated with a 1:1,000 dilution.
 (ii) Candida 1:1,000 (0·1 ml).
(iii) Trichophytin 1:1,000 (0·1 ml).
 (iv) Streptococcal antigens Varidase (Lederle) may be used at a concentration of 5 units streptokinase/0·1 ml.
       If negative, this should be repeated at a concentration of 40 units/0·1 ml.
  (v) Mumps skin test antigen (100 μg) (Eli Lilly).

Reactions should be read at 4 hours to assess any Arthus component in the reaction and at 24 and 48 hours for delayed hypersensitivity. The diameter of induration should be recorded rather than erythema. Other antigens are available to measure delayed hypersensitivity to bacteria, viruses, fungi and protozoa.

(b) *Active sensitization*

The only methods of active sensitization recommended are the application of a skin homograft, or sensitization with 2·4 dinitrochlorobenzene (DNCB). Keyhole limpet haemocyanin has been used in the past. However, this produces both humoral as well as cell-mediated immunity and could theoretically sensitize against shell fish. None of these procedures should be undertaken lightly. Homograft rejection and the sensitization site on which DNCB has been applied can leave unsightly scars. Thus these procedures are usually only used when the tests for pre-existing immunity are negative.

Sensitization to DNCB is usually with 0·05 ml 10% DNCB in acetone. Skin testing may then be performed 14 days later with 0·1% and 0·05% DNCB in equal volumes of acetone and olive oil. The area of sensitization and skin testing should be covered with a loose gauze dressing for 24 hours after skin test. Tests are read 48 hours after application of DNCB and are assessed as follows:

> 0 = no reaction
> + = erythema only
> + + = erythema and induration
> + + + = vesiculation
> + + + + = bullae and ulceration

Only + + or greater reactions are accepted as evidence of sensitization. If negative 14 days after sensitization, the patient should be re-tested 28 days later.

(c) *In vitro* tests of cell-mediated immunity

(i) *Lymphocyte transformation.* Peripheral blood lymphocytes from patients who are tuberculin positive can be induced to transform into lymphoblast-like cells when incubated with tuberculin *in vitro*. Lymphocyte transformation, as this phenomenon is known, can be assessed by counting under the microscope the proportion of such transformed cells in stained smears made directly from the cultures. Identification of transformed cells can be enhanced by inducing these cells to take up radioactive ^{3}H-thymidine added to the culture medium. Then autoradiographs can be prepared from the smears and the transformed cells can be identified far more readily, since they alone take up the radioactive label. A further development of this technique is to count the actual amount of radioactive label taken up directly, in a liquid scintillation counter.

Specifically sensitized lymphocytes can be induced to transformation *in vitro* by specific antigens. In these cases usually no more than 10% of the lymphocytes in the cultures become transformed. Phytomitogens such as phytohaemagglutinin (PHA) transform in the region of 80–90% of lymphocytes of normal people. However, there is a marked reduction under conditions where there is a reduction in the number of T-lymphocytes as in conditions of thymic hypoplasia. Thus the response of lymphocytes to PHA can be used as a marker of the presence of lymphocytes capable of partaking in a cell-mediated immune response. Reduction of PHA responsiveness occurs in a number of conditions where there may be reduced cell-mediated immunity. As well as in thymic hypoplasia, this may be found in certain neoplastic diseases, especially those of the reticuloendothelial system such as Hodgkin's disease and in certain chronic infections such as chronic mucocutaneous candidiasis, syphilis and leprosy. In many cases, reduced lymphocyte function may be shown to be associated with an inhibitory plasma factor rather than be as a direct result of deficient lymphocyte function.

(ii) *Migration inhibitory factor* (*MIF*)

The interaction between sensitized lymphocytes and antigen *in vitro* releases a number of chemical mediators of cell-mediated immunity. One of these will inhibit the migration of normal macrophages from capillary tubes. The release of migration inhibitory factor (MIF) is a good indicator of cell-mediated immunity. At present, the preferred technique involves the culture of peripheral blood lymphocytes with antigen for periods up to 3 days and addition of the concentrated cell-free supernatant to chambers containing the guinea pig macrophages in capillary tubes. Other workers use direct inhibition of migration of peripheral blood leucocytes from capillary tubes by antigen. However, the results of such cultures may vary from laboratory to laboratory.

So far, aside from these techniques, it has been difficult to assess the status of cell-mediated immunity in patients, as apart from the techniques mentioned above there are no readily available means of measuring lymphocyte function. These techniques do not have the precision of methods used to measure humoral antibodies, nor are they particularly easy to perform.

Proportions of T- and B-lymphocytes in the peripheral blood

T-cells can be recognized microscopically because they form rosettes with sheep erythrocytes (E-rosettes). B-lymphocytes form similar rosettes with erythrocytes coated with antibody and complement (EAC-rosettes) or can be recognized as having immunoglobulin on their surface by immunofluorescence techniques. The proportion of E-rosette and EAC-rosette forming lymphocytes in the peripheral blood can be determined. A decrease in E-rosettes can be found in a number of primary and secondary immunodeficiency states. In addition these techniques can be used to determine the cell type of a lymphatic leukaemia.

Investigation of Immunoglobulins and Humoral Antibodies

Qualitative determination of abnormalities in the different types of immunoglobulins is usually determined by paper or cellulose acetate electrophoresis. It is generally easier in the first place to detect the presence of a monoclonal band by straightforward zone electrophoresis than by immunoelectrophoresis in which the serum is electrophoresed in gel and the individual proteins developed by diffusing a polyvalent antiserum at right angles into the gel. Qualitative changes in the individual immunoglobulins can then be identified. A quantitative estimate of the level of IgG, IgA, IgM and β_{1C}/β_{1A} globulin can be determined using a single radial diffusion technique in which monospecific antisera are incorporated in gel and the serum is placed in a well in the plate. An area of precipitation then occurs in the gel and within certain limits the diameter of the circle of precipitation is proportional to the level of the particular protein in the serum. Each test should include at least three standard solutions in the plate. The volume of serum used in this technique is 10μl and it can detect concentrations of protein as low as 10 μg/ml. Results can usually be read within 24 hours. As discrepancies have occurred in the past in estimates from different laboratories, the World Health Organization have now made available standard reference preparations of the five immunoglobulins. It has been suggested that each laboratory now relate their own standards to the WHO standards.

Quantitation of immunoglobulins is mainly of value in suspected immunodeficiency disorders or in the diagnosis of myelomatosis. In other clinical conditions, knowledge of the level of immunoglobulins is of value but not diagnostic. Complement levels (β_{1C}/β_{1A} globulin) are of value in the diagnosis of immune complex diseases, especially those involving the kidney. Cryoglobulins may also be found in the serum of patients with immune complex diseases or in certain subacute or chronic infectious diseases (e.g. leprosy, syphilis, subacute bacterial endocarditis, streptococcal nephritis, *Mycoplasma pneumoniae* pneumonia and infectious mononucleosis). These may contain mixed immunoglobulins (e.g. IgG/IgM, IgG/IgA or IgG/IgA/IgM) and β_{1C} globulins. Estimation of immunoglobulins in the urine in certain diseases is also of use, especially Bence-Jones proteins. Bence-Jones proteins are light chains of immunoglobulins and their presence in the urine of patients with myelomatosis can be investigated using specific anti-κ and anti-λ light chain sera.

Detection of Autoimmune Phenomena

Certain autoimmune phenomena are of use in clinical diagnosis. These include the detection of the rheumatoid factor and the antinuclear factor. Rheumatoid factor may be detected by agglutination of sheep erythrocytes coated with rabbit antibody or by the agglutination of latex particles coated with human immunoglobulins. Report of the presence of one of these factors should always include the result of a serum titration.

The tests for the presence of antinuclear factor should include demonstration of LE cells which are mandatory if systemic lupus erythematosus is to be diagnosed. Antinuclear factor itself may be demonstrated by immunofluorescence. However, titres of 1:20 or lower may be found in 15% of normal elderly people. Organ-specific autoantibodies are of value in the diagnosis of thyroid disease.

A clinical immunology laboratory may find it of value to provide a service looking for other autoantibodies using fluorescent antibody techniques. These include:

(i) Non-specific mitochondrial autoantibodies which occur in over 90% of patients with primary biliary cirrhosis.

  (ii) Smooth muscle autoantibodies which are useful in the diagnosis of infectious hepatitis.

 (iii) Gastric parietal-cell antibodies in the diagnosis of megaloblastic anaemias.

 (iv) Antibodies against adrenal cortical cells, which are present in the serum of patients with idiopathic Addison's disease, but not in those due to tuberculosis of the adrenal cortex.

  (v) Striated muscle antibodies which occur in 50% of patients with myasthenia gravis, especially those associated with thymoma.

 (vi) Epidermal autoantibodies which can provide help in distinguishing pemphigus vulgaris from pemphigoid.

The Diagnosis of Immune-complex Diseases

One of the more important roles of the clinical immunologist in the future will be in the diagnosis of immune-complex disease. Immune-complex disease should be suggested wherever the symptom complex of skin rash (sometimes purpuric), arthritis, iridocyclitis or proteinuria is observed. These diseases, frequently termed in the past "collagen diseases" or "autoimmune diseases", may be due to the deposition of immune complexes in the tissues containing defined extrinsic antigens. Treatment should be directed towards the elimination of these antigens. However, in the majority of cases it is very difficult to detect them. The main tool for demonstrating the participation of immune complex in glomerulonephritis or the vasculitis of polyarteritis nodosa is the demonstration of immunoglobulin and β_{1c} globulin by immunofluorescence on tissue sections. The demonstration of a drop in total haemolytic complement or C3 is useful in determining whether there are circulating immune complexes. A drop in C4 would indicate that the classical pathway is involved, whereas a drop in C3PA would indicate activation of the alternative pathway. C3, C4 and C3PA can be estimated quantitatively by single radial immunodiffusion. Precipitation of Clq by sera can be demonstrated in some situations in which there are circulating immune complexes. A radioimmunoassay is also available for the detection of Clq binding. The ability to demonstrate antigen in the circulation of patients with immune-complex diseases could lead to more rational treatment of immune-complex disease which at the present time is somewhat empirical, using the purely symptomatic approach of steroids supplemented occasionally with azathioprine. So far, the demonstration of antigen in immune complexes deposited in the tissues has been remarkably unsuccessful in the majority of cases, probably because of the difficulty in demonstrating antigen already complexed with antibody. Many immune-complex diseases are associated with cryoglobulineamia, especially if chronic, and these could be investigated for the possible presence of an extrinsic antigen.

Transplantation Immunology

HLA tissue typing is now an accepted investigation before organ or bone marrow transplantation. However, many of the specific sera used for tissue typing are difficult to produce and may be restricted to local, national or provincial centres involved in a complex research programme. This means that, outside these centres, it will only be possible to perform an incomplete typing service for transplantation purposes. However with the commercial availability of sera for the more common serologically determined types at the A and B locus it is useful to screen patients for those antigens which have a high association with certain diseases, such as B27 and B8. The identification of antigens at the C and D loci will for the time being still be the function of a more specialized research laboratory.

Immunohaematology

This is a borderline territory between the clinical haematologist and the clinical immunologist. In many hospitals the investigation of haemolytic anaemias has been undertaken extremely successfully by the clinical haematologist. However, in a number of cases haemolytic anaemia, leucopenia and thrombocytopenia are only three aspects of a much deeper immunological disturbance. In this field there is much room for collaborative investigation between the haematologist and the immunologist.

The Role of the Clinical Immunologist in the Clinic and at the Bedside

As well as the recognition of conditions and syndromes with particular immunological connotations, there are certain clinical diagnostic procedures which may be performed by the immunologist in consultation with his colleagues. Many of these have been derived from the practice of clinical allergy. These include skin tests such as prick tests in the diagnosis of atopic allergy and patch tests for contact sensitivity. Intradermal tests for delayed hypersensitivity may be of value in certain infectious diseases, e.g. lepromin, leishmanin, coccidioidin, histoplasmin etc. Provocation tests by nasal, bronchial or ingestion challenge may be used in the confirmation of allergic conditions where these are not too dangerous.

However, the main value of the clinical immunologist will be to recognize when and how immunological processes initiate or influence disease. As the result of this, he can suggest or carry out therapeutic procedures designed to eliminate or modify immunological processes. Treatment of immunological disorders may be antigen-specific or generalized immunosuppression. In order to initiate antigen-specific therapy, it is necessary to identify the particular antigen involved. In anaphylactic allergy or chemical contact sensitivity treatment may be advice as to antigen avoidance. Hyposensitization by antigen adminis-tration is generally performed in allergy clinics in the prevention of anaphylactic disease, and where an allergy clinic does not exist this could be performed by the clinical immunologist. This will be especially so as some departments of clinical immunology will have developed on the basis of a pre-existing allergy department. It is likely that the process of antigen administration (hyposensitization) works by modifying the immune response deviating it to the production of IgG antibodies which have greater avidity for the antigen than IgE molecules. As a result of this immune complexes are formed which cause the antigen to be taken up preferentially by cells of the reticuloendothelial system. This would reduce the availability of free antigen to interact with IgE. Another way in which the immune response may be modified is by the development of immunological enhancement. Immunological enhancement may be induced by antigen administration producing "enhancing" antibody. A cell-mediated immune response in a second subject can then be modified by antibody administration using this enhancing antibody. A further way in which specific antibody administration can be used is to decrease the immune response to Rhesus antigen when administered to mothers of Rhesus incompatible babies.

Perhaps one of the major roles of the clinical immunologist is the control of immunosuppressive therapy. Many clinical immunologists take over the treatment of patients with conditions such as systemic lupus erythematosus, rheumatoid arthritis, polyarteritis nodosa, auto-immune haemolytic anaemia and glomerulonephritis where steroid therapy is supplemented by immonosuppressive drugs such as aza-thioprine or cyclophosphamide. This is especially important in situa-tions where antilymphocyte globulin is used. It is also particularly im-portant that a trained immunologist be a member of the team control-ling immunosuppression to prevent the rejection of organ grafts or bone marrow transplants, when there should be frequent assessments of residual immunological activity as well as the functioning of the grafted tissue. There is often a very narrow balance between suppression of the immune reaction towards the graft and the ability to withstand infec-tion, which needs frequent monitoring.

In treatment of infectious diseases the advice of the clinical immun-ologist will also be of value in fields other than active immunization and serotherapy. The clinical progress of patients with infectious diseases is frequently affected by immunological reactions against anti-gens derived from the infective organism, resulting in lesions due either to a cell-mediated immune process or to the deposition of soluble immune complexes in the tissues which may need temporary immuno-suppressive therapy. Hypersensitivity phenomena may aggravate diseases during actual immunization or more severe diseases may develop in a person who has been immunized previously to the particular infective organism.

The Training of a Clinical Immunologist

Clinical immunology flourishes as a research subject and cannot be divorced from research. The investigation of patients with immunological disorders leans very heavily on the knowledge obtained from basic immunological research. It is thus important for an individual who wishes to practise clinical immunology to receive some training in a department of basic immunology. Three years in a department studying such subjects as the basic mechanisms of lymphocyte function, hypersensitivity reactions, complement, transplantation or cancer immunology will give the basic knowledge that can later be applied to the investigation of clinical problems. Instruction should not be in the acquisition of techniques, which can always be learnt in passing, but in the development of a logical, controlled and critical approach to research. The production and investigation of hypersensitivity reactions under controlled standardized conditions in experimental animals is the only means of obtaining a deeper understanding of the mechanisms underlying similar processes in human disease. Following this, a further period of training is necessary in a department of clinical immunology where the knowledge obtained in the basic research department can be applied to the investigation of clinical problems. So far, the best results in the investigation of clinical immunological problems have been obtained from those departments which can put part of their energies into basic immunological research. Much of the know-how derived from basic research can be applied to the particular clinical problem that interests the unit. Considerable insight into basic immunological problems can be derived from the study of what have been called "experiments of nature" where naturally occurring immunological aberrations in man have led to major breakthroughs in basic knowledge. Cross-fertilization between the laboratory and the clinic are the lifeblood of immunology. Another facet, of which account should be taken, is that no single immunology unit can specialize in all aspects of the field of immunology. One laboratory may specialize in anaphylactic phenomena, another in immune-complex disorders, a third in aspects of transplantation immunology and a fourth in cancer immunology. Thus, to maintain as broad a front as possible, there must be continuous interaction between different groups. This means that no single department can provide a complete training programme. Finally, in judging the criteria for assessing whether an individual has completed a training programme, emphasis should be placed on his potential for critical investigation in a particular field rather than in the breadth of knowledge obtained. The main criteria in such a rapidly expanding field should be the ability to make a significant contribution to knowledge and to make the most use of the clinical material available to help work out some of the many unanswered questions.

Bibliography

Thompson, R. A. (1974), *The Practice of Clinical Immunology*. London: Edward Arnold.

Index